Clinical Therapy Research in the Inflammatory Diseases

Clinical Therapy Research in the Inflammatory Diseases

Ronald F van Vollenhoven
The Karolinska Institute, Sweden

World Scientific

NEW JERSEY • LONDON • SINGAPORE • BEIJING • SHANGHAI • HONG KONG • TAIPEI • CHENNAI

Published by

World Scientific Publishing Co. Pte. Ltd.

5 Toh Tuck Link, Singapore 596224

USA office: 27 Warren Street, Suite 401-402, Hackensack, NJ 07601

UK office: 57 Shelton Street, Covent Garden, London WC2H 9HE

Library of Congress Cataloging-in-Publication Data
Vollenhoven, Ronald van, author.
  Clinical therapy research in the inflammatory diseases / Ronald F. van Vollenhoven.
    p. ; cm.
  Includes bibliographical references and index.
  ISBN 978-9814656320 (hardcover : alk. paper)
  I. Title.
  [DNLM: 1. Autoimmune Diseases--therapy. 2. Inflammation--physiopathology. WD 305]
  RC600
  616.97'8061--dc23
                                        2015003152

British Library Cataloguing-in-Publication Data
A catalogue record for this book is available from the British Library.

Typeset by Stallion Press
Email: enquiries@stallionpress.com

CONTENTS

Foreword   ix
Contributing Authors   xiii

**PART 1   NOVEL THERAPEUTIC APPROACHES
            FOR THE INFLAMMATORY DISEASES**   1

CHAPTER 1 CLINICAL THERAPY RESEARCH IN THE
           INFLAMMATORY DISEASES — AN
           OVERVIEW   3
           Ronald F. van Vollenhoven

CHAPTER 2 FROM MOLECULAR MECHANISMS TO
           PERSONALIZED THERAPIES IN
           AUTOIMMUNE INFLAMMATORY DISEASES   15
           Helena Idborg and Per-Johan Jakobsson

CHAPTER 3 B CELL-DIRECTED THERAPIES FOR
           INFLAMMATORY DISEASES   31
           Thomas Dörner and Peter E. Lipsky

CHAPTER 4 CELL-BASED THERAPIES FOR
           AUTOIMMUNE DISEASES   61
           Per Marits, Christian Lundgren, Ola Winqvist

**PART 2   TREATMENT FOR SPECIFIC
           INFLAMMATORY DISEASES**   77

CHAPTER 5 ADVANCES IN THERAPIES FOR
           RHEUMATOID ARTHRITIS   79
           Katerina Chatzidionysiou

CHAPTER 6 ADVANCES IN THERAPIES FOR
           SPONDYLOARTHROPATHIES   109
           Irene E. van der Horst-Bruinsma

CHAPTER 7 ADVANCES IN THERAPIES FOR
           SYSTEMIC LUPUS ERYTHEMATOSUS   129
           Noémi Győri, Chiara Tani, and Marta Mosca

CHAPTER 8 ADVANCES IN THERAPIES FOR SYSTEMIC
           SCLEROSIS   165
           Vanessa Smith and Filip De Keyser

CHAPTER 9 ADVANCES IN THERAPEUTIC STRATEGIES
           FOR INFLAMMATORY BOWEL DISEASE   199
           Åsa Krantz and Sven Almer

CHAPTER 10 SKIN, A DISPLAY ORGAN FOR THE IMMUNE
           SYSTEM — AN UPDATE ON PUTATIVE
           THERAPY TARGETS   219
           Liv Eidsmo and Mona Ståhle

CHAPTER 11 ADVANCES IN THERAPY FOR CUTANEOUS
           LUPUS ERYTHEMATOSUS   237
           Annegret Kuhn and Aysche Landmann

CHAPTER 12 ADVANCES IN THERAPIES FOR
           INTERSTITIAL LUNG DISEASES   257
           Giovanni Ferrara and Magnus Sköld

CHAPTER 13 ADVANCES IN THERAPIES FOR MULTIPLE
SCLEROSIS AND RELATED INFLAMMATORY
DISEASES OF THE CNS   283
Fredrik Piehl

CHAPTER 14 CLINICAL THERAPY RESEARCH IN
ALLERGIC DISEASES   311
Raffaela Campana, Rudolf Valenta,
Jeanette Grundström, Carl Hamsten,
and Marianne van Hage

CHAPTER 15 FUTURE PROSPECTS FOR THE THERAPIES
OF INFLAMMATORY DISEASES   349
Ronald F. van Vollenhoven

Index   369

FOREWORD

What did the great French painter Pierre-Auguste Renoir, the Swedish playwright August Strindberg, and the 35th president of the United States John F. Kennedy have in common? *All three suffered from a chronic illness characterized by inappropriate inflammation in specific target organs.*

Renoir, during the final decades of his life, experienced severe pain and stiffness in the joints, accompanied by slowly progressive destructive changes that so severely impacted his manual dexterity that friends had to tape the pencil to his hand in order to allow him to continue painting. *The disease: rheumatoid arthritis.*

Strindberg suffered from severe and persistent inflammation in the skin, particularly of the hands, associated with thickening and scaling that was both cosmetically and practically a great concern. The diagnosis was made by a contemporary expert dermatologist and more recent examinations of photographs corroborate this conclusion: *Strindberg suffered from psoriasis.*

The nature of Kennedy's chronic complaints only became clear once the secrecy on many White House medical documents was lifted forty years after his death. It transpires that he had suffered during most of his adult life from chronic and recurring inflammation in the gut, associated with pain and diarrhea, *the hallmark symptoms of ulcerative colitis.*

The inflammatory diseases, also referred to by many other names such as "systemic inflammatory disorders", "autoimmune diseases", and "immune-mediated inflammatory diseases", are a large group of disorders characterized by inappropriately activated inflammatory mechanisms. Despite the common underlying mechanisms, these diseases may have little in common when seen from the patient's perspective, exhibiting very different symptoms and signs. They also require different kinds of medical specialists in order to correctly differentiate them from other diseases and to initiate the appropriate diagnostic work-up. However, similarities in the underlying mechanisms have over the past two decades begun to translate into specific immunomodulatory treatments with well-characterized mechanisms of action that are applicable to various inflammatory diseases, and into similar treatment strategies for these chronic conditions.

Unfortunately for the famous protagonists we discussed above and the millions of unknown patients suffering from inflammatory diseases in former times, there were only very limited treatment options available in most cases. Renoir may have been among the first patients with rheumatoid arthritis to be treated with acetyl-salicylic acid in high doses, a treatment that can have good symptom-relieving properties, albeit with major toxicities as well, but that cannot prevent the chronic destruction of the joints. Strindberg was perhaps treated topically with tar-preparations but systemic treatments would only become available a century later. Kennedy could be considered fortunate in that a very effective therapy for various inflammatory diseases was discovered during his lifetime: corticosteroids. There is little doubt that he was treated with these during the 1950s. Unfortunately, he also exemplifies the dreaded long-term adverse consequences of corticosteroid treatment: he was known to have developed Addison's syndrome which in this case clearly was iatrogenic; and all through his presidency he suffered from severe back pains, probably caused by corticosteroid-induced osteoporosis. On account of these he wore a stiff corset most of the time, including while riding in a motorcade in Dallas on November 22nd 1963. When Lee Harvey Oswald's first shot rang out and hit him, Kennedy was only lightly wounded, but the corset made it impossible for him to duck for cover. Oswald's third bullet then hit him in the head and killed him.

Fortunately, treatments for the inflammatory diseases have experienced major changes for the better over the past two decades: the development of biologics and other targeted therapies have made it possible to offer dramatically better prospects to many patients, but have also raised questions on the most optimal therapeutic strategies, the choice of medications, and the pharmaco-economic implications. For all these reasons, it is timely to present an overview of the field of therapeutics for the inflammatory diseases.

It gives me enormous pleasure to be able to offer you this book, where leading experts in a range of inflammatory diseases present the status of therapeutics in their specific area and their views both on the current status of the field and the future. The first four chapters of this book deal with treatment approaches and treatment categories. After the first introductory chapter, Idborg and Jakobsson present the promise that is offered by the emerging fields of genomics, proteomics and metabolomics in terms of achieving more personalized and thereby even more effective treatments. Next, Dörner and Lipsky discuss the role of B-cells in the inflammatory diseases and the treatments that specifically target these pathways, some of which have already contributed greatly to the treatment of many patients. Marits, Lundgren and Winqvist provide their insights into cell-based therapies, the large field emerging from advances in the transplantation of various types of stem-cells, including the recently renamed mesenchymal stromal cells. The subsequent chapters in this book describe the field of therapeutics for specific inflammatory diseases or closely related groups of diseases. Thus, Chatzidionysiou discusses advances in the treatment of rheumatoid arthritis, and Van der Horst-Bruinsma in the treatment of spondyloarthropathies. Györi, Tani and Mosca present the current field and future expectations for the treatment of the complex multisystem inflammatory disease systemic lupus erythematosus, and Smith and De Keyser do the same for the equally challenging disease progressive systemic sclerosis. The chapter by Krantz and Almer provides us with an overview of advances in the treatment of inflammatory bowel diseases, after which two chapters give us the latest update on inflammatory diseases of the skin: Eidsmo and Ståhle discuss psoriasis and related disorders, while Kuhn and Landmann shed light on cutaneous lupus erythematosus. Subsequently

Ferrara and Sköld discuss advances in the treatment of interstitial lung diseases; Piehl presents the latest on the treatment of multiple sclerosis and other inflammatory diseases of the central nervous system; and Campana, Valenta, Grundström, Hamsten, and Van Hage provide us with an overview of the latest in the treatment of allergic diseases.

Needless to say, the number of inflammatory diseases that *could have been* covered in this book is far greater than the number of those that are actually included. This reflects in part on practicalities, and certainly a more comprehensive textbook covering "all" inflammatory diseases could be on the wish list of any scholar in this field. But by focusing on a selection of important inflammatory diseases I believe this book provides a wealth of information, the overarching principles and many details of which are applicable to most other inflammatory diseases as well.

This book has pooled expertise from many individuals working in areas with great differences but with important similarities as well. It is my hope and belief that those of us working with, or with an interest in, the inflammatory diseases will become better equipped to treat patients, to study these diseases and their treatments, or to develop better therapies through benefitting from the combined expertise of the many contributors working in diverse fields of medicine but sharing a common hope: to provide for a better future for the patients suffering from inflammatory diseases.

Ronald F. van Vollenhoven
Editor
Stockholm, July 2015

CONTRIBUTING AUTHORS

Sven Almer, MD, PhD
(Chapter 9)
Professor
Unit for Clinical Therapy Research, Inflammatory Diseases (ClinTRID)
Department of Medicine
The Karolinska Institute
Gastrocentrum (Center for Digestive Diseases)
Karolinska University Hospital
Stockholm, Sweden
Email: sven.almer@ki.se

Raffaela Campana, PhD
(Chapter 14)
Division of Immunopathology
Department of Pathophysiology and Allergy Research
Center for Pathophysiology, Infectiology and Immunology
Medical University of Vienna
Vienna, Austria
Email: raffaela.campana@medunwien.ac.at

Katerina Chatzidionysiou, MD, PhD
(Chapter 5)
Unit for Clinical Therapy Research,
Inflammatory Diseases (ClinTRID)
Department of Medicine Solna

The Karolinska Institute
Rheumatology Clinic
Karolinska University Hospital
Stockholm, Sweden
Email: Aikaterini.chatzidionysiou@karolinska.se

Filip De Keyser, MD, PhD
(Chapter 8)
Professor
Department of Internal Medicine
Ghent University
Ghent, Belgium
Email: filip.dekeyser@ugent.be

Thomas Dörner, MD, PhD
(Chapter 3)
Professor
Deutsches Charité, Universitätsmedizin Berlin
Department of Medicine/Rheumatology and Clinical Immunology
Charite University Hospitals Berlin and DRFZ Berlin
Berlin, Germany

Liv Eidsmo, MD,
(Chapter 10)
Associate Professor
Dermatology Unit and Center for Molecular Medicine (CMM)
Department of Medicine Solna
The Karolinska Institute
Department of Dermatology and Venereology
Karolinska University Hospital
Stockholm, Sweden
Email: liv.eidsmo@ki.se

Giovanni Ferrara, MD, PhD
(Chapter 12)
Unit of Respiratory Medicine and Center
for Molecular Medicine (CMM)

Department of Medicine Solna
The Karolinska Institute
Stockholm, Sweden
Department of Internal Medicine
University of Perugia
Perugia, Italy
Email: giovanni.ferrara@ki.se

Jeanette Grundström
(Chapter 14)
Clinical Immunology and Allergy Unit
Department of Medicine Solna
The Karolinska Institute
Stockholm, Sweden
Email: jeanette.grundstrom@ki.se

Noémi Győri, MD
(Chapter 7)
Unit for Clinical Therapy Research Inflammatory Diseases
Department of Medicine Solna
The Karolinska Institute
Stockholm, Sweden
Email: noemi.gyori@ki.se

Carl Hamsten, PhD
(Chapter 14)
Clinical Immunology and Allergy Unit
Department of Medicine Solna
The Karolinska Institute
Karolinska University Hospital
Stockholm, Sweden
Email: carl.hamsten@ki.se

Helena Idborg, PhD
(Chapter 2)
Associate Professor
Rheumatology Unit

Department of Medicine Solna
The Karolinska Institute
Stockholm, Sweden
Email: helena.idborg@ki.se

Per-Johan Jakobsson, MD, PhD
(Chapter 2)
Professor
Rheumatology Unit
Department of Medicine Solna
The Karolinska Institute
Rheumatology Clinic
Karolinska University Hospital
Stockholm, Sweden

Åsa Krantz, MD
(Chapter 9)
Unit for Clinical Therapy Research,
Inflammatory Diseases (ClinTRID)
Department of Medicine
The Karolinska Institute
Gastrocentrum
Karolinska University Hospital
Stockholm, Sweden
Email: asa.krantz@karolinska.se

Annegret Kuhn, MD, MBA
(Chapter 11)
Professor
Interdisciplinary Center for Clinical Trials (IZKS)
University Medical Center Mainz
Mainz, Germany
Email: kuhn@izks-unimedizin-mainz.de

Aysche Landmann
(Chapter 11)
Division of Immunogenetics

German Cancer Research Center (DKFZ)
Heidelberg, Germany
Email: a.landmann@Dkfz-Heidelberg.de

Peter E. Lipsky, MD
(Chapter 3)
Charité — Universitätsmedizin Berlin
Department of Medicine, Rheumatology and Clinical Immunology
Deutsches Rheumaforschungszentrum Berlin
Berlin, Germany

Christian Lundgren
(Chapter 4)
Translational Immunology Unit
Department of Medicine Solna
The Karolinska Institute
Karolinska University Hospital
Stockholm, Sweden
Email: christian.lundgren@karolinska.se

Per Marits, MD, PhD
(Chapter 4)
Translational Immunology Unit
Department of Medicine Solna
The Karolinska Institute
Karolinska University Hospital
Stockholm, Sweden
Email: per.marits@karolinska.se

Marta Mosca, MD, PhD
(Chapter 7)
Associate Professor
Department of Clinical and Experimental Medicine
University of Pisa
Pisa, Italy
Email: marta.mosca@med.unipi.it

Fredrik Piehl, MD, PhD
(Chapter 13)
Professor
Neuroimmunology Unit
Department of Clinical Neuroscience
Karolinska Institutet
Karolinska University Hospital
Stockholm, Sweden
Email: fredrik.piehl@ki.se

C. Magnus Sköld, MD, PhD
(Chapter 12)
Professor
Division of Respiratory Medicine
Department of Medicine Solna
The Karolinska Institute
Lung-Allergy Clinic
Karolinska University Hospital
Stockholm, Sweden
Email: magnus.skold@ki.se

Vanessa Smith, MD, PhD
(Chapter 8)
Associate Professor
Faculty of Medicine and Health Sciences
Department of Internal Medicine
Ghent University
Department of Rheumatology
Ghent University Hospital
Ghent, Belgium
Email: vanessa.smith@ugent.be

Mona Ståhle, MD, PhD
(Chapter 10)
Professor
Dermatology Unit and Center for Molecular Medicine (CMM)
Department of Medicine Solna
Karolinska Institutet
Department of Dermatology and Venereology
Karolinska University Hospital
Stockholm, Sweden
Email: mona.stahle@ki.se

Chiara Tani, MD, PhD
(Chapter 7)
Department of Clinical and Experimental Medicine
University of Pisa
Pisa, Italy
Email: chiaratani78@gmail.com

Rudolf Valenta
(Chapter 14)
Division of Immunopathology
Department of Pathophysiology and Allergy Research
Center for Pathophysiology, Infectiology and Immunology
Christian Doppler Laboratory for Allergy Research
Medical University of Vienna
Vienna, Austria
Email: rudolf.valenta@meduniwien.ac.at

Irene E. van der Horst-Bruinsma MD, PhD
(Chapter 6)
Associate Professor
Department of Rheumatology
VU University Medical Centre
Amsterdam, The Netherlands
Email: IE.vanderHorst@vumc.nl

Marianne van Hage, MD, PhD
(Chapter 14)
Professor
Clinical Immunology and Allergy Unit
Department of Medicine Solna
The Karolinska Institute
Stockholm, Sweden
Email: marianne.van.hage@ki.se

Ronald F. van Vollenhoven, MD, PhD
(Chapters 1 and 15)
Professor
Unit for Clinical Therapy Research,
Inflammatory Diseases (ClinTRID)
Department of Medicine Solna
The Karolinska Institute
Rheumatology Clinic
Karolinska University Hospital
Stockholm, Sweden
Email: ronald.van.vollenhoven@ki.se

Ola Winqvist, MD, PhD
(Chapter 4)
Professor
Translational Immunology Unit
Department of Medicine Solna
The Karolinska Institute
Karolinska University Hospital
Stockholm, Sweden
Email: ola.winqvist@karolinska.se

PART 1

NOVEL THERAPEUTIC APPROACHES FOR THE INFLAMMATORY DISEASES

CHAPTER 1

CLINICAL THERAPY RESEARCH IN THE INFLAMMATORY DISEASES — AN OVERVIEW

Ronald F. van Vollenhoven

Introduction

- A 22-year-old man is seen by a specialist. For more than two years now he has been suffering from bouts of abdominal pain and diarrhea, associated with fever and weight loss. *After extensive investigations, the specialist diagnoses him with Crohn's disease.*
- A 32-year-old woman is seen because her skin disease is getting worse and worse. Large body surface areas are now covered with erythematous scaling lesions that have progressed despite various topical treatments. The impact on her personal life is disastrous. *There is no doubt that her disease, psoriasis, has progressed and requires more active treatment.*
- A 45-year-old woman seeks care from her doctor. For the past eight months, she has woken up feeling terribly stiff in her joints. The finger and wrists joints have become more and more swollen. She is having increasing difficulties doing her work. *After some blood tests, the physician concludes that she has rheumatoid arthritis.*

What do these three clinical cases have in common? On the surface, they describe very different patients, with completely different symptoms in different organ systems. If these individuals met they would probably not find much in common, other than that all three are impacted very severely by a long-lasting disease process. An important practical difference is also that they will most likely be taken care of by different specialists: a gastroenterologist, a dermatologist, and a rheumatologist. Nonetheless, they share very important commonalities between their diseases: all three suffer from one of the systemic *inflammatory diseases*, a group of diseases also frequently referred to as *autoimmune diseases*, and sometimes as *immune-mediated inflammatory diseases* or IMIDs. Included in this group are not only the inflammatory bowel diseases, psoriasis, and rheumatoid arthritis, as in our examples, but also a much larger number of diseases in the skin (for example, cutaneous lupus, pemphigus, bullous pemphigoid) and in the musculoskeletal system (the spondyloarthropathies, psoriatic arthritis, the inflammatory myopathies), as well as diseases in the central nervous system such as multiple sclerosis, inflammatory diseases in the lungs, allergic diseases, and conditions that by themselves can give rise to manifestations in many organs or organ systems, such as systemic lupus erythematosus and progressive systemic sclerosis. Inflammatory diseases are usually grouped according to the organ system affected and/or medical specialty area where the patient is usually seen. An overview is shown in Table 1.

The Inflammatory Diseases: Scope and Impact

Taken as a group, the inflammatory diseases represent a significant part of the overall medical needs in society. Depending on how the boundaries are drawn, 5–10% of the population may be affected by one of these diseases. And while most of these diseases are not immediately life-threatening, they all do impose very significant impacts on the patients' quality of life. Most of these diseases are chronic, although some may be self-limiting (sometimes after longer periods of disease activity) and many have notably undulating disease courses, with periods of intense inflammatory activity interspersed between periods of relative quiescence. These characteristics make the inflammatory diseases an important group of diseases: they have a very major impact on patients' lives, and because they

Table 1. Overview of the inflammatory diseases. Which diseases to include or not is subject to some debate; listed here is a selection of diseases where inflammation is believed to play an important part in the pathogenesis. In some the inflammation is low-grade (atherosclerosis); in others inflammation may only be present at a very early stage and not usually be amenable to intervention (type 1 diabetes).

- Rheumatology
  - Rheumatoid Arthritis
  - Ankylosing Spondylitis
  - Spondyloarthropathies
  - Psoriatic Arthritis
  - Juvenile Inflammatory Arthritis
  - Systemic Lupus Erythematosus
  - Behçet's Syndrome
  - Sjögren's Syndrome
  - Systemic Vasculitis
- Gastroenterology
  - Inflammatory Bowel Diseases
    - Crohn's Disease
    - Ulcerative Colitis
    - Microscopic Colitis
  - Primary Sclerosing Cholangitis
  - Chronic Autoimmune Hepatitis
- Dermatology
  - Psoriasis
  - Pyoderma Gangrenosum
  - Cutaneous Lupus
  - Lupus Pernio
  - Atopic Dermatitis
- Cardiovascular
  - Atherosclerosis
  - Idiopathic Myocarditis
- Endocrine
  - Type 1 (Autoimmune) Diabetes
- Pulmonary
  - Sarcoidosis
  - Asthma
  - Idiopathic Pulmonary Fibrosis
- Neurology
  - Multiple Sclerosis
- Ophthalmology
  - Chronic Uveitis

tend to be long-lasting or even life-long, this impact is amplified in time. In turn, this leads to very significant costs, both for the patients themselves, but also for society: it is estimated that the inflammatory diseases have an economic impact that is measured in the tens of billions of dollars or euros per year, both in terms of the actual costs of taking care of the patients' medical needs, but also the enormous loss of productivity and of participation in societies' many functions that are caused by the diseases (indirect costs). Therefore, finding better therapies for these diseases is a major healthcare priority.

For all their clinical variability, the inflammatory diseases share common pathophysiological mechanisms. Enormous advances in our understanding of the immune system and inflammatory pathways have clearly revealed the similarities, along with important differences, between many of these diseases. At the risk of some simplification, it can be said that the same inflammation when occurring in the gut causes inflammatory bowel disease; when in the joints, rheumatoid arthritis; and when in the brain, multiple sclerosis.

Developments in the Treatment of Inflammatory Diseases: The Advent of Biologics

In parallel with our increased understanding of these inflammatory pathways, another development has occurred that puts a completely new spotlight on inflammatory diseases: the development of very specific and targeted biological therapies for these diseases. Beginning with the development of interferon-beta as a biological response modifier that was proven effective in the treatment of multiple sclerosis,[1] the field exploded when specific inhibitors of tumor necrosis factor (TNF) were found to be highly effective medications for the treatment of RA[2,3] and Crohn's disease[4,5] in the early and mid-1990s, and subsequently for a long list of inflammatory diseases including ankylosing spondylitis[6-8] and other spondyloarthropathies, psoriatic arthritis,[9-11] juvenile inflammatory arthritis,[12,13] ulcerative colitis,[14] psoriasis,[15-17] pyoderma gangrenosum,[18] and even having efficacy in some studies and trials for unapproved indications such as uveitis[19-21] and Behçet's disease.[22] Buoyed by these successes, biotechnology industry working closely with academia and regulators developed many other biological agents with exquisite target specificity and in some cases very dramatic clinical efficacies. The interleukin-1 (IL-1) antagonist anakinra was developed with some efficacy in RA[23] and was later shown, along with canakinumab and rilonacept, to have extraordinary effectivity in certain rare autoinflammatory syndromes.[24–26] The anti-IL-6 receptor monoclonal tocilizumab was approved for RA[27] and several more IL-6 pathway inhibitors are being developed clinically at this time. An inhibitor of IL12/23 was found to be effective in psoriasis,[28] and several monoclonals targeting IL-17 have shown great promise in treating the same disease,[29–33] with a first one, secukinumab, having recently been approved in Europe. A biological agent, natalizumab, targeting α4-integrin was developed and exhibited very good efficacy in MS;[34] however, an important risk was subsequently identified in the form of the frequently fatal virus reactivation syndrome progressive multifocal leukoencephalopathy,[35] underscoring the two-sided nature of the development of biological therapies: along with sometimes dramatic efficacies, completely new toxicities and risks are also to be reckoned with. In an interesting further development, more selective anti-integrins that only target leucocyte trafficking to the gut have been developed and found to be very effective in IBD.[36,37]

Other biological agents with completely different mechanisms of action have also been developed and found specific clinical indications, such as the B-cell depleting anti-CD20 agents including rituximab with efficacy in rheumatoid arthritis[38,39] and vasculitis,[40,41] the T-cell costimulation modulator abatacept that is effective in RA,[42] the Blys/BAFF antagonist belimumab that became the first biologic approved for the treatment of SLE,[43] and developments continue including late-stage clinical trials of the anti-IL4 antagonist dupilumab with very promising results in asthma[44] and atopic dermatitis.[45] The biologics that are currently approved for rheumatoid arthritis are shown in Fig. 1.

The development of biological therapies has had several important implications:

(1) Having access to therapies with a well-defined target provided excellent opportunities for bedside-to-bench research, as opposed to the more usual bench-to-bedside paradigm, meaning that one uses clinical

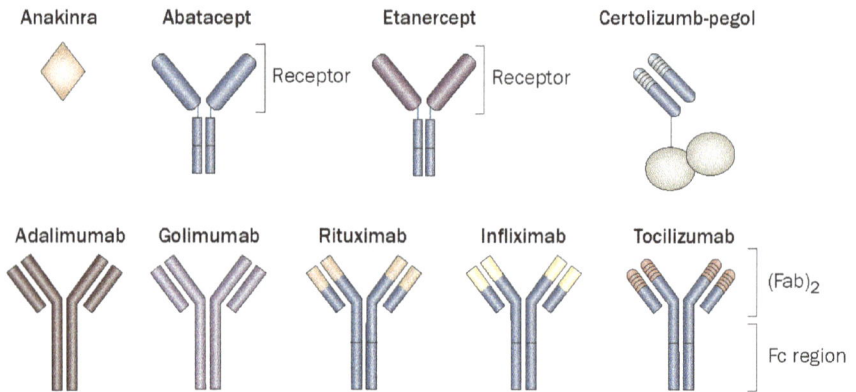

Figure 1. Nine biologics, with five distinct mechanisms of action, are currently approved for the treatment of rheumatoid arthritis. Many of these are approved for use in other diseases as well. Reproduced, with permission, from Ref. [52].

observations to generate new hypotheses. In contrast to conventional immunosuppressives, with broad mechanisms of action, the biologics very specifically target one molecule, so that clinical observations can be linked to the activities of that particular molecule or its downstream effects (Fig. 2). Thus, the effectiveness of the IL-1 antagonists in cryopyrin-associated syndromes helped elucidate the role of IL-1 in these diseases,[46] and the observation that TNF-blockade increases the risk for reactivation of latent tuberculosis[47] enhanced our understanding of the role of TNF and macrophages in the host response to *M. tuberculosis*.[48]

(2) The biologicals revolutionized therapies for many diseases but at a very high cost. Based on expensive biological production facilities, and having had costly development programs, these drugs were priced at levels that were sometimes several orders of magnitude higher than the most effective therapies for these diseases up to that point in time. The health-economic impacts of this have been large. In some societies, biological therapies have been available only to a very limited degree, and allocating these to the right patients has been a very hard task for those involved. In more fortunate societies biologics were frequently used, but costs for treatment escalated rapidly and resulted

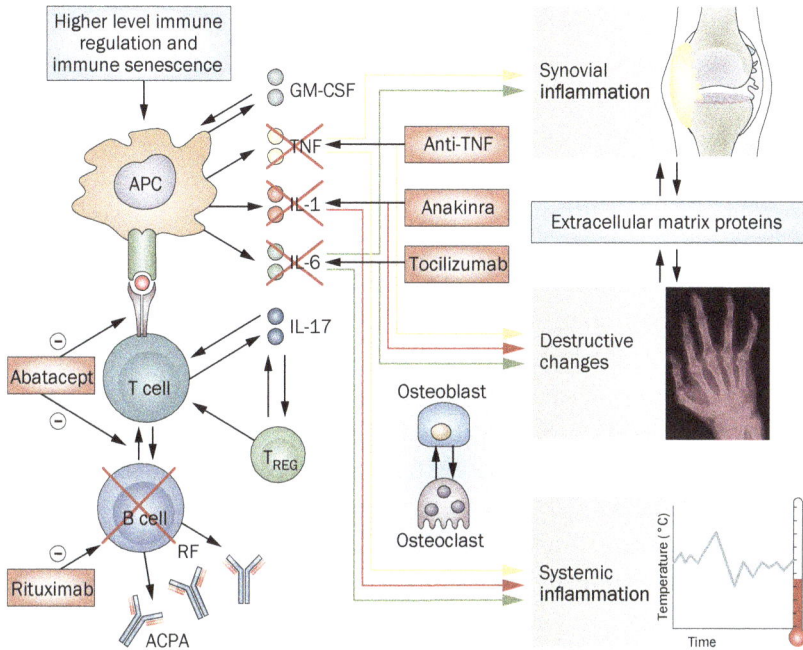

Figure 2. The biologics target precisely identified molecules or cell-types, thereby adding to our insights in the inflammatory process. Reproduced, with permission, from Ref. [53].

in increasing calls for regulation and oversight. The field of health-economics was strongly boosted by these issues, addressing questions of whether a treatment has to demonstrate a certain level of cost-effectiveness or cost-utility (the cost for each incremental improvement in health-related quality of life) in order to be "acceptable", but clear answers to most of these cannot easily be given and decisions on the use of biologics in clinical care remain the subject of a complex interplay between patients, physicians, healthcare administrators, drug regulators, and pharmaceutical companies.

(3) The biological therapies also helped break down some of the boundaries between medical specialties. From the examples at the beginning of this chapter it can be seen that patients understandably end up being seen by different specialists, in recognition of the highly divergent

nature of their symptoms and signs, and also because of each specialist's specific competence in evaluating symptoms from one specific organ system or another. But once the diagnosis of an inflammatory disease has been established, the treatments now at the specialists' disposal may very well be identical, and it stands to reason that important learning could take place between the specialists in these different areas of competence.

Thus, the advent of biological therapies spawned a surge in the investigation of these treatments: clinical therapy research. Many different kinds of research can be included under this moniker: the development of the drugs themselves; studies of their mechanisms and pharmacology; the evaluation of the drugs in clinical trial programs; and post-marketing studies of real-life efficacy and safety. All of these types of research are important, but a special interest has developed around comparative effectiveness research.[49] Whereas traditional drug development aims to determine whether a drug is effective at all, and therefore usually is compared to a placebo, the clinically more relevant question is whether drug A is more effective and/or safe than drug B, so that the clinician will know which of the two to choose. Studies required to resolve such important issues are difficult to do and very costly, and not always in the industry's interest. It has therefore become clear that investigator-initiated comparative trials are vitally necessary to further the fields of therapeutics for many groups of diseases, including the inflammatory diseases. Some good examples of such trials in rheumatoid arthritis have been published in recent years.[50,51]

In summary, inflammatory diseases represent a wide field in medicine that has expanded at a breath-taking pace, and clinical therapy research in these diseases has exploded over the past two decades. Owing to these advances, patients with inflammatory diseases are leading better lives today than they did yesterday, and it is very clear that the prospects for tomorrow will be better still.

References

1. (1993). Interferon beta-1b is effective in relapsing-remitting multiple sclerosis. I. Clinical results of a multicenter, randomized, double-blind, placebo-controlled trial. The IFNB Multiple Sclerosis Study Group. *Neurology*, **43**, 655–661.

2. Elliott, M.J., *et al.* (1994). Randomised double-blind comparison of chimeric monoclonal antibody to tumour necrosis factor alpha (cA2) versus placebo in rheumatoid arthritis. *Lancet*, **344**, 1105–1110.

3. Moreland, L.W., *et al.* (1997). Treatment of rheumatoid arthritis with a recombinant human tumor necrosis factor receptor (p75)-Fc fusion protein. *N Engl J Med*, **337**, 141–147.

4. D'Haens, G., *et al.* (1999). Endoscopic and histological healing with inflximab anti-tumor necrosis factor antibodies in Crohn's disease: A European multicenter trial. *Gastroenterology*, **116**, 1029–1034.

5. Schreiber, S., *et al.* (2005). A randomized, placebo-controlled trial of certolizumab pegol (CDP870) for treatment of Crohn's disease. *Gastroenterology*, **129**, 807–818.

6. Braun, J., *et al.* (2002). Treatment of active ankylosing spondylitis with infliximab: a randomised controlled multicentre trial. *Lancet*, **359**, 1187–1193.

7. Brandt, J., *et al.* (2003). Six-month results of a double-blind, placebo-controlled trial of etanercept treatment in patients with active ankylosing spondylitis. *Arthritis Rheum*, **48**, 1667–1675.

8. van der Heijde, D., *et al.* (2006). Efficacy and safety of adalimumab in patients with ankylosing spondylitis: Results of a multicenter, randomized, double-blind, placebo-controlled trial. *Arthritis Rheum*, **54**, 2136–2146.

9. Mease, P.J., *et al.* (2000). Etanercept in the treatment of psoriatic arthritis and psoriasis: a randomised trial. *Lancet*, **356**, 385–390.

10. Mease, P.J., *et al.* (2005). Adalimumab for the treatment of patients with moderately to severely active psoriatic arthritis: Results of a double-blind, randomized, placebo-controlled trial. *Arthritis Rheum*, **52**, 3279–3289.

11. Antoni, C., *et al.* (2005). Infliximab improves signs and symptoms of psoriatic arthritis: Results of the IMPACT 2 trial. *Ann Rheum Dis*, **64**, 1150–1157.

12. Ruperto, N., *et al.* (2007). A randomized, placebo-controlled trial of infliximab plus methotrexate for the treatment of polyarticular-course juvenile rheumatoid arthritis. *Arthritis Rheum*, **56**, 3096–3106.

13. Lovell, D.J., *et al.* (2003). Long-term efficacy and safety of etanercept in children with polyarticular-course juvenile rheumatoid arthritis: Interim results from an ongoing multicenter, open-label, extended-treatment trial. *Arthritis Rheum*, **48**, 218–226.

14. Probert, C.S., *et al.* (2003). Infliximab in moderately severe glucocorticoid resistant ulcerative colitis: A randomised controlled trial. *Gut*, **52**, 998–1002.

15. Chaudhari, U., *et al.* (2001). Efficacy and safety of infliximab monotherapy for plaque-type psoriasis: A randomised trial. *Lancet*, **357**, 1842–1847.

16. Gottlieb, A.B., *et al.* (2003). A randomized trial of etanercept as monotherapy for psoriasis. *Arch Dermatol*, **139**, 1627–1632; discussion 1632.

17. Gordon, K.B., *et al.* (2006). Clinical response to adalimumab treatment in patients with moderate to severe psoriasis: Double-blind, randomized controlled trial and open-label extension study. *J Am Acad Dermatol*, **55**, 598–606.

18. Brooklyn, T.N., *et al.* (2006). Infliximab for the treatment of pyoderma gangrenosum: A randomised, double blind, placebo controlled trial. *Gut*, **55**, 505–509.

19. Suhler, E.B., *et al.* (2005). A prospective trial of infliximab therapy for refractory uveitis: Preliminary safety and efficacy outcomes. *Arch Ophthalmol*, **123**, 903–912.

20. Smith, J.A., *et al.* (2005). A randomized, placebo-controlled, double-masked clinical trial of etanercept for the treatment of uveitis associated with juvenile idiopathic arthritis. *Arthritis Rheum*, **53**, 18–23.

21. Suhler, E.B., *et al.* (2013). Adalimumab therapy for refractory uveitis: Results of a multicentre, open-label, prospective trial. *Br J Ophthalmol*, **97**, 481–486.

22. Al-Rayes, H., *et al.* (2008). Safety and efficacy of infliximab therapy in active behcet's uveitis: An open-label trial. *Rheumatol Int*, **29**, 53–57.

23. Cohen, S., *et al.* (2002). Treatment of rheumatoid arthritis with anakinra, a recombinant human interleukin-1 receptor antagonist, in combination with methotrexate: Results of a twenty-four-week, multicenter, randomized, double-blind, placebo-controlled trial. *Arthritis Rheum*, **46**, 614–624.

24. Hawkins, P.N., Lachmann, H.J., Aganna, E. & McDermott, M.F. (2004). Spectrum of clinical features in Muckle-Wells syndrome and response to anakinra. *Arthritis Rheum*, **50**, 607–612.

25. Mueller, S.M., Itin, P. & Haeusermann, P. (2011). Muckle-Wells syndrome effectively treated with canakinumab: Is the recommended dosing schedule mandatory? *Dermatology*, **223**, 113–118.

26. Hashkes, P.J., *et al.* (2012). Rilonacept for colchicine-resistant or -intolerant familial Mediterranean fever: A randomized trial. *Ann Intern Med*, **157**, 533–541.

27. Emery, P., *et al.* (2008). IL-6 receptor inhibition with tocilizumab improves treatment outcomes in patients with rheumatoid arthritis refractory to anti-tumour necrosis factor biologicals: Results from a 24-week multicentre randomised placebo-controlled trial. *Ann Rheum Dis*, **67**, 1516–1523.

28. Leonardi, C.L., *et al.* (2008). Efficacy and safety of ustekinumab, a human interleukin-12/23 monoclonal antibody, in patients with psoriasis: 76-week results from a randomised, double-blind, placebo-controlled trial (PHOENIX 1). *Lancet*, **371**, 1665–1674.

29. Blauvelt, A., *et al.* (2014). Secukinumab administration by pre-filled syringe: Efficacy, safety and usability results from a randomized controlled trial in psoriasis (FEATURE). *Br J Dermatol.*
30. Papp, K.A., *et al.* (2012). Anti-IL-17 receptor antibody AMG 827 leads to rapid clinical response in subjects with moderate to severe psoriasis: Results from a phase I, randomized, placebo-controlled trial. *J Invest Dermatol*, **132**, 2466–2469.
31. Leonardi, C., *et al.* (2012). Anti-interleukin-17 monoclonal antibody ixekizumab in chronic plaque psoriasis. *N Engl J Med*, **366**, 1190–1199.
32. Reich, K. (2012). Anti-interleukin-17 monoclonal antibody ixekizumab in psoriasis. *N Engl J Med*, **367**, 274; author reply 275.
33. Wu, J.J. (2012). Anti-interleukin-17 monoclonal antibody ixekizumab in psoriasis. *N Engl J Med*, **367**, 274–275; author reply 275.
34. Miller, D.H., *et al.* (2003). A controlled trial of natalizumab for relapsing multiple sclerosis. *N Engl J Med*, **348**, 15–23.
35. Kleinschmidt-DeMasters, B.K. & Tyler, K.L. (2005). Progressive multifocal leukoencephalopathy complicating treatment with natalizumab and interferon beta-1a for multiple sclerosis. *N Engl J Med*, **353**, 369–374.
36. Wyant, T., *et al.* (2015). Vedolizumab affects antibody responses to immunisation selectively in the gastrointestinal tract: Randomised controlled trial results. *Gut*, **64**, 77–83.
37. Vermeire, S., *et al.* (2014). Etrolizumab as induction therapy for ulcerative colitis: A randomised, controlled, phase 2 trial. *Lancet*, **384**, 309–318.
38. Emery, P., *et al.* (2006). The efficacy and safety of rituximab in patients with active rheumatoid arthritis despite methotrexate treatment: Results of a phase IIB randomized, double-blind, placebo-controlled, dose-ranging trial. *Arthritis Rheum*, **54**, 1390–1400.
39. Tak, P.P., *et al.* (2011). Inhibition of joint damage and improved clinical outcomes with rituximab plus methotrexate in early active rheumatoid arthritis: the IMAGE trial. *Ann Rheum Dis*, **70**, 39–46.
40. Stone, J.H., *et al.* (2010). Rituximab versus cyclophosphamide for ANCA-associated vasculitis. *N Engl J Med*, **363**, 221–232.
41. Jones, R.B., *et al.* (2010). Rituximab versus cyclophosphamide in ANCA-associated renal vasculitis. *N Engl J Med*, **363**, 211–220.
42. Kremer, J.M., *et al.* (2006). Effects of abatacept in patients with methotrexate-resistant active rheumatoid arthritis: A randomized trial. *Ann Intern Med*, **144**, 865–876.
43. Furie, R., *et al.* (2011). A phase III, randomized, placebo-controlled study of belimumab, a monoclonal antibody that inhibits B lymphocyte stimulator,

in patients with systemic lupus erythematosus. *Arthritis Rheum*, **63**, 3918–3930.

44. Wenzel, S.E., Wang, L. & Pirozzi, G. (2013). Dupilumab in persistent asthma. *N Engl J Med*, **369**, 1276.

45. Beck, L.A., *et al.* (2014). Dupilumab treatment in adults with moderate-to-severe atopic dermatitis. *N Engl J Med*, **371**, 130–139.

46. Kone-Paut, I. & Piram, M. (2012). Targeting interleukin-1beta in CAPS (cryopyrin-associated periodic) syndromes: What did we learn? *Autoimmun Rev*, **12**, 77–80.

47. Cantini, F., Niccoli, L. & Goletti, D. (2014). Adalimumab, etanercept, infliximab, and the risk of tuberculosis: Data from clinical trials, national registries, and postmarketing surveillance. *J Rheumatol Suppl*, **91**, 47–55.

48. Beham, A.W., *et al.* (2011). A TNF-regulated recombinatorial macrophage immune receptor implicated in granuloma formation in tuberculosis. *PLoS Pathog*, **7**, e1002375.

49. Weinstein, M.C. & Skinner, J.A. (2010) Comparative effectiveness and health care spending — implications for reform. *N Engl J Med*, **362**, 460–465.

50. van Vollenhoven, R.F., *et al.* (2009). Addition of infliximab compared with addition of sulfasalazine and hydroxychloroquine to methotrexate in patients with early rheumatoid arthritis (Swefot trial): 1-year results of a randomised trial. *Lancet*, **374**, 459–466.

51. Moreland, L.W., *et al.* (2012). A randomized comparative effectiveness study of oral triple therapy versus etanercept plus methotrexate in early aggressive rheumatoid arthritis: The treatment of Early Aggressive Rheumatoid Arthritis Trial. *Arthritis Rheum*, **64**, 2824–2835.

52. van Vollenhoven, R.F. (2011). Unresolved issues in biologic therapy for rheumatoid arthritis. *Nat Rev Rheumatol*, **7**, 205–215.

53. van Vollenhoven, R.F. (2009). Treatment of rheumatoid arthritis: State of the art 2009. *Nat Rev Rheumatol*, **5**, 531–541.

CHAPTER 2

FROM MOLECULAR MECHANISMS TO PERSONALIZED THERAPIES IN AUTOIMMUNE INFLAMMATORY DISEASES

Helena Idborg and Per-Johan Jakobsson

Introduction

Today, advances in research have defined a multitude of biochemical pathways involved in inflammation and autoimmune diseases. However, disappointingly few of these recent advances have been implemented in the clinical care of patients. There are a number of recent reviews and books about involved pathways and the currently available drugs,[1–3] but we are still lacking clinical biomarkers to stratify patients and guide in the choice of drug.

In this chapter, we will focus on the importance of further characterization of inflammatory autoimmune diseases. We will discuss the advantage of biomarker panels as basis for diagnosis and identification of high-risk patient groups, the identification of biomarkers by technologies like proteomics and metabolomics, and how an increased knowledge of affected pathways in different subgroups of patients may allow for better diagnosis and treatment.

The aims are to identify:

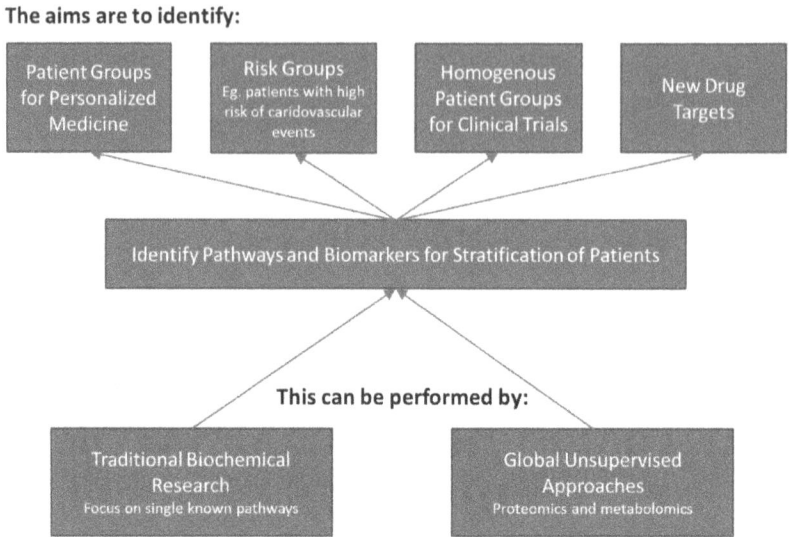

Figure 1.   Methods for reaching the aim of personalized medicine.

An Example of the Biocomplexity of Therapies in Autoimmune Diseases

The different drugs we currently have at our disposal treating rheumatoid arthritis and other rheumatic diseases can easily be short-listed and there are numerous reviews on their nature, clinical efficacies and main mechanisms of actions.[2] However, mechanistically it actually remains quite unclear how the individual DMARDs or biological drugs exert their actions. For instance, methotrexate, perhaps the most common DMARD used, may perform its action by inhibiting the biosynthesis of reduced folic acid or alternatively by influencing the release of adenosine or via other mechanisms like regulation of oxidative stress.[4] Likewise, TNF blocking agents on a group level reduces TNF, but what downstream and/or upstream events are in fact influenced? mTOR and NF-κB are two important pathways mediating TNF signaling.[5] In turn, there are several hundreds, possible thousands of NF-κB regulated proteins[6] which is also true for mTOR target genes.[7] To the number of all these genes regulated by NF-κB and mTOR, one needs to add the biological significance of all further downstream mediators and metabolites produced by the various enzymes within this large group of regulated proteins. From a biomarker point of view, these facts pose a problem that cannot be solved by any traditional clinical chemistry or immunology-based assays. Rather, omics technologies including appropriate biostatistics will be instrumental in unraveling novel biomarkers and affected pathways.

Stratification of Patients for Improved Clinical Care

Patient stratification may be defined as the use of biomarkers to differentiate patients into groups that will benefit more from a certain drug than others with the same diagnosis. It can also refer to the identification of patient groups that are more prone to develop certain side effects and toxicity. The most important advantage of patient stratification is of course the health effect for the patients but there are additional drivers. Financial interest is one main driver as society does not want to spend money on drugs that will not work in a certain patient group. There are regulatory drivers since we have an increasing intolerance to side effects of drugs where the majority of patients have low efficacy. An additional driver of patient stratification is that the development of data-rich technologies has made us aware of the possibility of subgrouping patients. Both physicians and patients are aware of long lists of medicines that are available for treatment and we need tools, *i.e.*, biomarkers, to make the right selection for each patient.

Patient groups for personalized medicine

We have always categorized patients into different subgroups, *i.e.* patients with different diseases, to assign them a certain treatment. However, this stratification has not been very specific and today we are aiming towards personalized medicine. There are many factors — *e.g.*, sex, genetic background and diet — that will affect the efficacy of the treatment and therapeutic strategies developed for one disease can also be applied to the treatment of other autoimmune diseases.

The knowledge of the pathology of RA has led to better therapies. The tumor-necrosis-factor (TNF) blocker is a biologic response modifier in RA as mentioned in the previous section. This drug suppresses the response of

TNF on a molecular level with antibodies and since this pathway is part of the inflammatory response, the drug might be used in other diseases where the TNF pathway is activated, *e.g.*, inflammatory bowel disease and psoriasis. In systemic lupus erythematosus (SLE), there is some evidence that the TNF pathway may in fact be activated in some patients; however observations on small numbers of patients using TNF blocking therapies in SLE have shown mixed results, and these treatments are usually avoided in SLE.[8] Nonetheless, if the correct SLE subgroup of patients with an activated TNF pathway could be identified, TNF blockers would possibly have a role also in the treatment of such SLE patients.

In RA, the use of TNF inhibitors has revolutionized the treatment and management of RA patients. However, there is still a substantial proportion (30%) of RA patients who do not responds to anti-TNF treatment and the use of these drugs is based on "trial and error".[9,10] Anti-TNF therapies are expensive and ineffective treatment is a disadvantage for both patient and society, so there is a great need for biomarkers of responders and non-responders enabling prescription of the correct drug to the right patients.

Identify patient risk groups

All therapies have drawbacks and for the safety of the patients, it is important to identify high-risk patient groups. In the case of anti-TNF treatment, there is an increased risk of infections and tumors.[11] Subgroups with increased risk of congestive heart failure should also be identified since TNF inhibitors might cause complications in this group of patients.[10] In general in inflammatory diseases, comorbidities such as cardiovascular events and cancer are important for risk stratification. By identification of risk groups, it is possible to add complementary treatment, monitor specific clinical signs or choose a different treatment.

Homogeneous patient groups for clinical trials

Stratification of patients is important in the choice of successful therapy as described above. However, it is just as important in the selection of patients for clinical trials. If a heterogeneous population is selected, it might be hard to show efficacy in a clinical trial and a drug that might be very potent in a subgroup of patients will never reach the market. For example, if it were possible to stratify for patients with TNF-driven disease as an inclusion criterion for a clinical trial of TNF inhibitors, the response to treatment would most likely be enhanced. Homogeneous patient groups are therefore crucial in clinical trials.

The fact of homogeneity is somewhat subjective. It can be a homogenous population based on sex, serological measurements or demographic factors. Therefore, it is important to define patient subgroups with suitable criteria or biomarkers. Well-defined biomarkers for disease activity and response measurements are highly important in clinical trials and in response to treatment.

Biomarker panels

Biomarkers are indicators of a certain biological state with different specificity and selectivity. CRP is, for example, an established but non-specific biomarker of inflammation frequently used in the clinic and there is a great need for additional and better biomarkers of inflammation. For RA, there are many biomarkers reported in the literature but most of those markers are limited by invasive sampling and have not reached the clinic.[12] These molecular markers can give insight into the pathogenesis of the disease and suggest possible drug targets but cannot be used to monitor the disease. For that purpose, biomarkers in serum, plasma or urine are preferable. Urine is the biological fluid that can be obtained least invasively. However, urine can be difficult to use since correct normalization strategies need to be applied to compensate for differences in water consumption and other physiological factors between patients.[13] In complex inflammatory autoimmune diseases, it has so far been difficult to find one single biomarker that will explain and predict diagnosis, disease activity etc. since for each individual, many different factors will influence the clinical outcome. Therefore, a combination of several biomarkers might be the solution in personalized medicine. One example is the development of a multi-biomarker disease activity (MBDA) test for RA.[14] These MBDA scores have shown significant correlation with DAS28 and could reflect disease activity over time.[15] Identification of new biomarkers is very important but a lot of effort is also needed to implement biomarkers in the clinic; therefore, translational science is crucial.

Current State of Identification of Biomarkers and Affected Pathways

Today, it is important to identify new specific biomarkers that can provide the basis for improved diagnosis and stratify patient into different subgroups as discussed in the previous section. Also, the pathogenesis and progression of the majority of the inflammatory diseases are not fully understood and affected pathways remain to be identified. In addition, such knowledge will give information about possible new drug targets. New drugs might be developed that can cure patients who can only get symptomatic relief or are treated with drugs that may cause side effects due to their less targeted mechanisms of action.

A lot is known today about affected pathways and these have been studied by a hypothesis-based approach and traditional biochemistry. As a

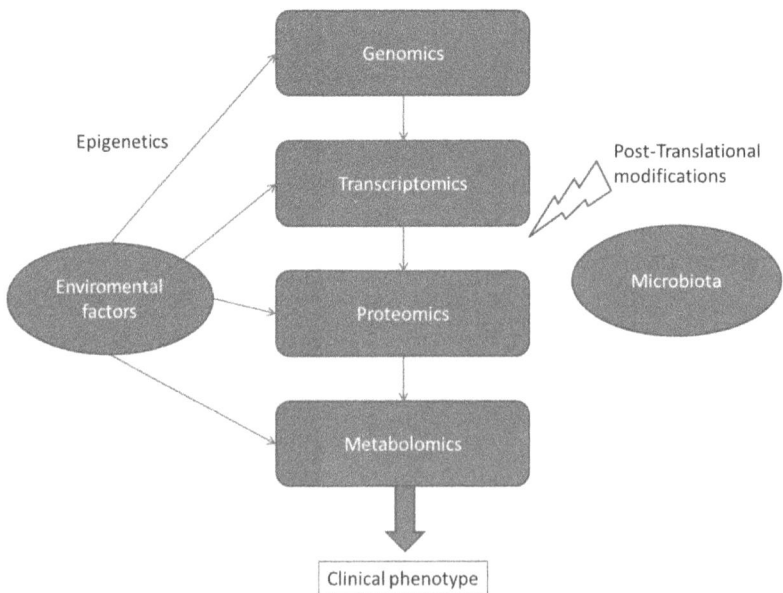

Figure 2.   Schemae of the hierarchy of different omics approaches.

complement to this approach, a data driven approach (discovery science) can be used. Methods like genomics, proteomics and metabolomics are then used to search for new biomarkers and affected pathways in a less supervised manner. We need both traditional biochemistry and omics approaches in order to achieve improved health.

Traditional biochemical approaches

Traditional biochemistry research is hypothesis driven and experiments are set up to test if a specific pathway/molecule is affected or not. Methods used are Western blot (WB), ELISA, enzyme activity assays, immunohistochemistry (IHC), 2D electrophoresis etc. These methods can of course also be used to validate results from the omics technologies. This targeted approach has generated biomarkers that are used in the clinic today.

Genomics and transcriptomics

In recent years, there have been significant improvements in the genomics and transcriptomics area that have had great impact on patient stratification and personalized medicine.[16] Genomics is the analysis of the genome, *i.e.*, the total DNA. DNA sequencing by microarrays can reveal differences in chromosome insertions and variations by single nucleotide polymorphisms (SNPs). Genes highly associated with different autoimmune diseases have been reported from several genome-wide association studies (GWAS).[17] In RA, more than 30 gene loci have been reported to influence the risk of RA but these only explain 20% of the total hereditary disease risk.[18] Therefore, in addition to genomics, proteins in general and autoantibodies such as rheumatoid factor in particular, are important for diagnostic purposes. Transcriptomics, *i.e.*, the universal detection of mRNA by microarrays will reflect the genes that are actively expressed at the time of sampling. However, it is the quantity of mRNA and not of expressed protein that is measured and proteomics will give further information about the protein expression.

Proteomics

Proteomics is an approach aiming for analysis of biological systems at the proteome level.[19,20] Proteomics is particularly informative for revealing pathways that drive inflammation and autoimmune reactions, since it can provide an integrated view of cellular processes and interactions at the protein level. In addition a vast majority of drug targets are proteins, especially membrane proteins.[21]

The suffix "-omic" refers to a holistic approach, *i.e.*, all proteins are studied. However, since it is not possible to detect all proteins in a system simultaneously, the moniker proteomics is also used when only a limited number of proteins are studied, targeted or non-targeted. Both targeted and untargeted proteomics approaches are important for screening the proteome in inflammatory diseases. Commonly used methods are mass spectrometry (MS) based[22] and affinity-based[23] proteomics. Several potential biomarkers have been suggested by a proteomics approach but few have been validated with additional methods and in larger cohorts. As pointed out for biomarkers of systemic sclerosis, the focus now must be on biomarker validation and panels of proteomic biomarkers for diagnosis/prognosis.[24]

Metabolomics

Metabolomics is a post-genomic research field for analysis of low molecular weight compounds in biological systems.[25,26] It is the youngest research field of the omics approaches. Analyzing metabolic differences between unperturbed and perturbed systems, such as healthy volunteers and patients with a disease, can lead to insights into the underlying pathogenic mechanisms.[27,28] The genome will give insight in what can happen, the proteome in what will happen and the metabolome in what has actually happened, taking into account posttranslational modifications etc. Therefore, the metabolome will give a better prediction of the expressed phenotype. However, the metabolome is much more complex, being highly influenced by environmental factors such as diet, and by the consistency in sample collection and storage. This approach will uncover pathways affected on the metabolite level and might be integrated with other omics approaches. Biomarkers identified by metabolomics within the field of rheumatology have been reported but not yet validated and implemented in the clinic.[29]

Data mining and biomarker validation

Through omics approaches, a wealth of experimental data is obtained and one challenge in discovery science is now how to handle "big data" and

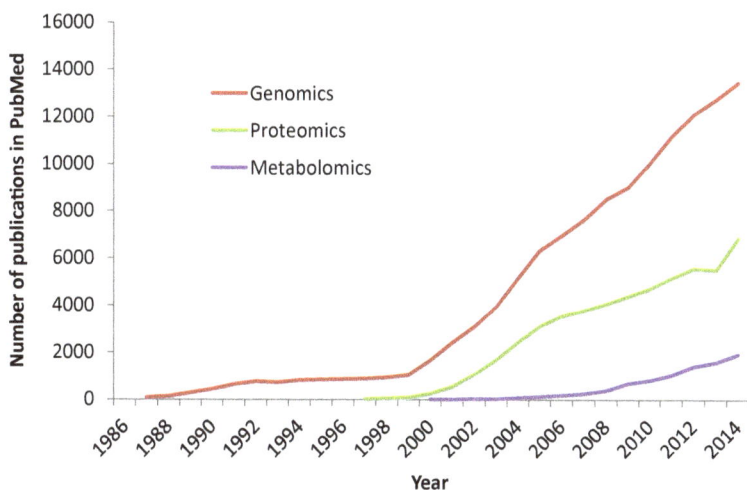

Figure 3. Metabolomics is the youngest omics science.

retrieve information that can be used in the clinic. Data mining is important as well as how the study is designed to collect the data.[30] Today, many biomarkers have been suggested but few have reached the clinic due to bad experimental design and lack of proper validation.[31] A possible biomarker or a set of biomarkers should be validated by complementary methods to show analytical validity and the biomarkers should be assigned biological relevance. Validation of prognostic biomarkers, *i.e.* biomarkers that will predict the outcome regardless of treatment, is relatively straightforward, but validation of predictive biomarkers, *i.e.* biomarkers that can predict the outcome in response to a certain therapy, is much more complex.[32] In both cases an appropriate clinical trial design, adequate biomarker assays and relevant outcome measurements must be selected.

Translational Science and Personalized Therapy

In this chapter, we have discussed the need for identifying new biomarkers for diagnosis and progression of disease and to stratify patients for personalized medicine. We have highlighted the need for identifying affected pathways in order to better understand the pathogenesis and be able to identify new drug targets. This is of course very important but it is just as

Table 1. Overview of technologies in biomarker discovery.

Biomarker technology	Strengths	Weaknesses	Opportunities	Techniques*
Traditional biochemistry	Focused methods where target is known. Methods are usually very sensitive. The experiment is designed to prove the hypothesis.	Only few parameters are taken into account although complex diseases are studied. Parameters of study are chosen based on prior knowledge and novel biomarkers are seldom discovered.	Most biomarkers used today have been identified by this approach. This approach can preferably be used complementarily to omics-approaches in the search for biomarkers.	Western blot ELISA Enzyme activity assays Immunohistochemistry 2D gel electrophoresis Various LC technologies with different types of detection, *e.g.*, UV or MS.
Genomics	Genetic biomarkers are conserved and stable.	Huge numbers of variables complicate the statistics and increase the probability of false positives. Genes only give information about what might happen in the biological system.	Understanding of etiology by epidemiological investigations and considering environmental factors. Drugs can be prescribed to specific subgroups characterized by a genetic modification.	DNA sequencing

Proteomics	The protein profile is more conserved than the metabolic profile but still more fine-tuned than the genetic profile. Proteomic techniques and data analysis tools are well-developed.	Post-translational modifications might be difficult to study. A lot of data is obtained and might be difficult to interpret and assign biological significance.	Many drug targets today are proteins and will most likely be so in the future. Proteins can be used as diagnostic and prognostic markers.	LC-MS Affinity-based protein/peptide arrays
Metabolomics	Metabolites are directly coding for the phenotype and will take everything into account including genetic modifications, post-translational modifications, environmental factors etc.	There are large fluctuations in the metabolic profile due to it being affected by diet etc., and homogenization of patient groups for studies of biomarkers is difficult to achieve.	A combination of metabolomic and proteomic targets might be the optimal biomarker panel to obtain a stable and, at the same time, specific response.	LC-MS, GC-MS, NMR

*Enzyme-linked immuno assay (ELISA), Liquid chromatography-mass spectrometry (LC-MS), Gas chromatography-mass spectrometry (GC-MS), Nuclear Magnetic resonance (NMR), Ultraviolet (UV).

important to validate suggested biomarkers, establish the biological relevance and implement biomarker panels in the clinic. Translational science, *i.e.*, taking knowledge from bench to bedside, must be the focus in the coming years.

The need for integrated clinical, molecular and serological classification of inflammatory diseases

It is not always the case that, for example, genomics results and proteomics results correlate. An up-regulated gene might not show a significant difference at the protein level. However, by applying several different omics approaches, pathways can be highlighted as affected in a certain disease and, in combination, the results can support each other. If so, the possibility for a real biomarker and not a biomarker by chance has increased.[30] To diagnose and predict prognosis, several markers should be combined in a multivariate manner, *i.e.*, combining several clinical and serological markers.

From science to medicine

Translational science merges basic and applied science and is evolving very rapidly,[33] but there is still a gap between basic and clinical research. If biomarker discoveries from basic science were set up to be validated in larger clinical cohorts and then implemented in the clinic, this could provide the basis for tailored medicine and therapeutic targets. But there are many obstacles in moving from bench to bedside.[34] Making sense of omics data in respect to bioinformatics and biological interpretation is crucial in accelerating the translation and is, today, the major bottle-neck. The interdisciplinary communication between biologists, bioinformatics specialists and clinical researchers must be improved.

References

1. Lipsky, P.E., Smolen, J.S., Informa, H. (2007). *Contemporary Targeted Therapies in Rheumatology*. New York: CRC Press.

2. Hahn, B.H., King, J.K. (2014). Chapter 80 — Treatment of autoimmune disease: established therapies. In: Mackay, N.R.R.R., editor. *The Autoimmune Diseases (Fifth Edition)*. Boston: Academic Press, p. 1209–1220.

3. Chatenoud, L. (2014). Chapter 81 — Treatment of autoimmune disease: biological and molecular therapies. In: Mackay, N.R.R.R., editor. *The Autoimmune Diseases (Fifth Edition)*. Boston: Academic Press, p. 1221–1245.

4. Cronstein, B.N. (2005). Low-dose methotrexate: a mainstay in the treatment of rheumatoid arthritis. *Pharmacol Rev*, **57**(2), 163–172.

5. Cejka, D., Hayer, S., Niederreiter, B., Sieghart, W., Fuereder, T., Zwerina, J., *et al.* (2010). Mammalian target of rapamycin signaling is crucial for joint destruction in experimental arthritis and is activated in osteoclasts from patients with rheumatoid arthritis. *Arthritis Rheum*, **62**(8), 2294–2302.

6. Available from: http://www.bu.edu/nf-kb/gene-resources/target-genes/.

7. Xu, K., Liu, P., Wei, W. (2014). mTOR signaling in tumorigenesis. *Biochim Biophys Acta*, **1846**(2), 638–654.

8. Aringer, M., Smolen, J.S. (2012). Therapeutic blockade of TNF in patients with SLE — Promising or crazy? *Autoimmun Rev*, **11**(5):321–325.

9. Verweij, C.L. (2011). Anti-TNF therapy in RA–towards personalized medicine? *Nat Rev Rheumatol*, **7**(3), 136.

10. Naguwa, S.M. (2005). Tumor necrosis factor inhibitor therapy for rheumatoid arthritis. *Ann New York Aca Sci*, **1051**(1), 709–715.

11. Aggarwal, B.B. (2003). Signalling pathways of the TNF superfamily: a double-edged sword. *Nat Rev Immunol*, **3**(9):745–756.

12. Prince, H.E. (2005). Biomarkers for diagnosing and monitoring autoimmune diseases. *Biomarkers*, **10**(Suppl 1), S44–S49. PubMed PMID: 16298911.

13. Warrack, B.M., Hnatyshyn, S., Ott, K.H., Reily, M.D., Sanders, M., Zhang, H., *et al.* (2009). Normalization strategies for metabonomic analysis of urine samples. *J Chromatogr B Analyt Technol Biomed Life Sci*, **877**(5–6):547–552. PubMed PMID: 19185549.

14. Centola, M., Cavet, G., Shen, Y., Ramanujan, S., Knowlton, N., Swan, K.A., *et al.* (2013). Development of a multi-biomarker disease activity test for rheumatoid arthritis. *PloS One*, **8**(4), e60635.

15. Hirata, S., Dirven, L., Shen, Y., Centola, M., Cavet, G., Lems, W.F., *et al.* (2013). A multi-biomarker score measures rheumatoid arthritis disease activity in the BeSt study. *Rheumatology*, **52**(7), 1202–1207. PubMed PMID: 23392591. Pubmed Central PMCID: 3685330.

16. Ginsburg, G.S., Willard, H.F. (2013). Preface. In: Willard, G.S.G.F., editor. *Genomic and Personalized Medicine (Second Edition)*: Academic Press, p. xi–xii.

17. Baranzini, S.E. (2013). Chapter 70 — Autoimmune Disorders. In: Willard, G.S.G.F., editor. *Genomic and Personalized Medicine (Second Edition)*: Academic Press, p. 822–838.
18. Plenge, R.M. (2013). Chapter 71 — Rheumatoid Arthritis. In: Willard, G.S.G.F., editor. *Genomic and Personalized Medicine (Second Edition)*: Academic Press, p. 839–852.
19. Ahrens, C.H., Qeli, E., Brunner, E., Basler, K., Aebersold, R. (2010). Generating and navigating proteome maps using mass spectrometry. *Nat Rev Mol Cell Biol*, **11**(11), 789–801.
20. Nilsson, T., Mann, M., Aebersold, R., Yates, r.J.R., Bairoch, A., Bergeron, J.J.M. (2010). Mass spectrometry in high-throughput proteomics: ready for the big time. *Nat Methods*, **7**(9), 681–685.
21. Lunn, C.A., Science, D. (2010). *Membrane Proteins as Drug Targets*. Amsterdam; Boston: Elsevier/Academic Press.
22. Mallick, P., Kuster, B. (2010). Proteomics: a pragmatic perspective. *Nat Biotechnol*, **28**(7), 695–709. PubMed PMID: 20622844.
23. Uhlen, M., Ponten, F., Kth, Proteomik, Skolan för b. (2005). Antibody-based proteomics for human tissue profiling. *Mol Cell Proteom*, **4**(4), 384–393.
24. Paul, Bln. (2014). Systemic sclerosis biomarkers discovered using mass-spectrometry-based proteomics: a systematic review. *Biomarkers*, **19**(5), 345–355.
25. van der Greef, J., Stroobant, P., van der Heijden, R. (2004). The role of analytical sciences in medical systems biology. *Curr Opin Chemical Biol*, **8**(5), 559–565.
26. Patti, G.J., Yanes, O., Siuzdak, G. (2012). Innovation: Metabolomics: the apogee of the omics trilogy. *Nat Rev Mol Cell Biol*, **13**(4), 263–269. PubMed PMID: 22436749. Pubmed Central PMCID: 3682684.
27. Fernie, A.R., Trethewey, R.N., Krotzky, A.J., Willmitzer, L. (2004). Innovation: Metabolite profiling: from diagnostics to systems biology. *Nat Rev Mol Cell Biol*, **5**(9), 763–769.
28. Madsen, R., Lundstedt, T., Trygg, J. (2010). Chemometrics in metabolomics — a review in human disease diagnosis. *Analytica Chimica Acta*, **659**(1–2), 23–33.
29. Julià, A., Alonso, A., Marsal, S. (2014). Metabolomics in rheumatic diseases. *Int J Clinical Rheumatol*, **9**(4), 353–369.
30. Ransohoff, D.F. (2005). Lessons from controversy: ovarian cancer screening and serum proteomics. *J Nat Cancer Inst*, **97**(4), 315–319.
31. Ioannidis, J.P.A. (2013). Biomarker failures. *Clin Chem*, **59**(1), 202.
32. Mandrekar, S.J., Sargent, D.J. (2010). Predictive biomarker validation in practice: lessons from real trials. *Clin Trials* (London, England), **7**(5), 567–573.

33. Palmer, A.M., Sundstrom, L. (2013). Translational medicines research. *Drug Discovery Today*, **18**(11–12), 503–505. PubMed PMID: 23454742.

34. Chin, L., Andersen, J.N., Futreal, P.A. (2011). Cancer genomics: from discovery science to personalized medicine. *Nat Med*, **17**(3):297–303. PubMed PMID: 21383744.

CHAPTER 3

B CELL-DIRECTED THERAPIES FOR INFLAMMATORY DISEASES

Thomas Dörner and Peter E. Lipsky

Introduction

The development of therapeutic monoclonal antibodies (mAb) has permitted targeted therapy of rheumatic autoimmune/inflammatory diseases (RAID). A number of approaches have been employed based on the prevailing view at the time of dominant cells initiating and perpertuating specific diseases. Traditional models of immune pathogenesis postulated a central role for CD4+ T cells and antigen presenting myeloid cells[1] and prompted efforts to treat RAID, such as rheumatoid arthritis (RA), with anti-CD4 mAb. The majority of these trials showed no clinical benefit and raised questions about the central role of CD4+ T cells. Recently, however, the successful treatment of RA by blocking T cell co-stimulation with CTLA4Ig (abatacept) has again implied a role for CD4+ T cells in RA pathogenesis.

Clinical application of anti-cytokine therapy in RA appears to be closely linked to blocking effector molecules of the innate immune system but also may have an impact on B cell and plasma cell differentiation and survival. Hence, this leaves the central role of B cells in RA pathogenesis unresolved. Moreover, trials of alemtuzumab targeting CD52 expressed on

T cells, B cells and other adaptive and innate immune cells have led to increased safety considerations with minimal efficacy,[2] questioning the role of the immune system in general in RA pathogenesis. Despite this, it has been accepted that autoantibodies play an important amplifying role in tissue (joint, vessel) inflammation and serve as diagnostic, classification and prognostic markers in RA and a number of other RAID. More recently, the success of B cell depleting therapy in ameliorating RA inflammation and inhibiting radiographic progression even after failure of TNF blockade[3] as well as in the induction of clinical benefit in ANCA vasculitides[4] has documented a role for B cells in the pathogenesis of these diseases.

Although animal models are very valuable for the identification of pathways potentially involved in the induction and perpetuation of specific RAID, ultimate proof for the efficacy and safety of an agent is only possible by clinical trials in humans. With the advent of different agents targeting specific parts of the immune system, clinical studies have begun to yield a plethora of lessons concerning the key immune mechanisms in individual RAID. Such examples will be discussed in this chapter with a main focus on anti-CD20 therapy, the anti-BLyS/BAFF agents belimumab, tabalumab, blisibimod and the anti-BLyS/BAFF/APRIL blocking agent atacicept. While some data may be influenced by limitations of the trial design and outcome measurements, one can arrive at the current conclusion that certain diseases such as RA and MS may depend more on CD20 B cell function, whereas the BAFF blocking agents inhibiting the survival of naive B cells and early plasma cells have a more substantial impact in SLE but not in RA or MS.

Role of B Cells in Immune Responses

B cells are an essential component of normal immune responses and are responsible for the maintenance of humoral protective memory.[5] The nature of the serologic component of memory is illustrated by the persisting protective antibody titers against a variety of microorganisms.[6] Interestingly, CD4+ T cells are important in instructing memory B cells to differentiate into long-lived plasma cells; these long-lived non-proliferating antibody-secreting cells survive independent of antigen and further direct interaction with antigen-specific T cells[7] in bone marrow niches.[8] While preclinical models[9] using B cell depleted mice provided evidence that T cell memory depends on IL-6 produced by B cells, antigen-non-specific interactions with T cells may also contribute to the survival of human B and plasma cells in secondary lymphoid organs.

Normal B cell development in health

In order to understand the role of B cells in autoimmunity and also to delineate possible points for therapeutic targeting, it is important to re-emphasize the role of these cells under normal conditions (Fig. 1). B cells follow a tightly regulated life cycle. In the bone marrow, B cells develop from stem cells through a series of precursor stages during which they rearrange their immunoglobulin genes to generate a wide range of unique antigen binding specificities and emigrate as immature CD20+ B cells, expressing surface IgM/IgD into the peripheral blood and differentiate through a series of maturational or transitional cell stages into mature naive B cells. These cells can migrate between blood and secondary lymphoid organs, react to the unique antigen they recognize, but only within secondary lymphoid organs after receiving the combination of specific B cell receptor stimulation and T cell help. It is now recognized that a specialized helper T cell residing within B cell follicles of secondary lymphoid nodules, the T follicular helper T cell (T_{FH}), provides the optimal help necessary for the induction of T cell-dependent B cell responses (Fig. 3).

T cell dependent (TD) B cell activation

After encountering their cognate antigen and receiving T cell help at the T cell-B cell interface in secondary lymphoid organs, B cells undergo germinal center (GC) reactions, during which antigen specific B cells clonally expand, somatically mutate their Ig genes to achieve avidity maturation, undergo Ig heavy chain class-switch recombination and mature either into memory B cells or Ig secreting plasma cells. Because of somatic hypermutation (SHM) and class-switch recombination (CSR), the avidity of the B cell immunglobulin receptor can be increased and the biologic function of secreted Ig altered. Important for the interaction with T cells and the

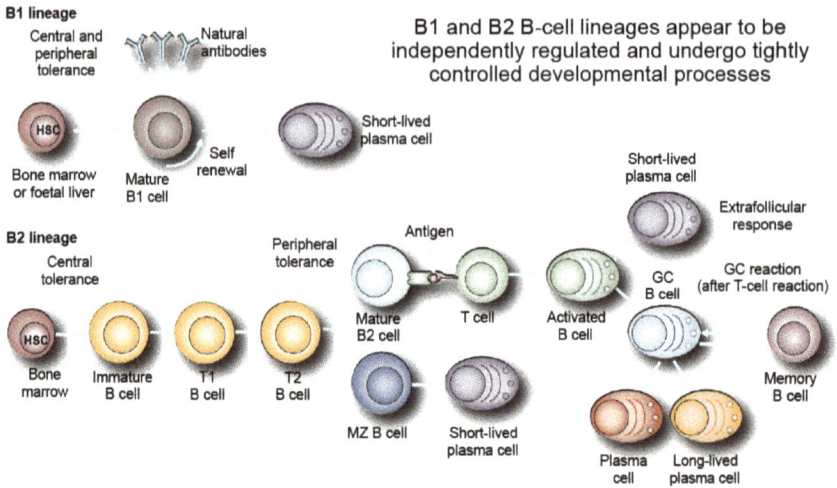

B1 lineage
Central and peripheral tolerance
Natural antibodies

Bone marrow or foetal liver

HSC

Mature B1 cell
Self renewal

Short-lived plasma cell

B1 and B2 B-cell lineages appear to be independently regulated and undergo tightly controlled developmental processes

Short-lived plasma cell

Extrafollicular response

B2 lineage
Central tolerance

Bone marrow

HSC

Immature B cell

T1 B cell

T2 B cell

Peripheral tolerance

Mature B2 cell

Antigen

T cell

Activated B cell

GC B cell

GC reaction (after T-cell reaction)

Memory B cell

MZ B cell

Short-lived plasma cell

Plasma cell

Long-lived plasma cell

HSC = haemopoietic stem cell; GC = germinal centre
MZ = marginal zone.

Adapted from Ref. [90]

Figure 1. A schematic of B-cell development. B1 and B2 B cell lineages appear to be independently regulated in the mouse and undergo tightly controlled developmental processes. (**a**) B1 B cells develop from HSCs in the bone marrow or fetal liver, are self-renewing and produce natural antibodies involved in self-defense. (**b**) B2 B cells develop from HSCs in the bone marrow. Following rearrangement of their B-cell-receptor chain genes and removal of autoreactive cells via central tolerance, immature (transitional) B2 B cells relocate to the spleen. Those immature B2 B cells that escape the processes of peripheral tolerance differentiate either into MZ B cells or mature follicular B2 cells. This dichotomous process is apparently regulated by fine tuned BCR complex related engagements where the strength of BCR activation appears to provide the important directive. Only follicular B2 cells develop into long-lived plasma cells or memory B cells upon T-cell-dependent activation. B1 B cells and MZ B cells are thought to be the main sources of short-lived plasma cells; the contribution of B2 B cells to this population has not been delineated. Abbreviations: GC, germinal center; HSC, hematopoietic stem cell; MZ, marginal zone.

generation of GC reactions are a series of ligand receptor interactions, including those mediated by CD154/CD40, CD28/CD80-CD86 and ICOS-L/ICOS. Defects in these interactions have been shown to lead to hyper-IgM syndrome resulting in impaired plasma cell and memory B cell generation and adult onset of common variable hypogammaglobulinemia, respectively. Some B cells can respond to specific antigens in a **T cell-independent manner (TI responses)**. TI responses largely induce IgM antibodies and do not generate classic post-switch memory B cells. In the mouse, these responses are thought to be restricted to CD1d+/IgM^{high} marginal zone B cells residing in the spleen that recognize polysaccharide antigens.

In addition, B cells are characteristically divided into two major lineages, B1 cells and B2 cells (Fig. 1). It is still a matter of debate whether B1 and B2 cells are similar in mice and humans.[10] In particular, the expression of CD5 used as marker of these cells in mice is not reliable in humans since the molecule is expressed during B cell activation and B cell maturation. **B1 cells** are considered to be self-renewing and long-lived, emerging early in development, and residing in the peritoneal and pleural cavities. In mice, B1 cells produce polyreactive IgM antibodies. The natural autoantibodies produced by B1 cells are important in the clearance of apoptotic material, senescent red blood cells and other cellular and subcellular debris. In mice the subset of B1 cells has, therefore, been considered to be a bridge between innate and adaptive immunity. **B2 cells** or conventional B cells comprise the adaptive portion of humoral immune responses. B2 cells participate preferentially in GC reactions, during which they can hypermutate their IgV gene rearrangements, switch Ig classes and differentiate into memory B cells and long-lived plasma cells. However, B2 cells can also be activated during TI responses, but in this circumstance they usually do not undergo SHM, CSR and do not generate either memory B cells or long-lived plasma cells. B2 cells are generated in the bone marrow where there are checkpoints for removal of autoreactive cells (central tolerance). The immature survivors with functional B-cell receptors leave the marrow where they are thought to be exposed to further negative selection to remove residual autoreactive clones (peripheral tolerance). Although it has not been fully delineated in humans, in mice, cells at this point are routed into **either a mature follicular B cell or a marginal zone B cell (MZ-B)** program.[11] However, ligation of the BCR complex, including CD22 and the strength of the BCR engagement[12] seem to determine whether B cells arriving in the spleen will develop into MZ or follicular B cells. This decision point may have directive/future consequences since

MZ B cells will have less or almost no further selection points in contrast to follicular B cells. Thus, the BCR specificity together with proper formation of the BCR complex defines the extent to which an autoreactive cell can escape complete selection. However, MZ B cells probably do not develop B cell memory but contribute to short-lived IgM/IgG.

Follicular B cells traffic throughout the secondary lymphoid organs,[13] whereas MZ-B cells are specialized to reside in a compartment in the spleen that samples the blood stream for pathogens. Both B1 and MZ-B cells are key parts of the adaptive immune system that can be activated rapidly and respond immediately to pathogens in the blood as well as the peritoneal and pleural cavities.[14] Responses by both cells occur independent of T cell help and they are thought to be excluded from undergoing GC reactions; they undergo CSR and SHM poorly and do not generate long-lived plasma cells or B cell memory. In contrast B2 cells respond to TD antigens, participate in GC responses, undergo extensive CSR and SHM and generate long-lived plasma cells and memory B cells.

In most autoimmune diseases, there are class-switched, high-affinity IgG autoantibodies likely resulting from the establishment of a fully formed T cell-dependent GC reaction. In some circumstance, T cell-dependent responses may occur in extra-follicular sites, although similar dependence of these responses on follicular helper T cells (T_{FH}), CD40/CD154 interactions and IL-21 suggests that they may be qualitatively similar.[15] There is little evidence that extra-follicular responses develop in humans with autoimmune diseases.[16] Importantly, pathogenic autoantibodies in SLE (anti-DNA[17]), RA (anti-CCP[18]), and pemphigus (anti-desmoglein 3[19]) are usually heavily mutated. Moreover, reversion of the mutations back toward the germline sequence nullifies autoantibody binding.[17–19] These results suggest that these autoantibodies may arise in GC where the mutational machinery is activated in humans, but also that the development of autoantibodies results from the mutational machinery operating on naive B cells that have no initial capacity to bind autoantigens, but rather recognise and are probably originally stimulated by exogenous antigen. These findings imply that despite many checkpoint abnormalities in autoimmune diseases,[20] the essential break in B cell tolerance may occur in the periphery and involve the lack of appropriate negative selection of B cells developing the capacity to recognize autoantigens as a result of GC reactions or the presence of abnormal positive selection owing to the abundance of apoptotic material present in the GC bound to FDC.[21] However, the detailed underlying mechanisms remain unclear.

Cytokines are also very important for B cell differentiation and maintenance. Although BLyS/BAFF is essential for the survival of naive B cells and contributes to the survival of some populations of plasma cells (PC),[22] there is recent evidence that this cytokine might also increase the lifespan of TLR-activated autoreactive B cells allowing them either to persist as antibody secreting effectors, or to enter ongoing GC reactions and be directed into the long-lived PC pool.[23] Consistent with this idea, plasmablasts and memory B cells upregulate one of the receptors for BLyS/BAFF (BCMA) in SLE patients, and BCMA stimulation might enhance the response to TLR9 stimulation.[24] Alternatively, BLyS/BAFF might enhance the ability of TLR-activated B cells to seed the memory B cell pool, since memory B cells are occasionally generated in response to TI antigens.[25]

The role of B cells in inflammatory diseases

B cells are directly and indirectly involved in the pathogenesis of certain RAID (Fig. 2) by their **differentiation into memory B cells and antibody-producing plasma cells** within the inflamed tissues **and formation of immune complexes** that activate the complement cascade and amplify local inflammation. Autoantibodies are usually taken as an indication of the breakdown of immune tolerance but are frequently determined by the genetic HLA class II background.[26] Importantly, the **induction of specific autoantibodies occurs before the disease onset** in both RA[27] and SLE,[28] as well as a number of other autoimmune diseases.

Other potential immunopathogenic functions of B cells. Antigen presentation mediated by MHC class II can be carried out by B cells. Memory B cells expressing high avidity BCR are particularly effective at taking up the antigen recognized by their unique BCR and presenting it to antigen specific CD4 T cells. In general, memory B cells are more effective antigen presenting cells for memory T cells, and thus may play a more important function in amplification and progression of autoimmunity after it has been initiated.

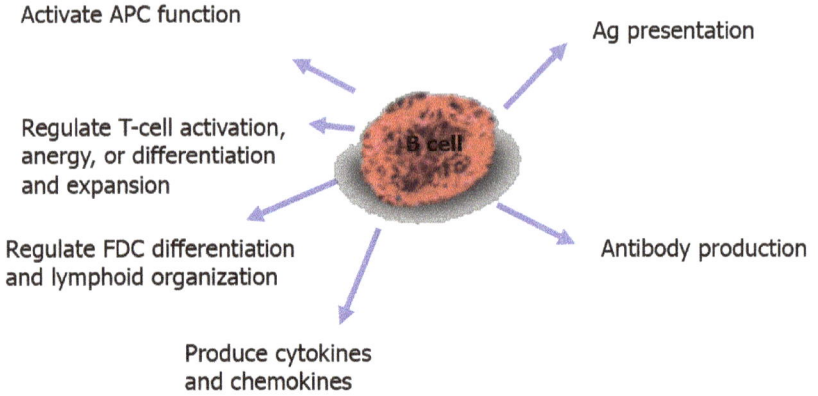

Figure 2. The various functions of B cells with implications for health and autoimmunity. APC: antigen presenting cell; FDC: follicular dendritic cell modified according to Ref. [5].

B cells are considered to produce **proinflammatory cytokines**, such as tumor necrosis factor (TNF) and interleukin (IL)-6, and immunoregulatory cytokines, such as IL-10. However, recent data show that B cells derived from patients with RA and SLE, respectively produce lesser amounts of cytokines and chemokines and this is inversely related to disease activity and normalized upon effective treatment (own data). These observations argue against the assumption that B cells are the major direct cytokine producers during active disease, although they still can indirectly activate T cells or DCs to enhance cytokine production globally. The normalization of cytokine production after effective treatment suggests that B cells may have potential regulatory functions which are substantially impaired during active disease. In this context, IL-10 as well as IL-35 producing B cells[29,30] have been shown in relevant animal models of EAE to control inflammation. Moreover, IL-10 production by human B cells with regulatory function is substantially reduced in patients with active SLE,[31,32] suggesting that there might be a parallel decline in the proinflammatory and regulatory cytokine production in lupus patients with active disease.

B cells **regulate follicular dendritic cell differentiation and the organization of the lymphatic architecture**. Mice that lack B cells do not develop antigen presenting M cells in the gut. B cells are also involved in the **regulation of T-cell activation, anergy, differentiation**, and the expansion of T cells. B cells play an important role in T-cell activation resulting in T_{FH} induction and induction of T_H memory cells. In humans, this conclusion is also supported by studies in patients with SLE that demonstrated a deactivation of T cells after selective B-cell depletion[33] and a reduction in T cell numbers.[34] Moreover, data from experiments in which synovial tissue was transplanted into immunodeficient scid/NOD mice[35,36] showed that B cell depletion by rituximab caused a substantial downregulation of T cell activation and reduction in IFNγ production. These data suggest that synovial B cells may be necessary for T cell activation.

Formation of ectopic germinal centers. It is known that memory B cells and plasma cells reside in affected tissues, such as in RA synovium, kidneys of lupus nephritis patients, in the spleen of immune thrombocytopenia patients[26] as well as in the brain of patients with multiple sclerosis,[37] often forming GC-like structures. Although it cannot be formally excluded since tissue resident B and plasma cells have migrated into the site of inflammation, the presence of these cells in affected organs likely reflects local generation in ectopic GC. Recent evidence has indicated that the tubulointerstitial infiltrate in lupus glomerulonephritis is composed of B cells, macrophages and plasma cells and is associated with the progression to end stage renal disease.[38,39] Blockade of BLyS/BAFF inhibited the progression of lupus nephritis in animal models and abolished the presence of inflammatory infiltrates in the kidneys despite the presence of pathogenic autoantibodies.[40]

In human lupus nephritis, local expression of BLyS/BAFF, but not serum levels, was found to be associated with the development of B cell infiltrates in the kidney (reviewed in Ref. [41]). This is consistent with the conclusion that local production of BLyS/BAFF in the kidney may play a specific role in driving the local inflammatory response and tissue damage, independent of the systemic role of this cytokine in B cell biology. It is notable, however, that BLyS/BAFF blockade with belimumab is associated with a significant increase in circulating memory B cells,[42] although the mechanism and clinical relevance of this finding are unknown.

Another important cytokine for B cell differentiation and plasma cell survival is IL-6, which, as a pleiotropic cytokine, is involved in the regulation of the crosstalk between haematopoietic and immune cells. Via

IL-6Ra, IL-6 signals by dimerized gp130 that stimulates JAK1 and TYK2 phosphorylation and subsequently leads to activation of STAT3 as a transcription factor. Both IL-6 and STAT3 appear to be central regulators of B cell differentiation and Th17 differentiation, including a positive feedback loop between IL-6, IL-17 and STAT3.[43] While there are positive reports for tocilizumab in an early SLE study,[44] a recent study using the IL-6 blocking monoclonal sirukumab in lupus nephritis[88] failed to meet its efficacy endpoints and was associated with an increased frequency of infectious complications.

The immune system is finely regulated via inhibitory and activating receptors. Innate immune cells such as monocytes, macrophages, immature DCs, mast cells and neutrophils constitutively express activating and inhibitory Fc receptors that contribute to a finely balanced innate immune response. By contrast, T cells upregulate inhibitory receptors (PD-1, CTLA-4 etc.) after activation via APC. Finally, B cells express both inhibitory (ICOS-L, FcRIIb, CD22) and activating receptors (FcRIIa, FcRIII, BCR). Although it remains to be further elucidated and translated into clinical application, B cells share a number of receptors expressed by cells of the innate immune system (including TLR, NLR, FcRIIb) and regulatory processes and therefore could be considered as a part of both the innate and adaptive immune systems, as well as being both immune-active and immune-regulatory. This is notable, since they simultaneously represent cells with a very sophisticated surface immunoglobulin receptor with the unique capacity to recognize the universe of antigens as well as cells that can autoregulate themselves through molecules such as FcRIIb and CD22 and cytokines such as IL-10 and also suppress other cells by producing IL-10 and inducing Treg activation.[31]

Antigen binding and subsequent stimulation involves the **activity of a fully functional BCR**. The BCR complex that comprises the BCR, CD22, CD21, CD74 is required for initial signal transduction. The nature of the BCR complex in SLE has not been fully delineated, whereas impaired TCR organization as well as localization into lipid rafts has been reported in SLE T cells.[45]

Until recently, the majority of research has focused on increased BCR signalling as a pathway to autoimmunity, with the demonstration that overexpression of molecules enhances the strength of BCR signalling, such as

CD19, or deletion/dysfunction of molecules which reduces BCR signalling, such as SHP-1 and FcγRIIb, leading to autoimmunity.[12] Enhanced BCR signalling capability implies that the same exposure to antigen will deliver a stronger signal to SLE B cells, and, as a result, there will be less tolerance of immature cells and more activation of mature B cells. This model further requires that the strength of BCR signalling differs at different stages of B cell development.[12]

In addition to defining the differentiation of B cells into MZ or follicular B cells, a number of recent reports suggest that diminished BCR signalling by B2 cells can also lead to autoimmunity. Given that negative selection depends on BCR signalling, it is expected that diminished signalling by self-reactive BCR permits B cells to escape negative selection. Evidence for this model was provided by studying B cells from patients with X-linked agammaglobulinemia (XLA) carrying defects in Bruton's tyrosine kinase (BTK), which is involved in BCR signalling.[46] Peripheral B cells from XLA patients were enriched with autoreactive BCRs indicating that diminished BCR signalling can result in increased autoreactivity within naive B cells.

B cells from lupus patients were found to have a higher frequency of autoreactive cells in the immature, transitional and naive B cell compartments compared to controls,[47] which is consistent with the idea that altered BCR signalling strength can result in autoimmunity. A recent genome-wide association study has found that alleles of the gene BLK are associated with lupus.[48] BLK is a mediator of BCR signalling, and the alleles associated with lupus risk correlate with decreased BLK expression, furthering the link between diminished BCR signalling as already reported for mouse lupus models.[12]

BCR signalling strength can also affect B cell fate after antigen activation. In mice transgenic for the heavy chain of an antibody to the hapten nitrophenyl (NP), B cells with low affinity BCRs participate in GC reactions and produce both memory and long-lived plasma B cells after antigen challenge, whereas B cells with high affinity BCRs differentiate into short-lived plasma cells and do not enter GC reactions.[12] This is of note because many pathogenic anti-DNA antibodies in lupus demonstrate class switch to IgG and affinity maturation, both of which are hallmarks of the GC reaction.

Recent Advances in Understanding GC Reactions and Considerations for Immune Therapeutics

GCs represent the functional site where clonal expansion, SHM, CSR and affinity-based selection resulting in high-affinity antibodies occur (Fig. 3). Intravital imaging allows further insight into GC biology, as reviewed recently.[20] The notable findings are that first, there is constant B cell trafficking between the distinct dark zone (DZ), composed of proliferating B cells, and light zone (LZ) composed of B cells that have previously undergone clonal expansion and are being exposed to selecting antigen bound to follicular dendritic cells (FDC), indicating that the GC reaction is an iterative one with repetitive rounds of proliferation and selection. Secondly, the chemokine receptor CXCR4 is important in controlling the

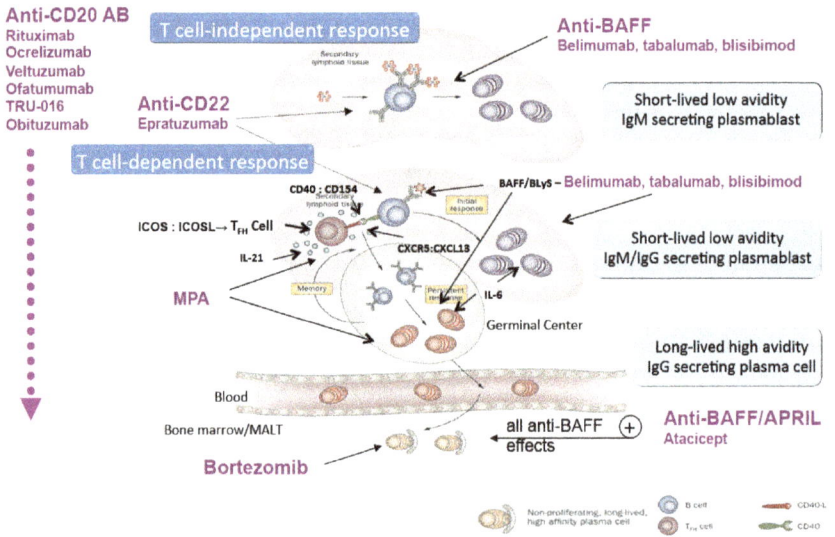

Figure 3. Direct (*i.e.* anti-CD20, CD22 therapies) and indirect (anti-BAFF/BLyS by belimumab, blisibimod or tabalumab and atacicept also affecting plasma cells) targeting of B cells including non-specific effects of drugs on B cells. These strategies interfere with different developmental stages of B cells within germinal centers and extrafollicular sites with certain effects on T cell-dependent and T cell-independent activation, and may also impact cellular survival and differentiation niches, while the less specific targeting strategies of MMF and bortezomib also have an impact on other immune cells. (modified according to Ref. [41]).

retention of B cells in the DZ of GC. Moreover, it was confirmed that re-expression of the BCR in the LZ is critical for positive selection on FDCs and presenting antigen to T_{FH} cells in LZ that provide survival signals via CD40-CD154 interaction. Proper function of GC requires establishment and maintenance of a precise microarchitecture requiring T follicular helper T cells (T_{FH}) expressing CXCR5, bcl-6, ICOS, PD1 and the adaptor molecule SAP. While there is evidence that there are subsets of T_{FH} cells, such as classical, extrafollicular, NK, γδTFH and T_{FR} regulatory cells,[49] the GC microarchitecture is at least partly under control of IL-6, BAFF, lymphotoxin-α and β, CXCL-13, -12, ICAM-1, VCAM-1 and these factors all contribute to GC function and localization of participating cells.

Very recently, the essential role of B cells in induction and maintenance of T_{FH} cells[50] has been clearly identified. The interaction of GC-B cells and T_{FH} cells depending on the availability of the stimulating antigen is apparent and emphasizes the critical role of B cells in orchestrating their microenvironment and the function of the T cells with which they interact. These findings have potential clinical implications. First, rituximab may not sufficiently deplete GC B cells[51] or total precursors,[52] and, thus, may have reduced impact on T-B collaboration at time of therapy. Similarly, treatment with belimumab led to a marked increase of memory B cells,[42] resulting in the possibility that an expanded population of autoantigen-committed memory B cell with the capacity to orchestrate GC responses might counter-balance the effect on naive B cell and plasma cell survival, and thereby thwart more effective clinical responses. These results suggest that more promising B cell-directed therapies should possibly focus more consistently on GC B cells and their interaction with T_{FH} cells. Potential candidates are therapeutics that block IL-21, ICOS/ICOS-L interactions, CD40/154 interactions, PD1/PD-L interactions, CXCR5/CXCL13 interactions, among others.

Besides classical GC, other forms of lymphoid structures may subserve the function of promoting B cell activation and differentiation.[15] In this regard, a recent study[16] identified two different lymphoid structures accommodating proliferating B cells in human spleen, classical GC and proliferative lymphoid nodules (PLN). The latter were characterized by proliferating Ki67+ B cells in close proximity to FDC, but lacked polarization into DZ and LZ and were composed of B cells and T cells that did not express the transcription factor bcl6, which is necessary for both the formation of GC and differentiation of T_{FH}.[53] Importantly, PLN of immune thrombocytopenia (ITP), not control spleens, were found to contain FDCs presenting the autoantigens glycoprotein (GP) IIb/IIIa and IV incorporated into immune complexes. Regulatory T cells were reduced within PLN of ITP spleens suggesting a defect of tolerance which is related to a loss of T cell regulation. These results suggest that unique PLN containing proliferating B cells are in direct contact with autoantigen bearing FDC, but lacking LZ, where negative selection normally occurs, and that a decreased frequency of Tregs may contribute to the persistent autoimmunity of ITP and, perhaps, RAID.

Pharmacologic Targeting of B Cells

There are different approaches to target B cells. These include depleting and non-depleting B cell-directed antibodies, modulation of B cell signalling, and manipulation of regulatory B cells[41] (Table 1). In addition, there are more indirect approaches to target B cell responses in GC, such as cytokine or ligand inhibition (IL-21, CTLA-4Ig, ICOS-L etc.) as well as blocking proteasome activity, intracellular kinases, inosine monophosphate dehydrogenase by mycophenolic acid or mycophenolate mofetil (MMF), TLR signaling (antimalarials, laquinimod), or certain metabolic pathways.

Direct targeting using mAB

Approval of rituximab, as a prototypic B cell depleting **anti-CD20** mAB, in patients with RA who are anti-TNF incomplete responders and recently anti-neutrophil cytoplasmic antibody-associated vasculitides was the first B cell-directed therapy for RAID. CD20 is a B-lymphocyte-specific antigen that is expressed by pre-B and mature B cells, but not fully differentiated plasma cells. It has a role in the regulation of cell-cycle initiation and differentiation of the B cell lineage. Rituximab is a chimeric monoclonal IgG1 antibody to CD20 that causes B cell depletion lasting from 6 to 12 months and is mediated through complement-dependent cytotoxicity and antibody-dependent cellular toxicity. Licensed for the treatment of non-Hodgkin lymphoma, RA and vasculitis, there are several case and registry reports of the use of rituximab in patients with diseases refractory to standard

Table 1. Direct and indirect B cell targeting therapies as well as therapies reported to impact on B cells in RAID (modified according to COR 2014).

Direct B cell targets	Example		Indirect B cell targets		Therapeutics that have been shown to co-impact on B /plasma cells
CD20	Rituximab	Depletion	BAFF/BLyS	Belimumab	Glucocorticoids
	Veltuzumab			Tabalumab	Methotrexate
	Ocrelizumab			Blisibimod	Etanercept
	Ofatumumab				Tocilizumab
	Obituzumab				Bortezomib
	SMIP SBI-087		BAFF/APRIL	Atacicept	
CD22	Epratuzumab	Modulation of B cell functions			TLR signalling by antimalarials
			Abatacept	Blockade of T-B interaction	Blockade of co-stimulation (CTLA4-Ig, ICOS-L etc.)
CD19	MD1342	Depletion			IVIG via FcRIIB inhibitory effects
CD19/ CD3	Blinatumomab	Depletion			mycophenolic acid
CD52	Alemtuzumab	Depletion			cyclophosphamide

treatments. Two major clinical trials in SLE (LUNAR, EXPLORER),[54,55] one trial in autoimmune myositis (RIM)[56] and one Sjögren's trial[57] have not met their endpoints.

The approval of rituximab in autoimmune indications has provided a stimulus for the development of additional depleting anti-CD20 mAB, including humanized (ocrelizumab, veltuzumab, obituzumab) or human (ofatumumab) mAB. An engineered polypeptide (humanized CD20-directed small modular immunopharmaceutical [SMIP]), SBI-087 is able to bind to CD20 and also results in B cell depletion. Although CD20 is uniquely expressed on mature B cells, rituximab binding has been reported on podocyte membranes[58] inducing remodelling of glomeruli that may explain an "off target" effect, namely the early impact on proteinuria in lupus nephritis before immune changes become effective.

Ocrelizumab has been intensively studied in SLE and RA but in both indications, phase III trials were discontinued in part because of safety concerns and, in the case of RA, insufficient benefit. However, the clinical development of ocrelizumab is continuing in multiple sclerosis. A phase II study in multiple sclerosis reported good efficacy and safety data, with no imbalance in serious infections between placebo and ocrelizumab. Phase III studies are underway.

Similar to anti-CD20, anti-CD19 and anti-CD52 (alemtuzumab) — that also targets T cells — lead to depletion by complement-dependent cytotoxicity (CDC) and antibody-dependent cell-mediated cellular cyto-toxicity (ADCC).

CD19 is also part of the BCR complex and is crucial for B cell development and activation. It is expressed from the early stages of B cell maturation onward, present on memory B cells, and — although substantially downregulated — expressed on a subset of plasma cells in the bone marrow which appears to be a precursor of CD19– cells.[59,60,89] Preliminary data could not find CD19 expression on PC in the tissues of autoimmune patients. This is of interest since overexpression of CD19 has been linked with development of autoimmunity,[61] possibly reflecting increased B cell activation, since autoimmunity is prevented by blocking BCR signalling. Depleting anti-CD19 mAB have been mainly investigated in the treatment of lymphoma and leukaemia. In this regard, a single-chain bispecific antibody to CD19 and CD3, blinatumomab, can cause lysis of human B cell lymphoma cells *in vivo* and has exhibited substantial clinical efficacy in clinical trials in patients with B cell lymphoma.[62] One phase I study using the human depleting nonfucosylated anti-CD19 mAB, MDX1342 has been completed in RA NCT00639834 (clinicaltrials.gov, accessed May 18th, 2015) and results are anticipated. Overall, available data indicate that there is a more comprehensive depletion of B and plasma cells with anti-CD19 as compared to anti-CD20 therapies but a substantial fraction of CD19-bone marrow plasma cells would not be affected by such therapy.

CD22 is a B-lymphocyte-specific transmembrane sialoglycoprotein. CD22 functions through the B cell receptor (BCR) complex by phosphorylation of three intracellular tyrosine-based inhibitory motifs. Phosphorylation initiates the recruitment of tyrosine phosphatase 1 that inhibits BCR signalling. CD22 is expressed to a higher extent on naive versus memory B cells,[63] and is also part of the CD19–CD21–CD22 BCR complex. Its function is to modulate BCR and CD19-mediated signal transduction, and it also provides essential B cell survival signals. As with CD20, cell-surface expression of CD22 is downregulated when mature B cells differentiate into plasma cells. Recently, CD22 has also been identified on the surface of normal DCs and pDC neoplasms[64] as well as on T cells by trogocytosis after *in vitro* co-culture.[65] However, the functional consequences of CD22 expression by non-B cells remain uncertain.

Epratuzumab, a humanized mAB to the B cell surface molecule, CD22, is thought to modulate B cell function, although a modest degree of peripheral B cell reduction likely based on redistribution of B cells into tissue can be observed after administration of this agent. Recent studies have shed new light concerning the mechanism by which epratuzumab alters B cell function. First, binding of epratuzumab changes the expression of adhesion molecules (downregulation of CD62L, β-7 integrin, upregulation of β-1 integrin) and modulates B cell migration,[63] a finding that may explain the 30% reduction of peripheral B cells after treatment of SLE patients[66,67] that is not related to cellular or complement mediated cytotoxicity. Since CD22 expression is more dense on naive versus memory B cells and more striking effects on adhesion and migration have been found for naive B cells, it is likely that these effects are related to CD22 density. Secondly, epratuzumab reduces intracellular kinase phosphorylation downstream of the BCR via the tyrosine protein kinase SYK and phospholipase C-γ2 (1-phosphatidylinositol 4,5-bisphosphate phosphodiesterase γ-2) and thereby modulates intracellular Ca^{2+} signalling.[68] Notably, these effects have been found for naive and memory B cells independent of the extent of CD22 expression. This is a first example of a non-depleting B cell-specific mAB that has an effect on BCR signalling. A recent study using liposomes with CD22 binding capacity were shown to have the autoantigen-specific potential to induce tolerance in a murine model of factor VIII deficiency based on inhibiting PI3K/Akt signalling.[69] Since a characteristic after CD22 binding is rapid internalization, these liposomes prevented internalization and simultaneously depleted autoreactive clones selectively.

An initial open-label clinical trial of epratuzumab in 14 patients with moderately active SLE showed that epratuzumab was well tolerated and improved BILAG scores by more than 50% in 77% of patients at 6 weeks, and in all patients at some point during the study period.[66] A subsequent study confirmed initial efficacy and safety data of epratuzumab,[70] including clinically meaningful and sustained improvements in PGA, PtGA and HRQOL as well as reductions in corticosteroid doses during open label extension.[71] A phase IIb study of epratuzumab in 227 patients with moderate to severe lupus showed that patients had a symptom reduction or absence of active disease within specific body systems, especially cardiorespiratory or neuropsychiatric systems.[72]

One study investigated epratuzumab in Sjögren's disease.[73] Overall, it appeared to be safe with the exception of one patient developing a severe infusion reaction.

Indirect B-cell targeting

A number of approaches can affect activation or survival of B cells and therefore — among other effects — substantially interfere with certain B-cell functions. This indirect targeting of B cells comprises blockade of cytokine pathways, such as those involving TNF, IL-6, IL-21, BLyS/BAFF and APRIL (also known as TNF ligand superfamily, member 13) (Table 1). A central aim of such approaches is to interfere with B-cell activation, maturation, survival, migration and/or differentiation, which can be achieved by blocking B-cell co-stimulation by T cells or APCs (via CTLA4–Ig, the inducible T-cell co-stimulator [ICOS]–ICOS-ligand, CD40-CD154 pathways or other receptor/ligand pairs within the CD28 family) as well as by blocking TLR activation, including downstream canonical NF-κB activation. For most of these approaches, the detailed impact on B cells has not been reported. However, blockade of CD40/CD154 and ICOS/ICOSL interaction have been identified to have potent inhibitory effects on generation of plasma cells and T_{FH}, respectively.[53,74]

The microenvironment in which B cells undergo maturation and differentiation and their maintenance in niches appears to be co-regulated by certain cytokines. There are a number of therapeutic effects on B cells by current treatments. It has been documented that the TNF/LTi, etanercept, is able to disrupt GC in tonsils of RA patients[75] whereas the specific TNFi, infliximab, normalizes peripheral B cell homeostasis in RA.[76] Normalization of T cell and B cell subsets has been shown following tocilizumab therapy of RA[77] as well as SLE.[78]

Based on the apparent role of the **BAFF–APRIL** family in autoimmune disease, blockade of the interactions between these molecules and their receptors became an area of intense interest. After approval of belimumab in SLE, other anti-BAFF mAB, such as tabalumab (LY2127399), are able to inhibit soluble and bound BAFF, and blisibimod (A-623) is in clinical development for SLE.

Recently, additional data on the impact of **belimumab** in SLE have been reported. Studies on the titers of antibodies to tetanus, influenza and *Pneumoccocus* over treatment periods of 52 weeks (BLISS-76 trial) showed no substantial declines compared to baseline.[79] A sub-study analyzing pneumococcal vaccination, as an example of TI B cell activation, indicated no impairment of responses. Since there is a decline of total serum IgM and IgG with belimumab therapy, these data are important to show that serologic memory appears to be preserved and specific long-term protective antibodies may not be affected. However, more long-term observational data are required since prolonged therapy may still have an impact on protective Ig. The combined impact of belimumab and immunosuppressive agents remains to be fully elucidated.

BAFF inhibitors represent a family of drugs with most ongoing or planned trials in SLE. Ongoing phase III trials are evaluating blisibimod in SLE as well as sucutaneous belimumab. Two trials of tabalumab failed their clinical endpoints recently and the program in SLE was discontinued (ref. press release INDIANAPOLIS, Oct. 2, 2014/PRNewswire/--Eli Lilly and Company). In contrast, tabalumab and belimumab did not show efficacy in RA.

The TACI-Ig fusion protein atacicept binds both BAFF and APRIL. Data of the impact of atacicept in six patients in a prematurely terminated trial of atacicept in lupus nephritis have been reported.[80,81] Three out of six patients developed IgG declines below 3 g/l. The occurrence of very serious infections in two patients with low IgG levels resulted in the discontinuation of the trial. Revisiting the data led to the hypothesis that initiation of MMF and high dose glucocorticoids may have amplified the effects of atacicept on Ig levels.[80] In this regard, a comprehensive analysis of 107 patients demonstrated that MMF substantially inhibits PC formation and B cell activation with modest Ig reduction, an effect that could be clearly differentiated from that of azathioprine.[82] Results of a post hoc analysis of the higher 150 mg dose of this trial have been published and indicated that atacicept might be effective at prevention of disease flare at this dose. This assumption needs further validation.

Regulatory B cells

B cells are typically considered to produce immunoglobulin, including autoantibodies, produce cytokines and act as APCs in certain circumstances. As with T cells, the B cell population also contains subsets capable of performing regulatory functions. Cytokines produced by B cells with regulatory function are IL-10, IL-35 and TGF-β, and they are also characterized by their potential ability to interact with pathogenic T cells to dampen harmful immune responses.[32,83–85] Investigations on the functions of regulatory B cells are at a very early stage of understanding, hence approaches to manipulate them are still in preclinical studies.

Inhibitors of certain B cell function

Bortezomib is a prototype of a number of proteasome inhibitors and provides an interesting possibility to interfere with this important subcellular structure while simultaneously targeting plasma cells and other immune cells. Encouraging preclinical data[86] in murine SLE models fuelled pioneering studies in refractory autoimmune patients.[87] However, the rather global blockade of the proteasome complex makes it very difficult to ascribe certain achievements unique to the B cell/PC system although the efficacy of bortezomib in myeloma clearly suggests this is certainly part of its action.

Perspective

B cells have many functions that could contribute to their role in initiating and perpetuating RAID, although their non-redundant function as precursors of antibody-secreting cells certainly contributes to the development of these diseases. Targeting B cells has shown promise as a therapeutic approach in some of these conditions, although the precise B cell subsets targeted and the functions inhibited have not been delineated and explanation of the failure of this approach in other inflammatory diseases is not forthcoming. Whether deleting B cells or modifying their function is a more appropriate option has not been defined. More recently, targeting specific functions of B cells, such as GC reactivity or interference with the BCR complex activity, rather than B cells in general has been considered. Whether this will provide more effective therapies has also not been confirmed. Targeting B cells in RAID has begun to contribute to a better understanding of normal human B cell function and the involvement of B cells in pathologic conditions, but in-depth knowledge of the role of B cells in specific diseases is still lacking, interfering with predictable application of B cell-directed therapy.

Reference

1. Panayi, G.S. (1993). The Immunopathogenesis of Rheumatoid-Arthritis (Reprinted from *Rheumatol Rev* Vol **1**, Pg 63–74, 1992). *Brit J Rheumatol*, **32**, 4–14.
2. Isaacs, J.D., Greer, S., Sharma, S., Symmons, D., Smith, M., Johnston, J., Waldmann, H., Hale, G., and Hazleman, B.L. (2001). Morbidity and mortality in rheumatoid arthritis patients with prolonged and profound therapy-induced lymphopenia. *Arthritis Rheum*, **44**, 1998–2008.
3. Cohen, S.B., Emery, P., Greenwald, M.W., Dougados, M., Furie, R.A., Genovese, M.C., Keystone, E.C., Loveless, J.E., Burmester, G.R., Cravets, M.W., Hessey, E.W., Shaw, T., and Totoritis, M.C., (2006). Rituximab for rheumatoid arthritis refractory to anti-tumor necrosis factor therapy — Results of a multicenter, randomized, double-blind, placebo-controlled, phase III trial evaluating primary efficacy and safety at twenty-four weeks. *Arthritis Rheum*, **54**, 2793–2806.
4. Jones, R.B., Tervaert, J.W.C., Hauser, T., Luqmani, R., Morgan, M.D., Peh, C.A., Savage, C.O., Segelmark, M., Tesar, V., van Paassen, P., Walsh, D., Walsh, M., Westman, K., and Jayne, D.R.W. (2010). Rituximab versus Cyclophosphamide in ANCA-Associated Renal Vasculitis. *N Eng J Med*, **363**, 211–220.
5. Lipsky, P.E. (2001). Systemic lupus erythematosus: an autoimmune disease of B cell hyperactivity. *Nat Immunol*, **2**, 764–766.
6. Amanna, I.J., Carlson, N.E., and Slifka, M.K. (2007). Duration of humoral immunity to common viral and vaccine antigens. *N Eng J Med*, **357**, 1903–1915.

7. Manz, R.A., Thiel, A., and Radbruch, A. (1997). Lifetime of plasma cells in the bone marrow. *Nature*, **388**, 133–134.

8. Tokoyoda, K., Hauser, A.E., Nakayama, T., and Radbruch, A. (2010). Organization of immunological memory by bone marrow stroma. *Nat Rev Immunol*, **10**, 193–200.

9. Barr, T.A., Shen, P., Brown, S., Lampropoulou, V., Roch, T., Lawrie, S., Fan, B., O'Connor, R.A., Anderton, S.M., Bar-Or, A., Fillatreau, S., and Gray, D. (2012). B cell depletion therapy ameliorates autoimmune disease through ablation of IL-6-producing B cells. *J Exp Med*, **209**, 1001–1010.

10. Griffin, D.O., Holodick, N.E., and Rothstein, T.L., (2011). Human B1 cells in umbilical cord and adult peripheral blood express the novel phenotype CD20(+)CD27(+)CD43(+)CD70(−). *J Exp Med*, **208**, 67–80.

11. Tarlinton, D., Radbruch, A., Hiepe, F., and Dorner, T. (2008). Plasma cell differentiation and survival. *Curr Opin Immunol*, **20**, 162–169.

12. Nashi, E., Wang, Y.H., and Diamond, B., (2010). The role of B cells in lupus pathogenesis. *Int J Biochem Cell Biol*, **42**, 543–550.

13. Giesecke, C., Frolich, D., Reiter, K., Mei, H.E., Wirries, I., Kuhly, R., Killig, M., Glatzer, T., Stolzel, K., Perka, C., Lipsky, P.E., and Dorner, T. (2014). Tissue distribution and dependence of responsiveness of human antigen-specific memory B cells. *J Immunol*, **192**, 3091–3100.

14. Dorner, T., Jacobi, A.M., and Lipsky, P.E. (2009). B cells in autoimmunity. *Arthritis Res Ther*, **11**.

15. Chang, A., Henderson, S.G., Brandt, D., Liu, N., Guttikonda, R., Hsieh, C., Kaverina, N., Utset, T.O., Meehan, S.M., Quigg, R.J., Meffre, E., and Clark, M.R. (2011). In situ B cell-mediated immune responses and tubulointerstitial inflammation in human lupus nephritis. *J Immunol*, **186**, 1849–1860.

16. Daridon, C., Loddenkemper, C., Spieckermann, S., Kuhl, A.A., Salama, A., Burmester, G.R., Lipsky, P.E., and Dorner, T. (2012). Splenic proliferative lymphoid nodules distinct from germinal centers are sites of autoantigen stimulation in immune thrombocytopenia. *Blood*, **120**, 5021–5031.

17. Winkler, T.H., Fehr, H., and Kalden, J.R. (1992). Analysis of immunoglobulin variable region genes from human-igg anti-dna hybridomas. *Eur J Immunol*, **22**, 1719–1728.

18. Amara, K., Steen, J., Murray, F., Morbach, H., Fernandez-Rodriguez, B.M., Joshua, V., Engstrom, M., Snir, O., Israelsson, L., Catrina, A.I., Wardemann, H., Corti, D., Meffre, E., Klareskog, L., and Malmstrom, V. (2013). Monoclonal IgG antibodies generated from joint-derived B cells of RA patients have a strong bias toward citrullinated autoantigen recognition. *J Exp Med*, **210**, 445–455.

19. Di Zenzo, G., Di Lullo, G., Corti, D., Calabresi, V., Sinistro, A., Vanzetta, F., Didona, B., Cianchini, G., Hertl, M., Eming, R., Amagai, M., Ohyama, B., Hashimoto, T., Sloostra, J., Sallusto, F., Zambruno, G., and Lanzavecchia, A. (2012). Pemphigus autoantibodies generated through somatic mutations target the desmoglein-3 cis-interface. *J Clin Invest*, **122**, 3781–3790.

20. Victora, G.D., and Nussenzweig, M.C. (2012). Germinal centers. *Annual Rev Immunol*, **30**, 429–457.

21. Gaipl, U.S., Munoz, L.E., Grossmayer, G., Lauber, K., Franz, S., Sarter, K., Voll, R.E., Winkler, T., Kuhn, A., Kalden, J., Kern, P., and Herrmann, M. (2007). Clearance deficiency and systemic lupus erythematosus (SLE). *J Autoimmun*, **28**, 114–121.

22. O'Connor, B.P., Raman, V.S., Erickson, L.D., Cook, W.J., Weaver, L.K., Ahonen, C., Lin, L.L., Mantchev, G.T., Bram, R.J., and Noelle, R.J. (2004). BCMA is essential for the survival of long-lived bone marrow plasma cells. *J Exp Med*, **199**, 91–97.

23. Oropallo, M.A., Kiefer, K., Marshak-Rothstein, A., and Cancro, M.P. (2011). Beyond transitional selection: New roles for BLyS in peripheral tolerance. *Drug Dev Rese*, **72**, 779–787.

24. Kim, J., Gross, J.A., Dillon, S.R., Min, J.K., and Elkon, K.B. (2011). Increased BCMA expression in lupus marks activated B cells, and BCMA receptor engagement enhances the response to TLR9 stimulation. *Autoimmunity*, **44**, 69–81.

25. Obukhanych, T.V., and Nussenzweig, M.C. (2006). T-independent type II immune responses generate memory B cells. *J Exp Med*, **203**, 305–310.

26. Wahren-Herlenius, M., and Dorner, T. (2013). Autoimmune rheumatic diseases 3 immunopathogenic mechanisms of systemic autoimmune disease. *Lancet*, **382**, 819–831.

27. Klareskog, L., Catrina, A.I., and Paget, S. (2009). Rheumatoid arthritis. *Lancet*, **373**, 659–672.

28. Arbuckle, M.R., McClain, M.T., Rubertone, M.V., Scofield, R.H., Dennis, G.J., James, J.A., and Harley, J.B. (2003). Development of autoantibodies before the clinical onset of systemic lupus erythematosus. *N Eng J Med*, **349**, 1526–1533.

29. Fillatreau, S., Sweenie, C.H., McGeachy, M.J., Gray, D., and Anderton, S.M. (2002). B cells regulate autoimmunity by provision of IL-10. *Nat Immunol*, **3**, 944–950.

30. Shen, P., Roch, T., Lampropoulou, V., O' Connor, R.A., Stervbo, U., Hilgenberg, E., Ries, S., Dang, V.D., Jaimes, Y., Daridon, C., Li, R., Jouneau, L., Boudinot, P., Wilantri, S., Sakwa, I., Miyazaki, Y., Leech, M.D., McPherson, R.C., Wirtz, S., Neurath, M., Hoehlig, K., Meinl, E.. Grützkau, A., Grün, J.R.,

Horn, K., Kühl, A.A., Dörner, T., Bar-Or, A., Kaufmann, S.H., Anderton, S.M., Fillatreau, S. (2014). IL-35-producing B cells are critical regulators of immunity during autoimmune and infectious diseases. *Nature*, **507**(7492), 366–370.

31. Blair, P.A., Norena, L.Y., Flores-Borja, F., Rawlings, D.J., Isenberg, D.A., Ehrenstein, M.R., and Mauri, C. (2010). CD19(+)CD24(hi)CD38(hi) B cells exhibit regulatory capacity in healthy individuals but are functionally impaired in systemic lupus erythematosus patients. *Immunity*, **32**, 129–140.

32. Mauri, C. (2010). Regulation of immunity and autoimmunity by B cells. *Curr Opin Immunol*, **22**, 761–767.

33. Tokunaga, M., Saito, K., Kawabata, D., Imura, Y., Fujii, T., Nakayamada, S., Tsujimura, S., Nawata, M., Iwata, S., Azuma, T., Mimori, T., and Tanaka, Y. (2007). Efficacy of rituximab (anti-CD20) for refractory systemic lupus erythematosus involving the central nervous system. *Ann Rheum Dis*, **66**, 470–475.

34. Melet, J., Mulleman, D., Goupille, P., Ribourtout, B., Watier, H., and Thibault, G. (2013). Rituximab-Induced T cell depletion in patients with rheumatoid arthritis association with clinical response. *Arthritis Rheum*, **65**, 2783–2790.

35. Takemura, S., Braun, A., Crowson, C., Kurtin, P.J., Cofield, R.H., O'Fallon, W.M., Goronzy, J.J., and Weyand, C.M. (2001). Lymphoid neogenesis in rheumatoid synovitis. *J Immunol*, **167**, 1072–1080.

36. Takemura, S., Klimiuk, P.A., Braun, A., Goronzy, J.J., and Weyand, C.M. (2001). T cell activation in rheumatoid synovium is B cell dependent. *J Immunol*, **167**, 4710–4718.

37. Serafini, B., Rosicarelli, B., Franciotta, D., Magliozzi, R., Reynolds, R., Cinque, P., Andreoni, L., Trivedi, P., Salvetti, M., Faggioni, A., and Aloisi, F. (2007). Dysregulated Epstein-Barr virus infection in the multiple sclerosis brain. *J Exp Med*, **204**, 2899–2912.

38. Chang, A., Henderson, S.G., Brandt, D., Liu, N., Guttikonda, R., Hsieh, C., Kaverina, N., Utset, T.O., Meehan, S.M., Quigg, R.J., Meffre, E., and Clark, M.R. (2011). In situ b cell-mediated immune responses and tubulointerstitial inflammation in human lupus nephritis. *J Immunol*, **186**, 1849–1860.

39. Hutloff, A., Buchner, K., Reiter, K., Baelde, H.J., Odendahl, M., Jacobi, A., Dorner, T., and Kroczek, R.A. (2004). Involvement of inducible costimulator in the exaggerated memory B cell and plasma cell generation in systemic lupus erythematosus. *Arthritis Rheum*, **50**, 3211–3220.

40. Ramanujam, M., Bethunaickan, R., Huang, W.Q., Tao, H.O., Madaio, M.P., and Davidson, A. (2010). Selective blockade of baff for the prevention and treatment of systemic lupus erythematosus nephritis in NZM2410 mice. *Arthritis Rheum*, **62**, 1457–1468.

41. Dorner, T., and Lipsky, P.E. (2014). B cells: depletion or functional modulation in rheumatic diseases. *Curr Opin Rheumatol*, **26**, 228–236.
42. Jacobi, A.M., Huang, W.Q., Wang, T., Freimuth, W., Sanz, I., Furie, R., Mackay, M., Aranow, C., Diamond, B., and Davidson, A. (2010). Effect of long-term belimumab treatment on b cells in systemic lupus erythematosus. *Arthritis Rheum*, **62**, 201–210.
43. Miossec, P., Korn, T., and Kuchroo, V.K. (2009). Mechanisms of disease: interleukin-17 and type 17 helper t cells. *N Eng J Med*, **361**, 888–898.
44. Illei, G.G., Shirota, Y., Yarboro, C.H., Daruwalla, J., Tackey, E., Takada, K., Fleisher, T., Balow, J.E., and Lipsky, P.E. (2010). Tocilizumab in systemic lupus erythematosus data on safety, preliminary efficacy, and impact on circulating plasma cells from an open-label phase I dosage-escalation study. *Arthritis Rheum*, **62**, 542–552.
45. Tsokos, G.C. (2011). Mechanisms of disease systemic lupus erythematosus. *N Eng J Med*, **365**, 2110–2121.
46. Ng, Y.S., Wardemann, H., Chelnis, J., Cunningham-Rundles, C., and Meffre, E. (2004). Bruton's tyrosine kinase is essential for human B cell tolerance. *J Exp Med*, **200**, 927–934.
47. Yurasov, S., Hammersen, J., Tiller, T., Tsuiji, M., and Wardemann, H. (2005). B-cell tolerance checkpoints in healthy humans and patients with systemic lupus erythematosus. *Hum Immunol Patient-Based Res*, **1062**, 165–174.
48. Hom, G., Graham, R.R., Modrek, B., Taylor, K.E., Ortmann, W., Garnier, S., Lee, A.T., Chung, S.A., Ferreira, R.C., Pant, P.V.K., Ballinger, D.G., Kosoy, R., Demirci, F.Y., . Kamboh, M.I, Kao, A.H., Tian, C., Gunnarsson, I., Bengtsson, A.A., Rantapaa-Dahlqvist, S., Petri, M., Manzi, S., Seldin, M.F., Ronnblom, L., Syvanen, A.C., Criswell, L.A., Gregersen, P.K., and Behrens, T.W. (2008). Association of systemic lupus erythematosus with C8orf13-BLK and ITGAM-ITGAX. *N Eng J Med*, **358**, 900–909.
49. Tangye, S.G., Ma, C.S., Brink, R., and Deenick, E.K., (2013). The good, the bad and the ugly — T-FH cells in human health and disease. *Nat Rev Immunol*, **13**, 412–426.
50. Baumjohann, D., Preite, S., Reboldi, A., Ronchi, F., Ansel, K.M., Lanzavecchia, A., and Sallusto, F. (2013). Persistent antigen and germinal center B cells sustain t follicular helper cell responses and phenotype. *Immunity*, **38**, 596–605.
51. Gong, Q., Ou, Q.L., Ye, S.M., Lee, W.P., Cornelius, J., Diehl, L., Lin, W.Y., Hu, Z.L., Lu, Y.M., Chen, Y.M., Wu, Y., Meng, Y.G., Gribling, P., Lin, Z.H., Nguyen, K., Tran, T., Zhang, Y.F., Rosen, H., Martin, F., and Chan, A.C.

(2005). Importance of cellular microenvironment and circulatory dynamics in B cell immunotherapy. *J Immunol*, **174**, 817–826.

52. Mei, H.E., Frolich, D., Giesecke, C., Loddenkemper, C., Reiter, K., Schmidt, S., Feist, E., Daridon, C., Tony, H.P., Radbruch, A., and Dorner, T. (2010). Steady-state generation of mucosal IgA(+) plasmablasts is not abrogated by B-cell depletion therapy with rituximab. *Blood*, **116**, 5181–5190.

53. Craft, J.E. (2012). Follicular helper T cells in immunity and systemic autoimmunity. *Nat Rev Rheumatol*, **8**, 337–347.

54. Merrill, J.T., Neuwelt, C.M., Wallace, D.J., Shanahan, J.C., Latinis, K.M., Oates, J.C., Utset, T.O., Gordon, C., Isenberg, D.A., Hsieh, H.J., Zhang, D., and Brunetta, P.G. (2010). Efficacy and safety of rituximab in moderately-to-severely active systemic lupus erythematosus the randomized, double-blind, phase ii/iii systemic lupus erythematosus evaluation of rituximab trial. *Arthritis Rheum*, **62**, 222–233.

55. Rovin, B.H., Furie, R., Latinis, K., Looney, R.J., Fervenza, F.C., Sanchez-Guerrero, J., Maciuca, R., Zhang, D., Garg, J.P., Brunetta, P., and Appel, G. (2012). Efficacy and safety of rituximab in patients with active proliferative lupus nephritis the lupus nephritis assessment with rituximab study. *Arthritis Rheum*, **64**, 1215–1226.

56. Aggarwal, R., Reed, A.M., Ascherman, D.P., Barohn, R.J., Feldman, B.M., Miller, F.W., Rider, L.G., Harris-Love, M., Levesque, M.C., and Oddis, C.V. (2012). Clinical and serologic predictors of response in rituximab-treated refractory adult and juvenile dermatomyositis (DM) and adult polymyositis (PM) — the RIM study. *Arthritis Rheum*, **64**, S682–S683.

57. St Clair, E.W., Levesque, M.C., Prak, E.T.L., Vivino, F.B., Alappatt, C.J., Spychala, M.E., Wedgwood, J., McNamara, J., Sivils, K.L.M., Fisher, L., and Cohen, P. (2013). Rituximab therapy for primary sjogren's syndrome: an open-label clinical trial and mechanistic analysis. *Arthritis Rheum*, **65**, 1097–1106.

58. Fornoni, A., Sageshima, J., Wei, C.L., Merscher-Gomez, S., Aguillon-Prada, R., Jauregui, A.N., Li, J., Mattiazzi, A., Ciancio, G., Chen, L.D., Zilleruelo, G., Abitbol, C., Chandar, J., Seeherunvong, W., Ricordi, C., Ikehata, M., Rastaldi, M.P., Reiser, J., and Burke, G.W. (2011). Rituximab targets podocytes in recurrent focal segmental glomerulosclerosis. *Sci Trans Med* 3.

59. Mei, H.E., Schmidt, S., and Dorner, T. (2012). Rationale of anti-CD19 immunotherapy: an option to target autoreactive plasma cells in autoimmunity. *Arthritis Res Ther*, 14.

60. Mei, H.E., and Dorner, T. (2013). B cells identified according to their expression of CD19 and surface ig are depleted from peripheral blood by rituximab in patients with rheumatoid arthritis: comment on the article by jones *et al.* *Arthritis Rheum*, **65**, 1132.

61. Sato, S., Ono, N., Steeber, D.A., Pisetsky, D.S., and Tedder, T.F. (1996). CD19 regulates B lymphocyte signaling thresholds critical for the development of B-1 lineage cells and autoimmunity. *J Immunol*, **157**, 4371–4378.

62. Bargou, R., Leo, E., Zugmaier, G., Klinger, M., Goebeler, M., Knop, S., Noppeney, R., Viardot, A., Hess, G., Schuler, M., Einsele, H., Brandl, C., Wolf, A., Kirchinger, P., Klappers, P., Schmidt, M., Riethmuller, G., Reinhardt, C., Baeuerle, P.A., and Kufer, P. (2008). Tumor regression in cancer patients by very low doses of a T cell-engaging antibody. *Science*, **321**, 974–977.

63. Daridon, C., Blassfeld, D., Reiter, K., Mei, H.E., Giesecke, C., Goldenberg, D.M., Hansen, A., Hostmann, A., Frolich, D., and Dorner, T. (2010). Epratuzumab targeting of CD22 affects adhesion molecule expression and migration of B-cells in systemic lupus erythematosus. *Arthritis Res Ther*, 12.

64. Reineks, E.Z., Osei, E.S., Rosenberg, A., Auletta, J., and Meyerson, H.J. (2009). CD22 expression on blastic plasmacytoid dendritic cell neoplasms and reactivity of anti-CD22 antibodies to peripheral blood dendritic cells. *Cytometry B Clin Cytometry*, **76B**, 237–248.

65. Rossi, E.A., Goldenberg, D.M., Michel, R., Rossi, D.L., Wallace, D.J., and Chang, C.H. (2013). Trogocytosis of multiple B-cell surface markers by CD22 targeting with epratuzumab. *Blood*, **122**, 3020–3029.

66. Dorner, T., Kaufmann, J., Wegener, W.A., Teoh, N., Goldenberg, D.M., and Burmester, G.R. (2006). Initial clinical trial of epratuzumab (humanized anti-CD22 antibody) for immunotherapy of systemic lupus erythematosus. *Arthritis Res Ther*, 8.

67. Jacobi, A.M., Goldenberg, D.M., Hiepe, F., Radbruch, A., Burmester, G.R., and Dorner, T. (2008). Differential effects of epratuzumab on peripheral blood B cells of patients with systemic lupus erythematosus versus normal controls. *Ann Rheum Dis*, **67**, 450–457.

68. Sieger, N., Fleischer, S.J., Mei, H.E., Reiter, K., Shock, A., Burmester, G.R., Daridon, C., and Dorner, T. (2013). CD22 ligation inhibits downstream B cell receptor signaling and Ca2+flux upon activation. *Arthritis Rheum*, **65**, 770–779.

69. Macauley, M.S., Pfrengle, F., Rademacher, C., Nycholat, C.M., Gale, A.J., von Drygalski, A., and Paulson, J.C. (2013). Antigenic liposomes displaying CD22 ligands induce antigen-specific B cell apoptosis. *J Clin Invest*, **123**, 3074–3083.

70. Wallace, D.J., Gordon, C., Strand, V., Hobbs, K., Petri, M., Kalunian, K., Houssiau, F., Tak, P.P., Isenberg, D.A., Kelley, L., Kilgallen, B., Barry, A.N., Wegener, W.A., and Goldenberg, D.M. (2013). Efficacy and safety of epratuzumab in patients with moderate/severe flaring systemic lupus erythematosus: results from two randomized, double-blind, placebo-controlled, multicentre studies (ALLEVIATE) and follow-up. *Rheumatology*, **52**, 1313–1322.

71. Strand, V., Petri, M., Kalunian, K., Gordon, C., Wallace, D.J., Hobbs, K., Kelley, L., Kilgallen, B., Wegener, W.A., and Goldenberg, D.M. (2014). Epratuzumab for patients with moderate to severe flaring SLE: health-related quality of life outcomes and corticosteroid use in the randomized controlled ALLEVIATE trials and extension study SL0006. *Rheumatology*, **53**, 502–511.
72. Wallace, D.J., Kalunian, K., Petri, M.A., Strand, V., Houssiau, F.A., Pike, M., Kilgallen, B., Bongardt, S., Barry, A., Kelley, L., and Gordon, C. (2014). Efficacy and safety of epratuzumab in patients with moderate/severe active systemic lupus erythematosus: results from EMBLEM, a phase IIb, randomised, double-blind, placebo-controlled, multicentre study. *Ann Rheum Dis*, **73**, 183–190.
73. Steinfeld, S.D., Tant, L., Burmester, G.R., Teoh, N.K.W., Wegener, W.A., Goldenberg, D.M., and Pradier, O. (2006). Epratuzumab (humanised anti-CD22 antibody) in primary Sjogren's syndrome: an open-label phase I/II study. *Arthritis Res Ther*, 8.
74. Grammer, A.C., Slota, R., Fischer, R., Gur, H., Girschick, H., Yarboro, C., Illei, G.G., and Lipsky, P.E. (2003). Abnormal germinal center reactions in systemic lupus erythematosus demonstrated by blockade of CD154-CD40 interactions. *J Clin Invest*, **112**, 1506–1520.
75. Anolik, J.H., Ravikumar, R., Barnard, J., Owen, T., Almudevar, A., Milner, E.C.B., Miller, C.H., Dutcher, P.O., Hadley, J.A., and Sanz, I. (2008). Cutting edge: Anti-tumor necrosis factor therapy in rheumatoid arthritis inhibits memory B lymphocytes via effects on lymphoid germinal centers and follicular dendritic cell networks. *J Immunol*, **180**, 688–692.
76. Souto-Carneiro, M.M., Mahadevan, V., Takada, K., Fritsch-Stork, R., Nanki, T., Brown, M., Fleisher, T.A., Wilson, M., Goldbach-Mansky, R., and Lipsky, P.E. (2009). Alterations in peripheral blood memory B cells in patients with active rheumatoid arthritis are dependent on the action of tumour necrosis factor. *Arthritis Res Ther*, 11.
77. Roll, P., Muhammad, K., Schumann, M., Kleinert, S., Einsele, H., Dorner, T., and Tony, H.P. (2011). *In vivo* effects of the anti-interleukin-6 receptor inhibitor tocilizumab on the b cell compartment. *Arthritis Rheum*, **63**, 1255–1264.
78. Shirota, Y., Yarboro, C., Fischer, R., Pham, T.H., Lipsky, P., and Illei, G.G., (2013). Impact of anti-interleukin-6 receptor blockade on circulating T and B cell subsets in patients with systemic lupus erythematosus. *Ann Rheum Dis*, **72**, 118–128.
79. Chatham, W.W., Wallace, D.J., Stohl, W., Latinis, K.M., Manzi, S., Mccune, W.J., Tegzova, D., Mckay, J.D., Avila-Armengol, H.E., Utset, T.O., Zhong, Z.J., Hough, D.R., Freimuth, W.W., and Migone, T.S. (2012). Effect of belimumab

on vaccine antigen antibodies to influenza, pneumococcal, and tetanus vaccines in patients with systemic lupus erythematosus in the BLISS-76 trial. *J Rheumatol*, **39**, 1632–1640.

80. Isenberg, D.A. (2012). Meryl Streep and the problems of clinical trials. *Arthritis Res Ther*, 14.

81. Ginzler, E.M., Wax, S., Rajeswaran, A., Copt, S., Hillson, J., Ramos, E., and Singer, N.G. (2012). Atacicept in combination with MMF and corticosteroids in lupus nephritis: results of a prematurely terminated trial. *Arthritis Res Ther*, 14.

82. Eickenberg, S., Mickholz, E., Jung, E., Nofer, J.R., Pavenstadt, H., and Jacobi, A.M. (2012). Mycophenolic acid counteracts B cell proliferation and plasmablast formation in patients with systemic lupus erythematosus. *Arthritis Res Ther*, 14.

83. Iwata, Y., Matsushita, T., Horikawa, M., DiLillo, D.J., Yanaba, K., Venturi, G.M., Szabolcs, P.M., Bernstein, S.H., Magro, C.M., Williams, A.D., Hall, R.P., St Clair, E.W., and Tedder, T.F. (2011). Characterization of a rare IL-10-competent B-cell subset in humans that parallels mouse regulatory B10 cells. *Blood*, **117**: 530–541.

84. Flores-Borja, F., Bosma, A., Ng, D., Reddy, V., Ehrenstein, M.R., Isenberg, D.A., and Mauri, C. (2013). CD19(+)CD24(hi)CD38(hi) B cells maintain regulatory T cells while limiting T(H)1 and T(H)17 differentiation. *Sci Trans Med*, 5.

85. Shen, P., Roch, T., Lampropoulou, V., O'Connor, R.A., Stervbo, U., Hilgenberg, E., Ries, S., Dang, V.D., Jaimes, Y., Daridon, C., Li, R., Jouneau, L., Boudinot, P., Wilantri, S., Sakwa, I., Miyazaki, Y., Leech, M.D., McPherson, R.C., Wirtz, S., Neurath, M., Hoehlig, K., Meinl, E., Grutzkau, A., Grun, J.R., Horn, K., Kuhl, A.A., Dorner, T., Bar-Or, A., Kaufmann, S.H.E., Anderton, S.M., and Fillatreau, S. (2014). IL-35-producing B cells are critical regulators of immunity during autoimmune and infectious diseases. *Nature*, **507**, 366–370.

86. Neubert, K., Meister, S., Moser, K., Weisel, F., Maseda, D., Amann, K., Wiethe, C., Winkler, T.H., Kalden, J.R., Manz, R.A., and Voll, R.E. (2008). The proteasome inhibitor bortezomib depletes plasma cells and protects mice with lupus-like disease from nephritis. *Nat Med*, **14**, 748–755.

87. Park, S.J., Cheong, H.I., and Shin, J.I., (2013). Antibody depletion by bortezomib through blocking of antigen presentation. *N Eng J Med*, **368**, 1364–1365.

88. van Vollenhoven, R., Aranov, C., Rovin, B., Wagner, C., Zhou, B., Gordon, R., Hsu, B. (2014). OP0047 a phase 2, multicenter, randomized, double-blind, placebo-controlled, proof-of-concept study to evaluate the efficacy and safety of sirukumab in patients with active lupus nephritis. *Ann Rheum Dis*, **73**(Suppl 2), 78.

89. Mei, H.E., Wirries, I., Frölich, D., Brisslert, M., Giesecke, C., Grün, J.R., Alexander, T., Schmidt, S., Luda, K., Kühl, A.A., Engelmann, R., Dürr, M., Scheel, T., Bokarewa, M., Perka, C., Radbruch, A., Dörner, T. (2015). A unique population of IgG-expressing plasma cells lacking CD19 is enriched in human bone marrow. *Blood*, pii: blood-2014-02-555169 [Epub ahead of print].

90. Dorner, T., Radburch, A., Burmester, G.R. (2009). B-cell-directed therapies for autoimmune disease. *Nat Rev Rheumatol*, **5**, 433–441.

CHAPTER 4

CELL-BASED THERAPIES FOR AUTOIMMUNE DISEASES

Per Marits, Christian Lundgren, and Ola Winqvist

Introduction

Cell-based therapies have been put forward as a coming, third therapeutic pillar in medicine, the first two being small-molecule drugs and biologicals.[1] In contrast to traditional drugs, cells are versatile therapeutic entities, capable of sensing and responding to environmental signals, as well as of directed migration, differentiation and/or proliferation. In addition, the longevity of cells provides long-term treatment with the potential to restore immunological imbalances and thus cure. Needless to say, standard pharmacokinetic and pharmacodynamic models will fall short when attempting to describe a cell-based therapy, which makes its testing and clinical implementation a challenge, both for researchers and regulatory authorities.

One of the most promising applications of cell-based therapy in clinical medicine today, is adoptive immunotherapy of cancer. This development has been based on a wealth of preclinical data, both from murine models and cancer patients, describing immune cell reactivity against different types of malignancies.[2] The therapy itself has undergone a fascinating and rapid evolution since the first trials with Lymphokine-Activated Killer

(LAK) cells in the 1980's, consisting of autologous mononuclear leukocytes from peripheral blood that had been cultured *in vitro* in the presence of interleukin-2 (IL-2) for three to four days followed by reinfusion into the patient. Today, T lymphocytes from peripheral blood can be genetically designed to express chimaeric antigen receptors with specificity for selected tumor antigens and may, in addition, be transduced with additional genes to modulate their cytokine profile or migratory properties.[3] Thus, a cell-based therapeutic can be tailored to suit its application thereby giving true meaning to the term "personalized medicine".

Cell-based Therapy to Suppress Unwanted Immune Responses?

The immune system has developed several regulatory mechanisms to limit tissue damage during desirable immune responses against pathogens in order to prevent autoreactivity and the development of autoimmune disease. Some of these mechanisms are cell-intrinsic, such as thymic negative selection of developing T cells displaying autoreactivity and Fas-mediated, activation-induced cell death (AICD) of T lymphocytes during the contraction phase of an immune response. However, these checkpoints are apparently not sufficient, since they are complemented by cell-extrinsic regulation in the form of immunosuppressive cell populations. Not surprisingly, these regulatory cell populations appear to be as diverse and complex as the immune system itself. Some regulatory subsets are characterized as more or less immature cells, whereas others appear as terminally differentiated cells, fully dedicated to an immunosuppressive mode of action.

In comparison with tumor immunotherapy, the therapeutic use of immune cells to accomplish suppression of an unwanted or excessive immune-response in immune-mediated inflammatory diseases (IMID), is less well explored. Nonetheless, promising candidate cell populations are now being tested in clinical trials with the aim to dampen and modulate the immune response in IMIDs. This review aims to give an overview of current applications of cell-based therapies in autoimmune and autoinflammatory conditions, collectively named immune-mediated diseases. Since the therapeutic potential of many regulatory cell subsets was first explored in the setting of hematopoietic stem cell and organ transplantation, some of these studies are discussed as well, in order to put the subsequent applications in an historical context. It is beyond the scope of this text to reproduce the cutting edge research regarding regulatory cell populations *in vivo*. Instead, the focus will be on the cell types that have been adopted for therapeutic purposes which, broadly speaking, can be divided into three categories: mesenchymal stromal cells, myeloid regulatory cells and regulatory T cells.

Mesenchymal Stromal Cells

Somewhat surprisingly, the most investigated regulatory cell in therapeutic clinical settings is not classified as an immune cell. Mesenchymal Stem Cells (MSCs) were first identified as stromal cells within the bone marrow equipped with the hallmarks of stem cells, *i.e.* self-renewal and differentiation potential of individual cells to form all the components of bone. Several decades after their initial discovery, MSCs were shown to inhibit T cell proliferation *in vitro* and to prolong allograft survival in animal models.[4] MSCs are isolated *in vitro* simply by plastic adherence and have been shown to be relatively easy to expand in cell cultures. These properties invoked considerable enthusiasm about their use for cell therapy. Well over 200 clinical trials have hitherto been registered with MSCs as the active intervention, and in about one fourth of these trials the main purpose has been immunomodulation.

MSCs have later been ascribed the potential to differentiate into other cells of mesodermal origin, primarily chondrocytes and adipocytes, but even some non-mesodermal cell lineages. Furthermore, cells with stem cell-like properties have been identified in other mesenchymal tissues and especially adipose tissue-derived MSCs have gained popularity due to their relative accessibility. However, at least bone marrow and adipose tissue-derived MSCs display distinct transcriptomes,[5] and could thus be considered as distinct cell types in a therapeutic setting. The apparent conceptual expansion of the term "MSCs" has led the International Society for Cellular Therapy (ISCT) to promote the alternative term Mesenchymal *Stromal* — instead of Stem — Cells. Minimal criteria for their definition include multilineage differentiation ability during standard culture conditions and expression of CD105, CD73 and CD90 with simultaneous lack of CD45, CD34, CD14, CD11b, CD79a and HLA-DR expression.[6] Another aspect that has been criticized is that the majority of studies on *in vitro* expanded MSCs only assessed the stem cell attributes in bulk cultures, as opposed to clonal cell populations. The observed multi-lineage differentiation capability may thus in some cases result from impure cell populations rather than reflecting true stem cell-ness.[7] Similarly, it is not known whether the immunoregulatory properties are common to all the different MSC-populations, nor is it known which subpopulations in these heterogeneous cell products are the most potent in this regard.

Nonetheless, there exists a substantial amount of data on the mechanisms behind MSC-mediated immunosuppression.[8] Apart from their opposing effects on T cell activation, MSCs have also been shown to inhibit innate immune activation, including Toll-like receptor signaling and macrophage and dendritic cell maturation. Overall, MSC-mediated immune interference seem to induce a shift in the T helper cell polarization and to promote regulatory T cell (Treg) differentiation. Importantly, MSCs do not appear to be spontaneously suppressive but rather acquire this function following exposure to pro-inflammatory mediators, notably interferon (IFN)-γ and TNF. This activation (or "licensing") induces the expression of several molecules that have been implicated in MSC-mediated immunosuppression, including indoleamine 2,3-dioxygenase, prostaglandin E-2, transforming growth factor (TGF)-ß and nitric oxide (NO). An additional appealing function of MSCs is their ability to migrate to sites of inflammation and, hence, to bring about their own licensing.

Acute graft-versus-host disease (GvHD) was the first immune-mediated disease in which the immunosuppressive capacity of MSCs was utilized. This devastating condition occurs after hematopoietic stem cell transplantation (HSCT), when alloreactive donor cells are activated against mismatched transplantation antigens in the host and is associated with high mortality and a lack of effective treatments. The regenerative ability of MSC had previously been used in the setting of HSCT, with the explicit goal to improve engraftment, and MSCs had been shown to dampen alloreactivity in animal models. In one of the first trials, 55 patients with severe, acute steroid-resistant GvHD received one or more infusions of bone marrow-derived MSCs and slightly more than half of the patients responded.[9] In this study, three of four MSC-preparations were derived

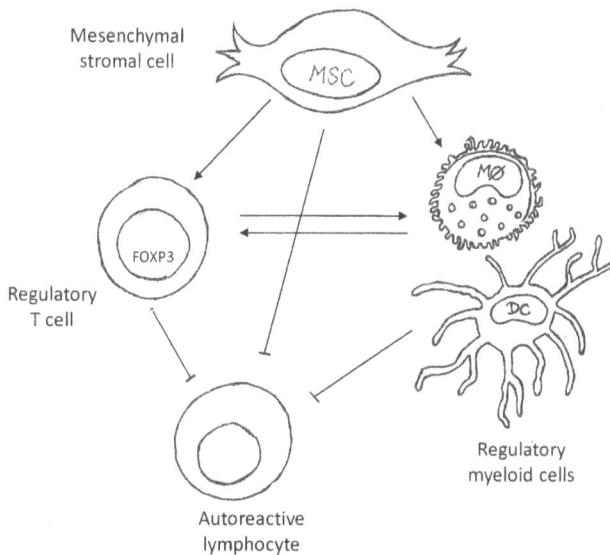

Figure 1. The complex *in vivo* interrelationship between the regulatory cell subsets used for therapy of autoimmune disease. Apart from an ability to directly suppress autoreactive effector cells, mesenchymal stromal cells (MSC) may regulate immune responses through regulatory myeloid cells, *i.e.* macrophages (MΦ) and dendritic cells (DC), and regulatory T cells (Tregs). The regulatory myeloid cell subsets and Tregs also exert direct suppressive effects on effector cells, as well as promote differentiation and expansion of each other.

from third-party HLA mismatched donors. Since the patient will be severely immunocompromised and the original donor might not be immediately available, a third-party donor will often be the only feasible alternative in GvHD, given the urgency of the condition.

MSCs are generally considered non-immunogenic by virtue of their low-level expression of MHC molecules and predominantly immunosuppressive phenotype. However, exposure to pro-inflammatory cytokines during licensing has been shown to upregulate MHC class I and class II expression *in vitro*. Even if MSC-mediated immunosuppression would effectively quench direct alloreactivity, there may still be a theoretical risk of indirect allorecognition, since antigens derived from apoptotic MSCs can be processed by host antigen-presenting cells and displayed to allo-reactive T cells. Indeed, in several animal models increased anti-donor T cell reactivity and antibody responses have been detected following infusions of allo-MSCs.[10] Whether this will be a clinical concern likely depends on the patient and condition being treated. It may not be so in the setting of acute GvHD, but when administering cells to an SLE-patient or to a future kidney recipient, the likelihood of immunization is higher and carries obvious clinical consequences. It is notable that assays to detect allo-responses against MSCs are not usually included in clinical study protocols.

In several animal models of autoimmune diseases, including rheumatoid arthritis, inflammatory bowel disease and experimental autoimmune encephalomyelitis (EAE), MSCs have shown efficacy.[11] Interestingly, *human*, that is xenogeneic, MSCs seem to be at least as efficacious as syngeneic cells in these animal models, which supports the common view that the MSCs do not need to engraft in order to exert their immunosuppressive effects. An observation worth considering, derived from a murine model of kidney transplantation, concerns the timing of MSC infusion. If the mice received MSCs prior to transplantation, the cells localized to lymphoid organs and induced Tregs, resulting in prolonged allograft survival, whereas cells infused post-transplantation localized inside the graft and were associated with neutrophil recruitment and graft dysfunction.[12] In autoimmunity, any therapeutic cell will invariably be administered after disease establishment and the therapeutic window will have to be defined for each indication.

Nevertheless, several trials have been conducted in human subjects with autoimmunity, including in conditions as diverse as Crohn's disease, systemic lupus erythematosus and multiple sclerosis (Table 1). The origin of the cells was similarly diverse, ranging from autologous bone-marrow-derived MSC to non-matched allogeneic cells from umbilical cord blood. In general, the therapy appears to be safe with no or minimal immediate side-effects and most authors have recorded signs of therapeutic benefit. However, the studies generally lack a control group and without randomization, such conclusions should not be drawn too hastily. A search on www.clinicaltrials.gov in December 2014 for MSC therapy and autoimmune disorders retrieved 31 relevant studies; 16 in multiple sclerosis and neuromyelitis optica, seven in type I diabetes, four in rheumatoid arthritis, two in Crohn's disease and one each in autoimmune hepatitis and primary biliary cirrhosis. Encouragingly, several of these

Table 1. Selected studies of MSC therapy in autoimmune disease.

Reference	Patient population	Source of cells	Patients (n)
Duijvestein *et al.* (2010)[13]	Crohn's disease	Autologous BM-derived	9
Cho *et al.* (2013)[14]	Crohn's disease	Autologous adipose tissue-derived	10
Forbes *et al.* (2014)[15]	Crohn's disease	Allogeneic BM-derived	16
Liang *et al.* (2010)[16]	SLE	Unmatched allogeneic BM-derived	15
Wang *et al.* (2014)[17]	SLE	Unmatched, allogeneic umbilical cord-derived	40
Wang *et al.* (2011)[18]	Poly- and dermatomyositis	Unmatched allogeneic BM-derived	10
Wang *et al.* (2013)[19]	Primary biliary cirrhosis	Unmatched, allogeneic umbilical cord-derived	7
Sengupta (2013)[20]	Idiopathic membranous nephropathy	Autologous BM-derived	12
Karussis *et al.* (2010)[21]	Multiple sclerosis	Autologous BM-derived, intrathecal injection	15 (MS)
Bonab (2012)[22]	Multiple sclerosis	Autologous BM-derived, intrathecal injection	25
Connick *et al.* (2012)[23]	Multiple sclerosis	Autologous BM-derived	10

Abbreviations: BM = Bone Marrow; SLE = Systemic Lupus Erythematosus

studies are equipped with a placebo arm and will therefore be informative on the actual efficacy of MSC therapy in these diseases. Thus, during the coming years the efficacy of MSC for the treatment of IMIDs will be evaluated.

Regulatory Myeloid Cells and Dendritic Cells

Suppressive cell populations of myeloid origin, with both distinct and overlapping characteristics, have emerged as an important component of normal immune homeostasis. First, one must recognize that most myeloid cells are primarily anti-inflammatory in the immature, resting state but this phenotype can be conserved or even enhanced upon activation in an immunosuppressive milieu. For example, tumor-infiltrating myeloid suppressor cells are a well-recognized phenomenon with documented negative impact on tumor immunity.[24] This is a heterogeneous cell population whose regulatory phenotype seem to be the result of exposure to tumor-derived substances, such as PGE2 and VEGF. Macrophages do exhibit an exhaustive diversity[25] and an effort to put this complexity in order is the simplistic view of monocyte differentiation into either classically (M1) or alternatively (M2) activated macrophages. The latter display an anti-inflammatory and wound-healing phenotype, although committed regulatory macrophages have been described as a third differentiation pathway, distinct from the M2 lineage. The dendritic cell (DC) is an additional cell type that is pivotal for productive antigen-presentation and activation of T cells. Consequently, DCs may acquire regulatory (or "tolerogenic") properties, in a similar manner as macrophages, and promote the expansion of Tregs rather than effector cells.[26]

For therapeutic purposes, there exist a large number of protocols that use various cytokines and other substances, such as rapamycin, to induce the differentiation of peripheral blood monocytes into regulatory macrophages or DCs.[27] Both tolerogenic DCs[28] and M2 macrophages[29] ameliorate diabetes in the NOD mouse and M2-differentiated microglia (resident macrophages of the central nervous system) have demonstrated efficacy in experimental autoimmune encephalomyelitis (EAE).[30] The tolerogenic DCs have even crossed the species barrier and been tested in a randomized phase I study.[31] In this study, autologous DCs were rendered tolerogenic with antisense oligonucleotides targeting the co-stimulatory molecules CD40, CD80 and CD86. Seven patients with type I diabetes received the autologous tolerogenic DC population and three patients received non-manipulated DCs. The therapy appeared safe, with no immediate side-effects but no discernible effect was observed on metabolic control. As for regulatory macrophages, protocols exist to induce differentiation of monocytes from patients with autoimmune diseases into functional M2 macrophages,[32] but the therapy still awaits clinical implementation. Moreover, pre-transplant immunosuppressive therapy with donor-derived regulatory macrophages ("Mregs") is being investigated in solid organ transplantation.[33] Although the transplantation setting is altogether different, these studies may still provide valuable information regarding the applicability of myeloid cell therapy for autoimmune disease.

Regulatory T cells

Both MSCs and myeloid regulatory cells exert their immunosuppressive effect partly through the induction of Tregs. Even if several distinct T cell subsets with regulatory properties have been described, such as the IL-10-producing Tr1 cell and $CD8^+$ $CD28^-$ T cells, the most studied cell in recent years is clearly the naturally occurring $CD4^+$ $CD25^+$ Tregs that express the transcription factor FOXP3. These cells have been the focus of intense research efforts since their description by Shimon Sakaguchi[34] and a full account for their biological properties is beyond the scope of this text. However, they do possess properties that make them appealing as a cellular immunosuppressant.

First, Tregs exhibit antigen-specificity by virtue of a unique T cell receptor (TCR). In order to be suppressive, a Treg must first be activated by TCR-induced signals but then regulates immune-responses in a non-specific manner, *i.e.* activated immune cells are affected irrespective of *their* antigen-specificity. In experimental models of alloreactivity, it has been demonstrated that antigen-specific Tregs are more potent than polyclonal Tregs in preventing injury to the graft.[35] Antigen-specific Tregs thus combine a means of "targeted drug delivery" to the site of (auto-) antigen expression and a more potent therapeutic.

Second, activated Tregs not only suppress nearby effector cells, but also catalyze the induction of new Tregs with broader specificities, a phenomenon termed "infectious tolerance",[36] which can be regarded as the reverse of "epitope spreading" often seen during the development of an autoimmune disease.

Third, T lymphocytes are long-lived cells and Tregs are no exception. If effective, adoptive Treg therapy may consequently result in prolonged protection against recurrence of disease.

However, there are some difficulties that have hampered the clinical introduction of Treg therapies. The major issue of Treg manufacturing is the balance between Treg numbers and purity. The CD4[+] CD25[+] Tregs comprise 5–10% of CD4+ T lymphocytes in peripheral blood, but this surface phenotype is shared with activated effector T cells. Since FOXP3 is an intracellular marker, it cannot be used to isolate cells for *in vitro* expansion, but the addition of CD127 can improve Treg purity by enabling the exclusion of CD4[+] T lymphocytes that simultaneously express high levels of both CD25 and CD127 (effector T cells).[37] Still, a minor contamination of non-Tregs may be a potential problem since effector cells are generally more prone to proliferate during *in vitro* cultures. On the other hand, the use of too stringent isolation criteria will compromise yield and likely therapeutic efficacy. In addition, it has been reported that repeated stimulation of Tregs in culture may result in loss of FOXP3 expression,[38] but whether this is due to the outgrowth of contaminating, conventional T cells or a destabilization of FOXP3 in "true" Tregs is a matter of debate. Nevertheless, a reliable means to address Treg purity after expansion seems to be necessary. Two possibilities have been suggested, either a functional assay of Treg suppressive ability or an epigenetic analysis of the FOXP3 locus, as an indication of Treg stability. A functional assay is informative regarding potency of the individual product, which may be indicated when using autologous cells, considering that Treg defects have been reported in patients with autoimmunity.[39] On the other hand, since Tregs potently suppress effector cells at a 1:4 ratio, a suppressive assay will tolerate a relatively large contamination of non-Tregs and is therefore insufficient to assess purity. Demethylation of certain CpG in the FOXP3 locus has been shown to indicate lineage specification of Tregs[40,41] and would fit the requirements for a purity assay. The degree of contaminating non-Tregs that can be tolerated will likely depend on the indication and suppressive potency of the Treg part of the cell product. The clinical experience of Treg therapy to date is mainly confined to GvHD, where a minor contamination of effector cells may be viewed as a contribution to the hematopoetic reconstitution. In the setting of autoimmunity, Treg therapy has been explored by Marek-Trzonkowska and colleagues.[42] In this study, CD4[+] CD25[+] CD127-Tregs were isolated by FACS from 10 patients with recently developed type I diabetes mellitus. After polyclonal *in vitro* expansion, 90–97% of the cells were FOXP3[+] and they were delivered as an i.v. infusion of 10–20×10^6 cells/kg. The therapy was not associated with any side-effects and at one-year follow-up insulin requirements were lower as compared to matched controls, with two children completely independent of exogenous insulin.[43] Desreumaux *et al.* have investigated the use of Tregs in 20 patients with treatment-refractory Crohn's disease.[44] These authors chose a different approach, where IL-10 producing ovalbumin-specific Treg cells (ova-Tregs) were isolated after stimulation of patients' peripheral blood mononuclear cells (PBMCs). Resulting cells were $CD4^+$ $CD25^+$ while FOXP3-expression was not analyzed, as these cells were classified as induced Tr1 cells. After re-stimulation with ovalbumin, the cells were administrated intravenously in doses ranging from 10^6–10^9 cells. The authors report that 8 of 20 patients had a clinical response as measured by CDAI at both weeks 5 and 8 after treatment.

These results indicate that different Treg populations may be therapeutic options for patients with IMIDs. Of note, most researchers employ polyclonal expansion of Tregs in order to obtain sufficient numbers. It has been suggested that partial lymphodepletion prior to transfusion, similar to the protocols used in adoptive tumor immunotherapy,[45] would reduce the number of Tregs needed to induce a response.[46] This reduced cell requirement might simultaneously make antigen-specific Treg therapy more feasible. Here, one can envision a development similar to that of tumor-specific T cells, where Tregs are genetically modified to express an autoantigen-specific TCR and equipped with additional properties of choice.

Concluding Remarks

As indicated above, there are several promising options for immunoregulatory cell therapy. However, most of the clinical experience in the field is derived from GvHD and organ transplantation. In autoimmunity, several unique issues have to be addressed such as the potential intrinsic defect of autologous regulatory cells versus the risk of allo-immunization against donor cells. Little knowledge exists on effective dosing and timing of cell infusion. Pre-treatment lymphodepletion has not been explored in this setting, but the beneficial effects of autologous bone marrow transplantation in multiple sclerosis indicate its applicability. However, the side-effects of lymphodepletion must clearly be balanced against potential benefits of the treatment. In addition, regulatory requirements need to be met before immunoregulatory cell therapy can become a part of standard care. First and foremost, standardized, clinical-grade preparation of cell products and defined release criteria consisting of functional and/or phenotypic assays must be established. Furthermore, clinical trials need to be conducted using standardized immunomonitoring and a randomized study design with comparison to best standard of care or placebo. In the field of organ transplantation, the ONE study embraces all these aspects in a combined effort to define effective cellular therapies. A similar initiative would be desirable in the field of immune mediated diseases.

References

1. Fischbach, M.A., Bluestone, J.A. and Lim, W.A. (2013). Cell-based therapeutics: the next pillar of medicine. *Sci Transl Med*, **5**(179), 179ps7.
2. Dunn, G.P., Old, L.J. and Schreiber, R.D. (2004). The three Es of cancer immunoediting. *Annu Rev Immunol*, **22**, 329–360.
3. Essand, M. and Loskog, A.S. (2013). Genetically engineered T cells for the treatment of cancer. *J Intern Med*, **273**(2), 166–181.
4. Bartholomew, A., *et al.* (2002). Mesenchymal stem cells suppress lymphocyte proliferation *in vitro* and prolong skin graft survival *in vivo*. *Exp Hematol*, **30**(1), 42–48.
5. Jaager, K., *et al.* (2012). RNA-seq analysis reveals different dynamics of differentiation of human dermis- and adipose-derived stromal stem cells. *PLoS One*, **7**(6), e38833.
6. Dominici, M., *et al.* (2006). Minimal criteria for defining multipotent mesenchymal stromal cells. The International Society for Cellular Therapy position statement. *Cytotherapy*, **8**(4), 315–317.
7. Bianco, P., *et al.* (2013). The meaning, the sense and the significance: translating the science of mesenchymal stem cells into medicine. *Nat Med*, **19**(1), 35–42.
8. English, K. (2013). Mechanisms of mesenchymal stromal cell immunomodulation. *Immunol Cell Biol*, **91**(1), 19–26.
9. Le Blanc, K., *et al.* (2008). Mesenchymal stem cells for treatment of steroid-resistant, severe, acute graft-versus-host disease: a phase II study. *Lancet*, **371**(9624), 1579–1586.

10. Griffin, M.D., *et al.* (2013). Anti-donor immune responses elicited by alloge-neic mesenchymal stem cells: what have we learned so far? *Immunol Cell Biol*, **91**(1), 40–51.
11. Lee, H.K., *et al.* (2014). Preclinical efficacy and mechanisms of mesenchy-mal stem cells in animal models of autoimmune diseases. *Immune Netw*, **14**(2), 81–88.
12. Casiraghi, F., *et al.* (2012). Localization of mesenchymal stromal cells dic-tates their immune or proinflammatory effects in kidney transplantation. *Am J Transplant*, **12**(9), 2373–2383.
13. Duijvestein, M., *et al.* (2010). Autologous bone marrow-derived mesenchy-mal stromal cell treatment for refractory luminal Crohn's disease: results of a phase I study. *Gut*, **59**(12), 1662–1669.
14. Cho, Y.B., *et al.* (2013). Autologous adipose tissue-derived stem cells for the treatment of Crohn's fistula: a phase I clinical study. *Cell Transplant*, **22**(2), 279–285.
15. Forbes, G.M., *et al.* (2014). A phase 2 study of allogeneic mesenchymal stromal cells for luminal Crohn's disease refractory to biologic therapy. *Clin Gastroenterol Hepatol*, **12**(1), 64–71.
16. Liang, J., *et al.* (2010). Allogenic mesenchymal stem cells transplantation in refractory systemic lupus erythematosus: a pilot clinical study. *Ann Rheum Dis*, **69**(8), 1423–1429.
17. Wang, D., *et al.* (2014). Umbilical cord mesenchymal stem cell transplanta-tion in active and refractory systemic lupus erythematosus: a multicenter clinical study. *Arthritis Res Ther*, **16**(2), R79.
18. Wang, D., *et al.* (2011). Efficacy of allogeneic mesenchymal stem cell trans-plantation in patients with drug-resistant polymyositis and dermatomyositis. *Ann Rheum Dis*, **70**(7), 1285–1288.
19. Wang, L., *et al.* (2013) Pilot study of umbilical cord-derived mesenchymal stem cell transfusion in patients with primary biliary cirrhosis. *J Gastroenterol Hepatol*, **28 Suppl 1**, 85–92.
20. Sengupta, U., *et al.* (2013). Infusion of autologous bone marrow mononu-clear cells leads to transient reduction in proteinuria in treatment refractory patients with Idiopathic membranous nephropathy. *BMC Nephrol*, **14**, 262.
21. Karussis, D., *et al.* (2010). Safety and immunological effects of mesenchy-mal stem cell transplantation in patients with multiple sclerosis and amyotrophic lateral sclerosis. *Arch Neurol*, **67**(10), 1187–1194.
22. Bonab, M.M., *et al.* (2012). Autologous mesenchymal stem cell therapy in progressive multiple sclerosis: an open label study. *Curr Stem Cell Res Ther*, **7**(6), 407–414.

23. Connick, P., *et al.* (2012). Autologous mesenchymal stem cells for the treatment of secondary progressive multiple sclerosis: an open-label phase 2a proof-of-concept study. *Lancet Neurol*, **11**(2), 150–156.

24. Poschke, I. and Kiessling, R. (2012). On the armament and appearances of human myeloid-derived suppressor cells. *Clin Immunol*, **144**(3), 250–268.

25. Mosser, D.M. and Edwards, J.P. (2008). Exploring the full spectrum of macrophage activation. *Nat Rev Immunol*, **8**(12), 958–969.

26. Steinman, R.M., Hawiger, D. and Nussenzweig, M.C. (2003). Tolerogenic dendritic cells. *Annu Rev Immunol*, **21**, 685–711.

27. Riquelme, P., Geissler, E.K. and Hutchinson, J.A. (2012). Alternative approaches to myeloid suppressor cell therapy in transplantation: comparing regulatory macrophages to tolerogenic DCs and MDSCs. *Transplant Res*, **1**(1), 17.

28. Machen, J., *et al.* (2004). Antisense oligonucleotides down-regulating costimulation confer diabetes-preventive properties to nonobese diabetic mouse dendritic cells. *J Immunol*, **173**(7), 4331–4341.

29. Parsa, R., *et al.* (2012). Adoptive transfer of immunomodulatory M2 macrophages prevents type 1 diabetes in NOD mice. *Diabetes*, **61**(11), 2881–2892.

30. Zhang, X.M., *et al.* (2014). Adoptive transfer of cytokine-induced immunomodulatory adult microglia attenuates experimental autoimmune encephalomyelitis in DBA/1 mice. *Glia*, **62**(5), 804–817.

31. Giannoukakis, N., *et al.* (2011). Phase I (safety) study of autologous tolerogenic dendritic cells in type 1 diabetic patients. *Diabetes Care*, **34**(9), 2026–2032.

32. Mia, S., *et al.* (2014). An optimized protocol for human M2 macrophages using M-CSF and IL-4/IL-10/TGF-beta yields a dominant immunosuppressive phenotype. *Scand J Immunol*, **79**(5), 305–314.

33. Hutchinson, J.A., *et al.* (2011). Cutting Edge: Immunological consequences and trafficking of human regulatory macrophages administered to renal transplant recipients. *J Immunol*, **187**(5), 2072–2078.

34. Sakaguchi, S. (2004). Naturally arising CD4+ regulatory t cells for immunologic self-tolerance and negative control of immune responses. *Annu Rev Immunol*, **22**, 531–562.

35. Sagoo, P., *et al.* (2011). Human regulatory T cells with alloantigen specificity are more potent inhibitors of alloimmune skin graft damage than polyclonal regulatory T cells. *Sci Transl Med*, **3**(83), 83ra42.

36. Kendal, A.R. and Waldmann, H. (2010). Infectious tolerance: therapeutic potential. *Curr Opin Immunol*, **22**(5), 560–565.

37. Liu, W., *et al.* (2006). CD127 expression inversely correlates with FoxP3 and suppressive function of human CD4+ T reg cells. *J Exp Med*, **203**(7), 1701–1711.
38. Hoffmann, P., *et al.* (2009). Loss of FOXP3 expression in natural human CD4+CD25+ regulatory T cells upon repetitive in vitro stimulation. *Eur J Immunol*, **39**(4), 1088–1097.
39. Long, S.A. and Buckner, J.H. (2011). CD4+FOXP3+ T regulatory cells in human autoimmunity: more than a numbers game. *J Immunol*, **187**(5), 2061–2066.
40. Janson, P.C., *et al.* (2008). FOXP3 promoter demethylation reveals the committed Treg population in humans. *PLoS One*, **3**(2), e1612.
41. Polansky, J.K., *et al.* (2008). DNA methylation controls Foxp3 gene expression. *Eur J Immunol*, **38**(6), 1654–1663.
42. Marek-Trzonkowska, N., *et al.* (2012). Administration of CD4+CD25high CD127- regulatory T cells preserves beta-cell function in type 1 diabetes in children. *Diabetes Care*, **35**(9), 1817–1820.
43. Marek-Trzonkowska, N., *et al.* (2014). Therapy of type 1 diabetes with CD4(+)CD25(high)CD127-regulatory T cells prolongs survival of pancreatic islets — results of one year follow-up. *Clin Immunol*, **153**(1), 23–30.
44. Desreumaux, P., *et al.* (2012). Safety and efficacy of antigen-specific regulatory T-cell therapy for patients with refractory Crohn's disease. *Gastroenterology*, **143**(5), 1207–1217 e1–2.
45. Dudley, M.E., *et al.* (2002). Cancer regression and autoimmunity in patients after clonal repopulation with antitumor lymphocytes. *Science*, **298**(5594), 850–854.
46. Tang, Q. and Bluestone, J.A. (2013). Regulatory T-cell therapy in transplantation: moving to the clinic. *Cold Spring Harb Perspect Med*, **3**(11).

PART 2

TREATMENT FOR SPECIFIC INFLAMMATORY DISEASES

CHAPTER 5

ADVANCES IN THERAPIES FOR RHEUMATOID ARTHRITIS

Katerina Chatzidionysiou

Introduction

Rheumatoid Arthritis (RA) is a chronic, systemic, inflammatory disease of unknown etiology which is generally thought to be autoimmune in nature. It typically affects the small and medium joints and causes synovial inflammation which can lead to cartilage and bone destruction if untreated. The landscape of RA treatment has unquestionably changed dramatically during the last decade. A deeper understanding of the pathophysiological and immunological mechanisms in RA has led to the development and introduction to daily clinical practice of a new class of anti-rheumatic drugs, the so-called biologic therapies, as well as earlier and more aggressive treatment, has contributed to this treatment revolution. To date, nine biologic agents and the first janus kinase inhibitor have been approved for the treatment for RA. More molecules with distinct mechanisms of action are currently being tested in laboratories and in clinical trials. In many cases, very good clinical efficacy and safety were documented in large, randomized, controlled clinical trials leading to regulatory approval. Despite the dramatic improvement, there are still unmet needs, with a significant number of patients being refractory to currently available treatments and many patients losing efficacy or not tolerating biologic agents. More optimal use of the currently available treatments and better treatment strategies are needed.

Biologic DMARDs

The emergence and establishment of biologic disease modifying antirheumatic drugs (DMARDs) in everyday clinical practice was perhaps the most important factor that contributed to the dramatic change of the field of RA treatment during the past decade. To date, nine biologic agents have been approved for treatment of RA: five inhibitors of tumor necrosis factor (TNF: *i.e.* infliximab, etanercept, adalimumab, golimumab and certolizumab pegol), the interleukin (IL)-1 blocker anakinra, IL-6 blocker tocilizumab, B cell depleting agent rituximab and T-cell co-stimulation inhibitor abatacept.[1] In addition, more molecules with similar and distinct mechanisms of action are currently being tested in laboratories and in phase II and III clinical trials (Table 1). In most cases, very good clinical efficacy and safety were documented in trials that led or can lead to regulatory approval.

TNF inhibition

Cytokines in general are molecules involved in signaling between cells during immune responses. Pro-inflammatory cytokines are important mediators of active RA, promoting the activation of the adaptive immune system and "communication" between cells. T cells, macrophages and stromal cells are the main source of cytokines in early and established RA. TNF (initially named TNF-α in order to be differentiated from TNF-β, now known as lymphotoxin) is produced primarily by macrophages but from other cells as well, such as the macrophage-like synoviocytes, and has many functions in the development of inflammation and the activation of other leukocytes. It is prothrombotic and promotes leukocyte adhesion and migration. It has an important role in macrophage activation and differentiation, it regulates hematopoiesis, lymphocyte development and induces other cytokines as well. It is therefore a perfect target for RA, as has also been proven in clinical practice.

Table 1. Biologic DMARDs that have been approved for the treatment of RA according to their mechanism of action.

Target	Biologic DMARD	Molecule	Administration, usual starting dose
	Infliximab	Chimeric anti-TNF monoclonal antibody	Intravenous, 3 mg/kg every 8 weeks*
	Etanercept	Fusion protein composed of the constant end of the IgGl antibody to the TNF receptor	Subcutaneous, 50 mg once weekly
TNF	Adalimumab	Human anti-TNF monoclonal antibody	Subcutaneous, 40 mg every other week
	Golimumab	Human anti-TNF monoclonal antibody	Subcutaneous, 50 mg once every 4 weeks
	Certolizumab pegol	PEGylated Fab fragment of humanized anti-TNF monoclonal antibody	Subcutaneous, 200 mg every other week or 400 mg once every 4 weeks
IL-1	Anakinra	IL-1 receptor antagonist	Subcutaneous, 100 mg once daily
IL-6	Tocilizumab	Humanized anti-IL6 receptor monoclonal antibody	Intravenous, 8 mg/kg once every 4 weeks Subcutaneous, 162 mg once weekly
B-cell	Rituximab	Chimeric anti-CD20 monoclonal antibody	Intravenous, 1000 mg × 2 (with 2 weeks interval), variable retreatment rate**
T-cell costimulation	Abatacept	Fusion protein composed of the Fc region of the IgGl fused to the extracellular domain of CTLA-4	Intravenous, 500–1000 mg once monthly or subcutaneous 125 mg once every week

* 3 mg/kg at 0, 2 and 6 weeks, then every 8 weeks. Some patients may benefit from increasing the dose up to 10 mg/kg or shortening the interval to as short as every 4 weeks.
** Retreatment after clinical flare or at fixed interval, for example every 6 months.

Table 2. Biologic DMARDs that have not been approved for the treatment of RA but have recently been or are currently in phase II/III trials.

Target	Biologic DMARD	Molecule	Administration
IL-6	Olokizumab	Humanized anti-IL6 monoclonal antibody	Subcutaneous (Phase II)*
	Sarilumab	Human anti-IL6 receptor monoclonal antibody	Subcutaneous (Phase II)
	Sirukumab	Human anti-IL6 monoclonal antibody	Subcutaneous (Phase II)
	Clazakizumab	Humanized anti-IL6 monoclonal antibody	Intravenous (Phase II)*
IL-17	Secukinumab	Human anti-IL-17A monoclonal antibody	Subcutaneous; the 150 mg and 300 mg doses have been approved for psoriasis
	Ixekizumab	Humanized monoclonal antibody against IL-17	Subcutaneous (Phase II)*
	Brodalumab	Human anti-IL17 RA monoclonal antibody	Subcutaneous (Phase II)*
B cell	Ofatumumab	Human anti-CD20 monoclonal antibody	Subcutaneous: the 700 mg dose has been approved in hematology; Intravenous: phase II for RA*
GM-CSF	Mavrilimumab	Human anti-granulocyte-macrophage colony-stimulating factor receptor (GM-CSF) monoclonal antibody	Subcutaneous (Phase II)

* Development of brodalumab, secukinumab and ixekizumab, is currently focused on psoriatic arthritis and ankylosing spondylitis. Phase II trials demonstrated modest efficacy of these agents in RA without significant difference between the active drug and the placebo groups. The RA clinical trial programs of olokizumab, clazakizumab and ofatumumab are not currently active.

There are five TNF inhibitors available today for the treatment of RA. Although they all target the same cytokine, there are important differences in their molecular structure, pharmacodynamics and pharmacokinetics (Table 1). The first three TNFis that received approval for the treatment of RA were infliximab, etanercept and adalimumab. Infliximab is a human murine chimeric monoclonal antibody that binds both soluble and membrane bound

TNF. It is approved at a dose of 3 mg/kg given at week 0, 2, 6 and thereafter every 8 weeks intravenously. Etanercept is a recombinant TNF receptor that is fused to a human Fc molecule. It is administered as a subcutaneous injection of 50 mg once a week. Adalimumab is a fully human monoclonal antibody against TNF. The approved dose is 40 mg once every other week. The newer TNFs are golimumab and certolizumab pegol. Golimumab is a fully human IgG1 monoclonal antibody specific for both circulating and bound TNF. It is given subcutaneously once every month at a dose of 50 mg and in combination with methotrexate (MTX) (or another synthetic DMARD). Certolizumab pegol differs from the other antibodies as it consists of a recombinant antigen-binding fragment (Fab´) of a humanized antibody against TNF, conjugated to a polyethylene glycol (PEG) moiety. It is approved at a dose of 200 mg subcutaneous injection every 2 weeks or 400 mg every month both in combination with synthetic disease modifying antirheumatic drugs (DMARDs) and as monotherapy. The doses given above are the usual starting doses of these biologic DMARDs.

Several studies have demonstrated the efficacy and safety of these TNF inhibitors in RA patients who are naive to synthetic DMARDs (who in practical terms often equate to newly diagnosed patients). These trials have generally provided clear evidence of the superiority of the combination of biologics with MTX over MTX alone in such patients. In a small (20 patients), randomized, double-blind, placebo-controlled trial, Quinn *et al.* showed significantly greater clinical, functional and radiological benefit of combination treatment with MTX plus infliximab in early RA compared to MTX alone.[2] It is interesting that one year after stopping induction therapy with infliximab, 70% of patients had a sustained response. In a larger study by St. Clair *et al.* patients with RA of ≤3 years of duration achieved significantly better clinical efficacy with infliximab plus MTX than with MTX monotherapy.[3] Similar results were shown in large, randomized, controlled trials for etanercept and adalimumab, as well as for the newer TNFi golimumab.[4–6] All of the above-mentioned studies were based on a population of patients with early RA (disease duration from 6.5 to 10.8 months) who had not received prior MTX, and they all demonstrated that the combination of a biologic agent and MTX can yield better clinical, functional and radiographic outcome than MTX alone. However, it is worth noting that a substantial proportion of patients in these trials responded well to MTX monotherapy. Thus, one should

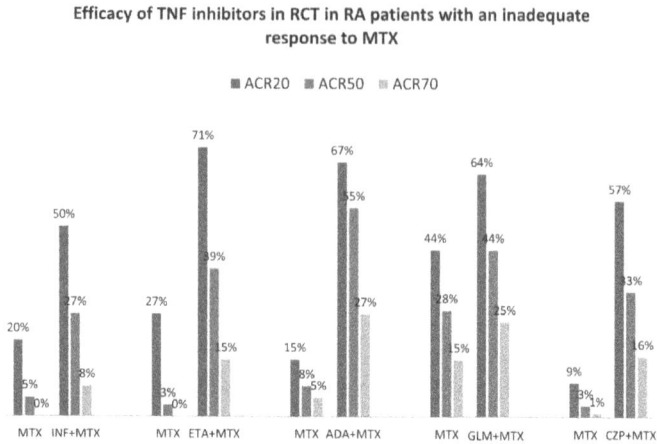

Figure 1. Efficacy of TNF inhibitors in RCT in RA patients with an inadequate response to MTX

■ ACR20   ■ ACR50   ▪ ACR70

Figure 1. Efficacy of the five TNF inhibitors approved today for RA, as demonstrated in five large RCTs in RA patients who had previously failed methotrexate (MTX).

INF: infliximab, ETA: etanercept, ADA: adalimumab, GLM: golimumab, CZP: certolizumab pegol

keep in mind that in the combination groups, there are patients who would have responded to MTX monotherapy as well.[7]

The most clearly established and best documented role for biologics in the treatment for RA, however, is in those patients who have failed to respond adequately to one or more conventional DMARD, usually including MTX. Double-blind, placebo-controlled, randomized trials for all nine biologic agents available today have been conducted and have established the efficacy of these drugs in patients with RA with inadequate response to MTX. The clinical responses after six months of therapy with all five TNFis plus MTX versus placebo plus MTX are summarized in Figure 1.[8-12] All these biologic agents seem to have comparable efficacy in the MTX non-responder population and significantly greater efficacy than placebo.

IL-6 inhibition

Interleukin 6 (IL-6) is another pleiotropic cytokine which plays a central role in RA pathogenesis. It contributes to B and T cell activation, synovio-cyte stimulation, osteoclast maturation and production of acute-phase proteins. Tocilizumab, a humanized anti-IL6 receptor, is approved for the treatment of active RA as monotherapy or in combination with a synthetic DMARD. Its efficacy and safety has been studied both in synthetic DMARD non-responders as well as in RA patients who have already failed TNF inhibition.[13,14] A recently published study demonstrated the superiority of tocilizumab compared to adalimumab as monotherapy in patients who did not tolerate MTX.[15] Four new biologic DMARDs targeting IL6 and IL6 receptor have emerged (Table 2). Olokizumab, a humanized anti-IL6 monoclonal antibody, was associated with significantly greater reductions in DAS28 (CRP) compared to placebo, in RA patients who had previously failed TNF inhibitor therapy.[16] Olokizumab was given as a subcutaneous injection every two or every four weeks in four different dosing regimens in this phase II study. Its efficacy was comparable to tocilizumab. Sarilumab is a human monoclonal antibody targeting IL6-R. The efficacy and safety of sarilumab has been studied in a phase II study on a MTX non-responders RA population.[17] The study met its primary endpoint with the sarilumab groups achieving significantly greater ACR20 responses at week 12 (72% for sarilumab 150 mg qw, 67% for sarilumab 150 mg q2w and 200 mg q2w) compared to placebo. Subcutaneous sirukumab, an anti-IL6 monoclonal antibody, also proved to be effective and safe in a recently published phase II trial.[18] All the above agents seem to have an acceptable safety profile similar to that of tocilizumab. A fifth IL-6 blocking agent, clazakizumab, given intravenously at day 1 and week 8, has also been associated with rapid and significant improvements in disease activity in patients with an inadequate response to MTX.[19]

One or more of these biologic agents targeting IL-6 may soon be available. The next question is whether a patient who fails to respond adequately to one of these agents can achieve a better response to another anti-IL6 monoclonal antibody. As will be discussed below with TNF inhibitors, differences in molecular structure, route of administration and immunogenicity make switching between biologics with similar mechanism of action rational. That remains to be studied further with IL-6 antagonists.

IL-1 inhibition

Anakinra is a recombinant, human IL-1 receptor antagonist. It has been shown that anakinra is associated with worse efficacy compared to TNF inhibitors.[20] The limited efficacy in combination with the inconvenient administration (one subcutaneous injection daily, due to the drug's short half-life) makes anakinra one of the less used biologic DMARDs in RA. In contrast, anakinra as well as canakinumab, an anti-IL-1 monoclonal antibody, are effective for the treatment of autoinflammatory diseases.[21] Autoinflammatory diseases are a group of diseases characterized by an abnormal activation of the innate immune system leading to increased levels of acute-phase reactants and clinical inflammation. Periodic fever diseases such as familial Mediterranean fever and TNF-receptor associated periodic syndrome (TRAPS) are typical examples of autoinflammatory diseases.

Inhibition of other cytokines

Mavrilimumab is a human monoclonal antibody targeting the alpha subunit of the granulocyte-macrophage colony-stimulating factor (GM-CSF) receptor. GM-CSF acts as a pro-inflammatory cytokine. A recent phase II trial in RA showed rapid and significant efficacy with generally mild or moderate adverse events.[86] Phase III trials are currently being planned.

IL17 is a cytokine that has received a lot of interest during recent years, and several studies assessing the efficacy of antibodies blocking IL17 are in phase II/III. Secukinumab is a fully human anti-IL17A antibody that has achieved greater ACR20 responses than placebo in a phase II trial, although the differences were not significant and the primary endpoint was not achieved.[22] Phase III trials are ongoing. Ixekizumab is a humanized IgG4 mAb against IL-17, which when added to background DMARD therapy in biologic-naive RA patients produced a statistically significant dose-related response.[23] Brodalumab is a fully human IgG2 anti-IL17R monoclonal antibody. In a randomized, double-blind, placebo-controlled phase II trial, a total of 252 patients with active RA despite MTX treatment who were biologic naive were randomized to receive brodalumab 70, 140, or 210 mg subcutaneously or placebo at weeks 0, 1, 2, 4, 6, 8, and 10 (Pavelka *et al.*). The primary endpoint was ACR50 at week 12, which was achieved by 10–16% of patients in the brodalumab groups compared with 13% of those in the placebo group. Mean changes from baseline in DAS28 also did not differ significantly between brodalumab and placebo groups. Development of brodalumab, as well as ixekizumab, is currently focused on psoriatic arthritis and ankylosing spondylitis.

B cell Depletion

B cells play a key role in RA pathogenesis. Their multifaceted role made them a very promising target for the treatment of RA. Today only one B cell depleting agent is approved for the treatment of RA, rituximab. Rituximab (RTX) is a genetically engineered, chimeric anti-CD20 monoclonal antibody. CD20 is a membrane-associated phosphoprotein that regulates the early steps in B cell activation. Its expression is restricted to B cells. Treatment with RTX causes rapid depletion of certain B cells within the first treatment infusions and the effects can last for 6 to 9 months. CD20 positive B cell precursors, transitional B cells and naive B cells are most susceptible to deletion by RTX, while B1, marginal zone and germinal center B cells are more resistant.

It is hypothesized that RTX works through numerous candidate mechanisms, such as antibody dependent cell-mediated cytotoxicity (ADCC), where an antibody coated target cell is directly killed by an effector cell expressing Fc receptors, complement activation through the classical pathway which leads to the formation of the membrane attack complex (MAC) and consequently cell lysis and induction of apoptosis.[24] Which mechanism of action takes place is influenced by host factors — genetic background and disease specific factors such as the availability of an intact complement pathway and the magnitude of B cell survival signals. One other possible mechanism through which RTX might work is the immune complex decoy hypothesis, whereby the binding of RTX-IgG molecules to B cells forms immune complexes that efficiently attract and bind Fc gamma receptor-expressing effector cells, which diminishes recruitment of these effector cells at sites of immune complex deposition and, therefore, reduces inflammation and tissue damage.[25]

By depleting B cells and modulating the immune system, RTX leads to reduced antigen presentation, proinflammatory cytokine production and autoantibody production, thus efficiently reducing the severity of B cell-mediated autoimmune diseases, like RA.

Initially it was shown that although depletion of B cells in the periphery was observed in all RTX-treated patients, not all responded to therapy.[26] A possible explanation could be the presence of residual B cells in lymph nodes and in the synovium. Another explanation might be the sensitivity of measurement of B cells in the periphery. Indeed, more recent studies have shown a correlation between the depth of B cell depletion both in the circulation and synovium and clinical response.[27,28] Persistence of B cells is associated with poorer response.[29]

RTX is shown to be more efficacious than placebo in randomized controlled trials with an acceptable safety profile. In the SERENE trial both RTX doses (1000 mg × 2 and 500 mg × 2) achieved significantly greater responses compared to placebo in RA patients with background MTX who had not responded adequately to MTX.[30] No significant differences in efficacy or safety between the two dose groups were observed. The objective of the MIRROR study was to determine if initiating treatment with RTX 2 × 500 mg followed by a repeat treatment at 24 weeks with 2 × 500 mg was different from repeat treatment with a higher dose of 2 × 1000 mg. The study was also designed to compare the efficacy and safety of RTX 2 × 500 and 2 × 1000 mg over 48 weeks with a fixed repeat treatment at Week 24.[31] Similar to the SERENE trial, no significant differences in response rates were shown. In the IMAGE trial, which was conducted in DMARD-naive RA patients, both doses of RTX were associated with significant clinical improvement (in some comparisons the improvement was slightly higher numerically for the 1000 mg x 2 group but not significantly higher), but only the higher dose of RTX was proven effective in inhibiting progression of joint damage as assessed by the change in total Genant-modified Sharp score (mTSS) from baseline to week 52.[32] The lower dose of RTX could also slow the progression but the change in score compared to MTX monotherapy did not achieve statistical significance.

In the DANCER trial RTX proved to be effective in patients who had not previously responded to DMARD treatment, including biologic DMARDs.[33] Both RTX dosages were effective, with 54–55% of patients achieving an ACR20 response by week 24, and a high proportion achieving ACR50 or ACR70 responses. No dose-response relationship was established, based on the ACR20 criteria, for the two RTX doses studied. There were, however, trends to indicate that the dosage may influence the achievement of high-level response (*i.e.*, ACR70 response and good EULAR response). Similarly, in the REFLEX study RTX yielded significant ACR responses compared to placebo in patients with longstanding disease who did not respond to TNFis.[34] In an indirect comparison, one could observe that the efficacy of RTX is best in DMARD-naive patients and reduced in patients who have already failed at least one biologic agent.

All the above studies assessed the safety of RTX in a systematic way. The most common adverse effects of RTX are infusion reactions (common with the first infusion), increased risk for infections (upper respiratory tract infection, urinary tract infection, and nasopharyngitis) and reactivation of viral infections. Hitherto few cases of progressive multifocal leukoencephalopathy (PML) have been reported in RA. In a pooled analysis of safety data from patients treated with RTX in combination with MTX in a global clinical trial program, the overall rate of adverse events was 357 events per 100 patient-years (95% CI 354.4; 364.9). The rate of adverse events seems to decline with time. Hypogammaglobulinemia is an expected finding in RTX-treated patients. IgM levels decrease with multiple courses of RTX, but this does not appear to be associated with increased risk for serious infections. IgG is the most important among serum immunoglobulins for protective immunity. In some RTX-treated patients, levels of IgG can also be decreased but less frequently so compared to IgM. No obvious differences in the rate of adverse events have been observed between the higher and lower dose RTX.

Regarding prognostic factors of response, there is evidence that patients who are seropositive, especially anti-CCP positivity, have a greater chance of responding to RTX than seronegative ones (Fig. 2).[35]

Some other B cell depleting agents have been tested in RA. Ofatumumab, a fully human anti-CD20 monoclonal antibody, which is approved for the treatment of chronic lymphocytic leukemia, significantly improved all clinical outcomes in biologic-naive RA patients in a randomized, double-blind, placebo controlled trial.[36] No unexpected safety signals were seen. In contrast, ocrelizumab, a humanized anti-CD20 monoclonal antibody, was associated with a significant risk for serious infections and in particular with opportunistic infections in RA, and therefore the clinical trial program was terminated.

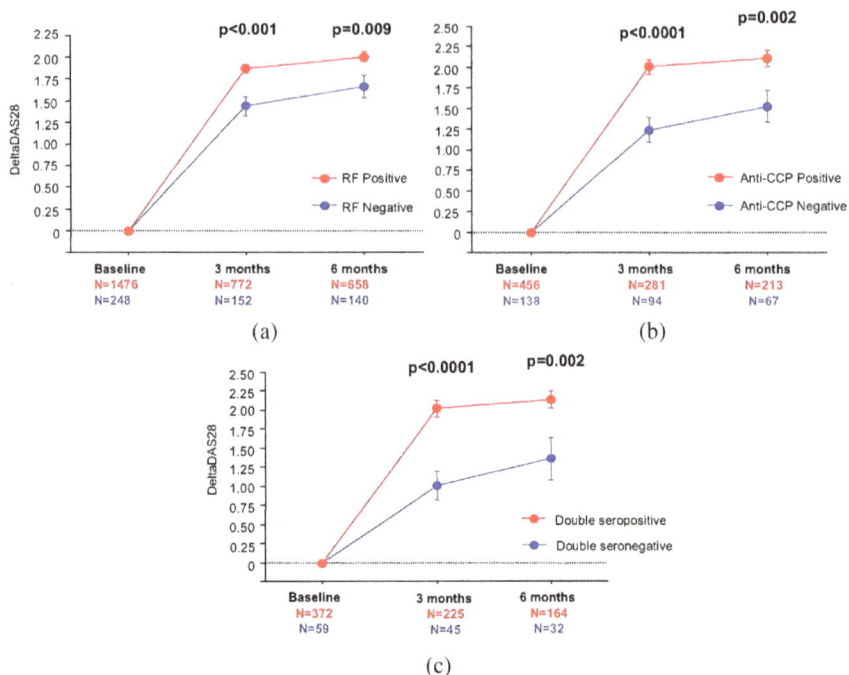

Figure 2. Mean DAS28 improvement (bars: SEM) during the first 6 months of treatment with rituximab for seropositive and seronegative RA patients. At 3 and 6 months, RF positive patients (A) as well as anti-CCP positive (B) and double positive patients (C) achieved significantly larger reductions of DAS28 compared to RF negative, anti-CCP negative and double negative patients, respectively.[35]

DAS28: disease activity score based on 28 joints, RF: rheumatoid factor, anti-CCP: anti-cyclic citrullinated peptide

(This figure has been reused with the permission of *Annals of the Rheumatic Diseases*)

Modulation of T cell co-stimulation

Abatacept is a fully human, recombinant, soluble fusion protein comprising the extracellular domain of human CTLA-4 (cytotoxic T lymphocyte-associated antigen-4). CTLA-4 is a naturally occurring inhibitory molecule which acts as a negative regulator of CD28-mediated T cell costimulation, as it has a markedly greater affinity for CD80 or CD86 than CD28.[37] Abatacept has been proven effective in patients with RA, including in MTX-naive patients with early RA and poor prognostic factors[38] and in patients with established RA and an inadequate response to either MTX or anti-TNF therapy.[39,40] In the AMPLE trial, subcutaneous abatacept plus MTX is non-inferior to subcutaneous adalimumab plus MTX in patients with active RA who are naive to biological therapy and have an inadequate response to MTX.[41]

Emerging Small Molecules

Tofacitinib is the first JAK (janus kinase) inhibitor to be approved in the USA and many other countries but not yet in the EMA (European Medicines Agency) countries for the treatment of RA. JAKs are nonreceptor tyrosine kinases. In mammals, this family of tyrosine kinases has four members: JAK1, JAK2, JAK3 and TyK2.[42] JAKs mediate signaling via surface receptors for several proinflammatory cytokines involved in the pathogenesis of RA. JAK inhibitors prevent signaling of JAK enzymes and thus, interrupt signal transduction of cytokines. Tofacitinib is a selective inhibitor of JAK1 and JAK3. JAK1 is expressed in lymphoid cells and in the nervous system, while JAK3 is found at high levels in hematopoietic tissues, myeloid cells, NK cells, and activated B and T cells.[43] JAK1 binds to the beta-subunit of several cytokine receptors such as IL-2, IL-4, IL-7, IL-9, IL-15 and IL-21, while JAK3 binds to the common gamma-chain of these receptors.[44] When one of these cytokines binds to its receptor, JAK1 and JAK3 undergo autotransphosphorylation, which leads to the binding and activation of STAT proteins. These STAT proteins are subsequently translocated to the nucleus where they regulate transcription of several genes critical for the immune response. Over recent years, JAKs have emerged as attractive targets for the treatment of autoimmune diseases.

Several phase II clinical trials suggested that tofacitinib is a promising new drug for the treatment of active RA.[45,46] In a phase III, double-blind, placebo-controlled, parallel-group, 6-month clinical trial, the efficacy and safety of two different doses of tofacitinib were assessed.[47] A total of 611 patients who had previously failed at least one non-biologic or biologic DMARD were randomly assigned, in a 4:4:1:1 ratio, to tofacitinib 5 mg twice daily (b.i.d.), tofacitinib 10 mg b.i.d., placebo for three months followed by tofacitinib 5 mg b.i.d., or placebo for three months followed by tofacitinib 10 mg b.i.d., respectively. The ACR20 primary endpoint was met, with a total of 59.8% of the patients in the tofacitinib 5 mg group and

65.7% in the 10 mg group, as compared with 26.7% in the combined placebo groups, achieving an ACR20 response ($p < 0.001$ for both comparisons). Significant differences were also observed for ACR50 and ACR70 responses. The results of this phase III trial suggested that tofacitinib monotherapy was more efficacious than placebo in reducing inflammatory activity and in improving physical function in patients with active RA. This result has important clinical implications, since a significant number of patients do not tolerate MTX, and most biologic DMARDs available today are approved in combination with MTX.

In another recently published phase III randomized clinical trial, tofacitinib was compared to adalimumab.[48] Seven hundred and seventeen biologic-naive RA patients with an inadequate response to MTX were assigned to one of five arms: tofacitinib 5 mg b.i.d., tofacitinib 10 mg b.i.d., adalimumab 40 mg administered by subcutaneous injection once every two weeks, placebo for three or six months followed by tofacitinib 5 mg b.i.d., and placebo for three or six months followed by tofacitinib 10 mg b.i.d.. This design, with the inclusion of an active comparator arm with a TNF inhibitor, allowed an estimate of the efficacy and safety of tofacitinib relative to an established biologic therapy. The three primary endpoints were ACR20 response, HAQ-DI improvement and disease remission rate at six months. All three endpoints were met. The efficacy outcomes for tofacitinib were numerically similar to those seen with adalimumab, suggesting that, at least as far as the clinical efficacy is concerned, these agents are comparable.

Another phase III trial demonstrated the efficacy and safety of tofacitinib in a population of RA patients who had previously failed TNF inhibition.[49] Both when used as monotherapy or with background MTX, tofacitinib was associated with an increased rate of infections (upper respiratory tract infection, urinary tract infection, bronchitis and herpes zoster virus), increases in low-density lipoprotein levels and aminotransferase levels, cytopenias (neutropenia, anemia and thrombocytopenia), small increase in the creatinine levels and gastrointestinal adverse events. Few cases of tuberculosis have been reported.

Several other JAK inhibitors are currently in development. Bariticinib is a selective blocker of JAK1 and JAK2 with promising efficacy in phase II trials and, perhaps surprisingly, no major problems with cytopenias.

VX-509, a selective JAK3 inhibitor, showed a dose-dependent increase in ACR20 versus placebo in a phase II monotherapy trial.

Syk is a spleen tyrosine kinase expressed on macrophages, neutrophils, mast cells and osteoclasts, and associates directly with the B cell- and Fcgamma-receptor. Fostamatinib is a novel inhibitor of Syk that has been shown to improve inflammation in RA.[50] Adverse events include neutropenia, elevated liver enzymes, diarrhea and hypertension. However, in another phase II study with RA patients who previously failed TNF inhibition therapy, no significant differences were shown between fostamatinib and placebo at month 3, with the ACR20 response rates being 38% in the fostamatinib 100 mg b.i.d. group versus 37% in the placebo group.[51] No significant differences were achieved in the ACR50 or ACR70 response levels either.

Apremilast is an oral PDE4 inhibitor that is approved for the treatment of psoriasis and psoriatic arthritis. While effective in an animal model,[52] a recent trial in RA was negative.[85]

Treatment Strategies — Optimizing the use of DMARDs

As is obvious from the above, the armamentarium of highly effective antirheumatic drugs is increasing. The question that arises next is how these drugs can be optimally used in the clinical setting. There are still many aspects about the optimal use of biologic DMARDs that remain elusive today. Some of these aspects will be discussed below.

When is it the right time to start a biologic DMARD?

Data from epidemiological studies suggest that about 30–40% of RA patients respond very well to MTX. That means that the remaining percentage, which is more than half of all RA patients do not achieve the goal of treatment, which is remission. There are two main treatment strategies after the failure of MTX: adding a biologic agent or adding other synthetic DMARDs, the so called triple therapy which consists of MTX, sulphasalazine and hydroxychloroquine. So far, only a few clinical trials have made a direct comparison of these two treatment options. In the SWEFOT trial, patients with early RA with an inadequate response to MTX after three months, defined as lack of achievement of low disease activity, were randomly allocated to addition of either sulfasalazine and hydroxychloroquine or infliximab.[53] The latter group had significantly greater responses after 12 months of therapy, with 39% of patients achieving the primary endpoint EULAR good response compared to 25% in the former group ($p = 0.016$). However, after two years, the clinical difference was smaller and no longer statistically significant.[54] Radiological progression was, however, greater with conventional therapy than with the biologic agent. In the BeSt trial, it was shown that initial combination therapy with initial high-dose prednisone followed by a gradual prednisone-dose reduction or with infliximab provided earlier clinical improvement than sequential monotherapy and conventional combination therapy.[55] After two years, patients in all four treatment groups had approximately the same improvement in disease activity and functional status irrespective of initial treatment, probably because of tight control and frequent treatment adjustments. However, the more aggressively treated patients had less radiological progression of joint damage, and during the second year, more of them could be treated successfully with monotherapy, suggesting that the initial aggressive therapy did result in some long-term gains.

In the Treatment of Early Aggressive RA (TEAR) trial, patients with early RA were randomized to one of four groups: MTX monotherapy followed by triple therapy in case of insufficient response ($n = 124$); MTX followed by the addition of etanercept ($n = 255$); immediate triple therapy ($n = 132$); or immediate MTX plus etanercept ($n = 244$).[56] Rather surprisingly, at 1-year follow-up none of the four strategies was superior clinically, and only small differences were observed in radiographic progression. Both TEAR and SWEFOT were early-RA studies. In a recently published double-blinded, randomized clinical trial, patients ($n = 353$) with established RA with an average disease duration of five years who had been receiving MTX in at least one year but despite that had still active disease, were randomized to receive either triple therapy (MTX, sulphasalazine and hydroxychloroquine) or MTX + etanercept.[57] The main result was that triple therapy was non-inferior to the addition of a biologic agent to MTX. The difference in average 28-joint disease activity score (DAS28) at 24 weeks almost achieved significance ($p =$ 0.06), but was smaller than the non-inferiority margin. Thus, one could summarize the result by saying that triple therapy might be a little bit less effective than the addition of an anti-TNF agent in the event of inadequate response to traditional DMARD therapy, but the difference is not clinically relevant.[58]

Treatment strategies after the failure of the first TNF inhibitor

Switching between TNF inhibitors

In clinical reality, the first biologic DMARD is almost always a TNF inhibitor in combination with a synthetic DMARD, unless there are contraindications. It has been shown that a significant number of patients discontinue this treatment for various reasons, mainly due to inefficacy or intolerance. Indeed, a number of studies indicate that as many as 50% of all patients discontinue TNF inhibitor during the first three years of therapy.[59,60] Different TNF inhibitors might target the same cytokine but differ substantially in their molecular structure, pharmacokinetics and immunogenicity. This is the rationale behind switching between different TNF inhibitors. This issue was investigated in the randomized double-blinded GO-AFTER study, in which after failure of a prior TNF inhibitor, patients who received golimumab showed significantly greater responses than those who received placebo.[61] In the REALISTIC study, the efficacy of certolizumab pegol after the failure of one or more TNFis was demonstrated.[62] In addition, results from many observational studies support switching between TNF inhibitors, as a substantial proportion of patients can benefit from this strategy.[60,63–68] Cohort study data also suggest a gradual loss of efficacy after a greater number of switches. Thus, a first switch might provide significant improvement, whereas the effect is much less profound at the second or third switch.[69]

A large cohort study based on the Swedish national register demonstrated, in line with previous studies, that switching to a second TNFi may lead to significant clinical improvements.[70] Almost 40% of patients achieved low disease activity or remission, regardless of the specific TNFi. However, switching strategy might also be important. When the

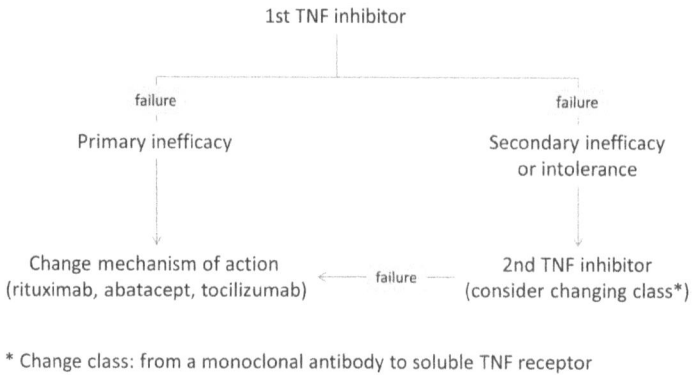

```
                        1st TNF inhibitor


        failure                                    failure
   Primary inefficacy                      Secondary inefficacy
                                               or intolerance


Change mechanism of action                      2nd TNF inhibitor
(rituximab, abatacept, tocilizumab)    failure   (consider changing class*)
```

* Change class: from a monoclonal antibody to soluble TNF receptor

Figure 3. Proposed algorithm on switching biologic DMARDs after the failure of the first TNF inhibitor. The reason of failure should be taken into consideration, as well as the type of the first TNF inhibitor (monoclonal antibody, soluble TNF receptor). When the reason for switching is primary inefficacy, then switching to a biologic DMARD with different mechanism of action can yield to better results.

effectiveness of switching was assessed as a function of the 1st TNFi, overall better results were observed when patients were switched from a monoclonal antibody (adalimumab or infliximab) to etanercept while worse results were observed for those switching from etanercept to adalimumab. When the reason for discontinuation of the 1st TNFi was taken into consideration, better results (rate of low disease activity/remission) at 6 months were observed with the 2nd TNFi when the reason for switch was loss of efficacy or intolerance. Patients who switched due to lack of efficacy (primary inefficacy) achieved worse results.

To conclude, switching between TNF inhibitors can yield clinically meaningful results, which is very important for both treating rheumatologists and patients, but the type of switching (switching class of TNF inhibitor from a monoclonal antibody to a TNF receptor) and reason for switch should be taken into consideration (Fig. 3).

Switching mechanism of action

Another possible treatment strategy after the failure of TNF inhibition (with a single or multiple agents), is change of mechanism, which might be more logical than trying different regimens of the same drug class.

Large trials have proved the efficacy of RTX, abatacept and tocilizumab versus placebo after TNF treatment.[14,40,71] Superiority of RTX over placebo was observed in the REFLEX trial.[34] Abatacept demonstrated acceptable safety and clinically meaningful efficacy in patients who failed TNF inhibitor treatment in the ATTAIN trial.[72] Additionally, in the RADIATE trial, tocilizumab-treated patients achieved significantly better results than those who received placebo during the first six months of therapy.[14] But are these biologic agents with a different mechanism of action better than an alternative TNF inhibitor? Again, no randomized clinical trial has provided us with hard evidence to answer this question. On the other hand, observational studies have compared the two treatment options. In the Swiss Clinical Quality Management program for RA (SCQM-RA) registry, patients with inadequate response to TNF inhibitor treatment achieved greater reductions in DAS28 when switching to RTX than to an alternative TNF blocker.[73] In a sub-analysis of the same population, it was shown that the superiority of RTX over an alternative TNF inhibitor was observed for the subgroup of patients who discontinued previous TNF inhibitor therapy because of primary or secondary inefficacy.[74] Newer data from the British Society for Rheumatology Biologics Register suggest that switching to RTX may be of more benefit than switching to an alternative anti-TNF therapy after failing the first anti-TNF therapy in RA patients.[75]

In a prospective observational study from Spain, no difference in the reduction of DAS28 was observed during the first year of treatment between RTX and TNFi groups, but there was a significant difference between adalimumab/infliximab and RTX in a sub-analysis.[76] Interestingly, our data from the Stockholm biologic RA register yielded similar results.[77] Two hundred and fifty-nine patients who switched to a 2nd TNFi and 69 who switched to RTX after the failure of a 1st TNFi were identified. Both treatments yielded significant results during the first six months of therapy. The mean (SD) DAS28 improvement was significantly lower for infliximab and adalimumab (group of TNFi monoclonal antibodies) compared to RTX and etanercept. When the effectiveness of switch was examined as a function of the type of the 1st TNFi, we observed a significantly greater EULAR Good response rate for RTX (36.9%) compared to mAb (11.1%) ($p = 0.001$) after the failure of etanercept. After the failure of mAb, RTX and ETA yielded similar EULAR Good/Moderate response rates (no statistical difference was observed) that were numerically higher than mAB.

Discontinuation of DMARDs — a feasible goal?

After the achievement of low disease activity or remission, the next goal is the "biologic-free remission", which is important with respect to long-term safety issues, patient comfort and health economics. In various settings, the possibility has been investigated of discontinuing the biologic agent whilst maintaining the patient in remission on a conventional DMARD. As part of the ATTRACT study,[78] 17 patients in a single center in the United Kingdom received infliximab and all 17 experienced flare-ups after discontinuation of the biologic therapy after two years, with a mean time of 13.5–15.0 weeks at the end of therapy. Of importance, reintroduction of infliximab after disease flare was associated with comparable responses without any safety issues. Whereas patients included in the ATTRACT study had longstanding disease (mean disease duration, 11 years), Quinn *et al.* addressed the same question in a randomized, double-blind, placebo-controlled trial in a population of patients with early RA, with symptom duration of <12 months.[2] These authors showed that induction of remission with infliximab plus MTX in early, poor prognosis RA provided not only significant reduction in synovitis and erosions at 1 year (shown by magnetic resonance imaging) but also sustained functional and quality-of-life benefits for 70% of the patients at 2 years despite infliximab withdrawal. More recently, Tanaka *et al.* determined the possibility of discontinuing infliximab after attaining DAS-guided low disease activity in patients with RA in the remission induction by infliximab in RA (RRR) study.[79] Of 102 patients, 56 (55%) maintained DAS28 < 3.2 and 44 (43%) reached remission (DAS28 < 2.6) one year after the discontinuation of infliximab. The mean disease duration in this study was 5.9 years, which suggests that discontinuation of infliximab would be possible not only in patients with early RA but also in patients with more established disease. In a post hoc analysis from the BeSt study, it was shown that significantly more patients who received initial combination therapy with infliximab and MTX achieved sustained DAS ≤ 2.4 and were able to discontinue infliximab, compared with those with delayed introduction of the biologic agent (56% vs. 29%, *p* = 0.008).[80] It was also shown in the BeSt study that the shorter the symptom duration, the higher the likelihood of a biologic-free, and even a drug-free, remission.[81] In the OPTIMA trial, RA patients with early RA who achieved stable low disease activity on adalimumab plus MTX who withdrew adalimumab mostly maintained their good responses.[82] Even in more established RA, discontinuation of adalimumab can be feasible but mainly for patients in deep remission, as shown in the HONOR study.[83] The results of a systematic review and meta-analysis showed that patients with established RA who stopped treatment with synthetic DMARDs had a significantly higher risk of disease flare or deterioration than those who continued treatment.[84] In this analysis, however, patients had RA of more than two years of duration.

From the results of the above studies, one can draw several conclusions. First, biologic-free remission might be possible after achieving remission or low disease activity in a considerable proportion of patients. Second, the duration of disease until the introduction of the biologic treatment might be negatively associated with the risk of deterioration after discontinuation of treatment, thus suggesting that earlier initiation of biologic treatment not only leads to better results but also increases the possibility of withdrawal of biologic agents with maintenance of remission. Third, if a patient has had a remission for a long time, it is more likely that the patient will remain in remission.

Future Perspectives — What to Hope for, What to Expect

Despite the dramatic progress in the treatment of RA, there are still important issues that remain unsolved. A significant number of patients are refractory to the available treatments. With many new drugs emerging, there is hope for this group of patients. The biggest challenge however for rheumatologists and clinical researchers is to optimize the use of all these highly effective, but at the same time, expensive and potentially harmful drugs. Identification of prognostic factors of response to each DMARD or group of DMARDs (depending on the target) could lead to a more individualized therapy approach based, perhaps, on genetic or immunological profile. Direct comparison of therapeutic strategies could lead to better guidelines about the sequential use of DMARDs. Optimal dose, right time of introduction and feasibility of dose-reduction or discontinuation of a DMARD, even combination of DMARDs with distinct mechanism of action, are other clinically significant issues that remain to be further elucidated. It has been a revolutionary decade for RA but an even more exciting future is ahead of us.

References

1. van Vollenhoven, R.F. (2013). Rheumatoid arthritis in 2012: Progress in RA genetics, pathology and therapy. *Nat Rev Rheumatol,* **9**(2), 70–72.
2. Quinn, M.A., Conaghan, P.G., O'Connor, P.J., *et al.* (2005). Very early treatment with infliximab in addition to methotrexate in early, poor-prognosis rheumatoid arthritis reduces magnetic resonance imaging evidence of synovitis and damage, with sustained benefit after infliximab withdrawal: Results from a twelve-month randomized, double-blind, placebo-controlled trial. *Arthritis Rheum,* **52**(1), 27–35.
3. St Clair, E.W., van der Heijde, D.M., Smolen, J.S., *et al.* (2004). Combination of infliximab and methotrexate therapy for early rheumatoid arthritis: A randomized, controlled trial. *Arthritis Rheum,* **50**(11), 3432–3443.
4. Emery, P., Breedveld, F.C., Hall, S., *et al.* (2008). Comparison of methotrexate monotherapy with a combination of methotrexate and etanercept in active, early, moderate to severe rheumatoid arthritis (COMET): A randomised, double-blind, parallel treatment trial. *Lancet,* **372**(9636), 375–382.
5. Breedveld, F.C., Weisman, M.H., Kavanaugh, A.F., *et al.* (2006). The PREMIER study: A multicenter, randomized, double-blind clinical trial of combination therapy with adalimumab plus methotrexate versus methotrexate alone or adalimumab alone in patients with early, aggressive rheumatoid arthritis who had not had previous methotrexate treatment. *Arthritis Rheum,* **54**(1), 26–37.
6. Emery, P., Fleischmann, R.M., Moreland, L.W., *et al.* (2009). Golimumab, a human anti-tumor necrosis factor alpha monoclonal antibody, injected subcutaneously every four weeks in methotrexate-naive patients with active rheumatoid arthritis: Twenty-four-week results of a phase III, multicenter, randomized, double-blind, placebo-controlled study of golimumab before methotrexate as first-line therapy for early-onset rheumatoid arthritis. *Arthritis Rheum,* **60**(8), 2272–2283.
7. Chatzidionysiou, K., van Vollenhoven, R.F. (2011). When to initiate and discontinue biologic treatments for rheumatoid arthritis? *J Internal Med,* **269**(6), 614–625.

8. Maini, R., St Clair, E.W., Breedveld, F., *et al.* (1999). Infliximab (chimeric anti-tumour necrosis factor alpha monoclonal antibody) versus placebo in rheumatoid arthritis patients receiving concomitant methotrexate: A randomised phase III trial. ATTRACT Study Group. *Lancet,* **354**(9194), 1932–1939.

9. Weinblatt, M.E., Kremer, J.M., Bankhurst, A.D., *et al.* (1999). A trial of etanercept, a recombinant tumor necrosis factor receptor:Fc fusion protein, in patients with rheumatoid arthritis receiving methotrexate. *N Eng J Med,* **340**(4), 253–259.

10. Weinblatt, M.E., Keystone, E.C., Furst, D.E., *et al.* (2003). Adalimumab, a fully human anti-tumor necrosis factor alpha monoclonal antibody, for the treatment of rheumatoid arthritis in patients taking concomitant methotrexate: The ARMADA trial. *Arthritis Rheum,* **48**(1), 35–45.

11. Keystone, E., Genovese, M.C., Klareskog, L., *et al.* (2010). Golimumab in patients with active rheumatoid arthritis despite methotrexate Therapy: 52-week results of the GO-FORWARD study. *Ann Rheum Dis,* **69**(6), 1129–1135.

12. Smolen, J., Landewe, R.B., Mease, P., *et al.* (2009). Efficacy and safety of certolizumab pegol plus methotrexate in active rheumatoid arthritis: The RAPID 2 study. A randomised controlled trial. *Ann Rheum Dis,* **68**(6), 797–804.

13. Genovese, M.C., McKay, J.D., Nasonov, E.L., *et al.* (2008). Interleukin-6 receptor inhibition with tocilizumab reduces disease activity in rheumatoid arthritis with inadequate response to disease-modifying antirheumatic drugs: The tocilizumab in combination with traditional disease-modifying antirheumatic drug therapy study. *Arthritis Rheum,* **58**(10), 2968–2980.

14. Emery, P., Keystone, E., Tony, H.P., *et al.* (2008). IL-6 receptor inhibition with tocilizumab improves treatment outcomes in patients with rheumatoid arthritis refractory to anti-tumour necrosis factor biologicals: Results from a 24-week multicentre randomised placebo-controlled trial. *Ann Rheum Dis,* **67**(11), 1516–1523.

15. Gabay, C., Emery, P., van Vollenhoven, R., *et al.* (2013). Tocilizumab monotherapy versus adalimumab monotherapy for treatment of rheumatoid arthritis (ADACTA): A randomised, double-blind, controlled phase 4 trial. *Lancet,* **381**(9877), 1541–1550.

16. Genovese, M.C., Fleischmann, R., Furst, D., *et al.* (2014). Efficacy and safety of olokizumab in patients with rheumatoid arthritis with an inadequate response to TNF inhibitor therapy: Outcomes of a randomised Phase IIb study. *Ann Rheum Dis,* **73**(9), 1607–1615.

17. Huizinga, T.W., Fleischmann, R.M., Jasson, M., *et al.* (2014). Sarilumab, a fully human monoclonal antibody against IL-6Ralpha in patients with rheumatoid arthritis and an inadequate response to methotrexate: Efficacy and

safety results from the randomised SARIL-RA-MOBILITY Part A trial. *Ann Rheum Dis,* **73**(9), 1626–1634.

18. Smolen, J.S., Weinblatt, M.E., Sheng, S., *et al.* (2014). Sirukumab, a human anti-interleukin-6 monoclonal antibody: A randomised, 2-part (proof-of-concept and dose-finding), phase II study in patients with active rheumatoid arthritis despite methotrexate therapy. *Ann Rheum Dis,* **73**(9), 1616–1625.

19. Mease, P., Strand, V., Shalamberidze, L., *et al.* (2012). A phase II, double-blind, randomised, placebo-controlled study of BMS945429 (ALD518) in patients with rheumatoid arthritis with an inadequate response to methotrexate. *Ann Rheum Dis,* **71**(7), 1183–1189.

20. Singh, J.A., Christensen, R., Wells, G.A., *et al.* (2009). A network meta-analysis of randomized controlled trials of biologics for rheumatoid arthritis: A Cochrane overview. *Canadian Medical Assoc J,* **181**(11), 787–796.

21. Sandborg, C., Mellins, E.D. (2012). A new era in the treatment of systemic juvenile idiopathic arthritis. *N Eng J Med,* **367**(25), 2439–2440.

22. Genovese, M.C., Durez, P., Richards, H.B., *et al.* (2013). Efficacy and safety of secukinumab in patients with rheumatoid arthritis: A phase, I.I., dose-finding, double-blind, randomised, placebo controlled study. *Ann Rheum Dis,* **72**(6), 863–869.

23. Genovese, M.C., Greenwald, M., Cho, C.S., *et al.* (2014). A phase II randomized study of subcutaneous ixekizumab, an anti-interleukin-17 monoclonal antibody, in rheumatoid arthritis patients who were naive to biologic agents or had an inadequate response to tumor necrosis factor inhibitors. *Arthritis Rheumatol,* **66**(7), 1693–1704.

24. Weiner, G.J. (2010). Rituximab: Mechanism of action. *Sem Hematol,* **47**(2), 115–123.

25. Taylor, R.P., Lindorfer, M.A. (2007). Drug insight: The mechanism of action of rituximab in autoimmune disease — the immune complex decoy hypothesis. *Nat Clin Pract Rheumatol,* **3**(2), 86–95.

26. Breedveld, F., Agarwal, S., Yin, M., *et al.* (2007). Rituximab pharmacokinetics in patients with rheumatoid arthritis: B-cell levels do not correlate with clinical response. *J Clin Pharmacol,* **47**(9), 1119–1128.

27. Thurlings, R.M., Vos, K., Wijbrandts, C.A., *et al.* (2008). Synovial tissue response to rituximab: Mechanism of action and identification of biomarkers of response. *Ann Rheum Dis,* **67**(7), 917–925.

28. Teng, Y.K., Levarht, E.W., Hashemi, M., *et al.* (2007). Immunohistochemical analysis as a means to predict responsiveness to rituximab treatment. *Arthritis Rheum,* **56**(12), 3909–3918.

29. Dass, S., Rawstron, A.C., Vital, E.M., *et al.* (2008). Highly sensitive B cell analysis predicts response to rituximab therapy in rheumatoid arthritis. *Arthritis Rheum,* **58**(10), 2993–2999.
30. Emery, P., Deodhar, A., Rigby, W.F., *et al.* (2010). Efficacy and safety of different doses and retreatment of rituximab: A randomised, placebo-controlled trial in patients who are biological naive with active rheumatoid arthritis and an inadequate response to methotrexate (Study Evaluating Rituximab's Efficacy in MTX iNadequate rEsponders (SERENE)). *Ann Rheum Dis,* **69**(9), 1629–1635.
31. Rubbert-Roth, A., Tak, P.P., Zerbini, C., *et al.* (2010). Efficacy and safety of various repeat treatment dosing regimens of rituximab in patients with active rheumatoid arthritis: Results of a Phase III randomized study (MIRROR). *Rheumatol,* **49**(9), 1683–1693.
32. Tak, P.P., Rigby, W.F., Rubbert-Roth, A., *et al.* (2011). Inhibition of joint damage and improved clinical outcomes with rituximab plus methotrexate in early active rheumatoid arthritis: The IMAGE trial. *Ann Rheum Dis,* **70**(1), 39–46.
33. Mease, P.J., Revicki, D.A., Szechinski, J., *et al.* (2008). Improved health-related quality of life for patients with active rheumatoid arthritis receiving rituximab: Results of the Dose-Ranging Assessment: International Clinical Evaluation of Rituximab in Rheumatoid Arthritis (DANCER) Trial. *J Rheumatol,* **35**(1), 20–30.
34. Keystone, E.C., Cohen, S.B., Emery, P., *et al.* (2012). Multiple courses of rituximab produce sustained clinical and radiographic efficacy and safety in patients with rheumatoid arthritis and an inadequate response to 1 or more tumor necrosis factor inhibitors: 5-year data from the REFLEX study. *J Rheumatol,* **39**(12), 2238–2246.
35. Chatzidionysiou, K., Lie, E., Nasonov, E., *et al.* (2011). Highest clinical effectiveness of rituximab in autoantibody-positive patients with rheumatoid arthritis and in those for whom no more than one previous TNF antagonist has failed: Pooled data from 10 European registries. *Ann Rheum Dis,* **70**(9), 1575–1580.
36. Ostergaard, M., Baslund, B., Rigby, W., *et al.* (2010). Ofatumumab, a human anti-CD20 monoclonal antibody, for treatment of rheumatoid arthritis with an inadequate response to one or more disease-modifying antirheumatic drugs: Results of a randomized, double-blind, placebo-controlled, phase I/II study. *Arthritis Rheum,* **62**(8), 2227–2238.
37. Korhonen, R., Moilanen, E. (2009). Abatacept, a novel CD80/86-CD28 T cell co-stimulation modulator, in the treatment of rheumatoid arthritis. *Basic Clin Pharmacol Toxicol,* **104**(4), 276–284.

38. Westhovens, R., Robles, M., Ximenes, A.C., *et al.* (2009). Clinical efficacy and safety of abatacept in methotrexate-naive patients with early rheumatoid arthritis and poor prognostic factors. *Ann Rheum Dis,* **68**(12), 1870–1877.
39. Schiff, M., Keiserman, M., Codding, C., *et al.* (2008). Efficacy and safety of abatacept or infliximab vs placebo in ATTEST: A phase II.I., multi-centre, randomised, double-blind, placebo-controlled study in patients with rheumatoid arthritis and an inadequate response to methotrexate. *Ann Rheum Dis,* **67**(8), 1096–1103.
40. Genovese, M.C., Becker, J.C., Schiff, M., *et al.* (2005). Abatacept for rheumatoid arthritis refractory to tumor necrosis factor alpha inhibition. *N Eng J Med,* **353**(11), 1114–1123.
41. Weinblatt, M.E., Schiff, M., Valente, R., *et al.* (2013). Head-to-head comparison of subcutaneous abatacept versus adalimumab for rheumatoid arthritis: Findings of a phase IIIb, multinational, prospective, randomized study. *Arthritis Rheum,* **65**(1), 28–38.
42. Yamaoka, K., Saharinen, P., Pesu, M., *et al.* (2004). The Janus kinases (Jaks). *Genome Biol,* **5**(12), 253.
43. Leonard, W.J., O'Shea, J.J. (1998). Jaks and STATs: Biological implications. *Ann Rev Immunol,* **16**:293–322.
44. Rochman, Y., Spolski, R., Leonard, W.J. (2009). New insights into the regulation of T cells by gamma(c) family cytokines. Nature reviews. *Immunol,* **9**(7), 480–490.
45. Kremer, J.M., Bloom, B.J., Breedveld, F.C., *et al.* (2009). The safety and efficacy of a JAK inhibitor in patients with active rheumatoid arthritis: Results of a double-blind, placebo-controlled phase IIa trial of three dosage levels of CP-690,550 versus placebo. *Arthritis Rheum,* **60**(7), 1895–1905.
46. Tanaka, Y., Suzuki, M., Nakamura, H., *et al.* (2011). Phase II study of tofacitinib (CP-690,550) combined with methotrexate in patients with rheumatoid arthritis and an inadequate response to methotrexate. *Arthritis Care Res,* **63**(8), 1150–1158.
47. Fleischmann, R., Kremer, J., Cush, J., *et al.* (2012). Placebo-controlled trial of tofacitinib monotherapy in rheumatoid arthritis. *N Eng J Med,* **367**(6), 495–507.
48. van Vollenhoven, R.F., Fleischmann, R., Cohen, S., *et al.* (2012). Tofacitinib or adalimumab versus placebo in rheumatoid arthritis. *N Eng J Med,* **367**(6), 508–519.

49. Burmester, G.R., Blanco, R., Charles-Schoeman, C., *et al*. (2013). Tofacitinib (CP-690,550) in combination with methotrexate in patients with active rheumatoid arthritis with an inadequate response to tumour necrosis factor inhibitors: A randomised phase 3 trial. *Lancet,* **381**(9865), 451–460.

50. Weinblatt, M.E., Kavanaugh, A., Burgos-Vargas, R., *et al*. (2008). Treatment of rheumatoid arthritis with a Syk kinase inhibitor: A twelve-week, randomized, placebo-controlled trial. *Arthritis Rheum,* **58**(11), 3309–3318.

51. Genovese, M.C., Kavanaugh, A., Weinblatt, M.E., *et al*. (2011). An oral Syk kinase inhibitor in the treatment of rheumatoid arthritis: A three-month randomized, placebo-controlled, phase II study in patients with active rheumatoid arthritis that did not respond to biologic agents. *Arthritis Rheum,* **63**(2), 337–345.

52. McCann, F.E., Palfreeman, A.C., Andrews, M., *et al*. (2010). Apremilast, a novel PDE4 inhibitor, inhibits spontaneous production of tumour necrosis factor-alpha from human rheumatoid synovial cells and ameliorates experimental arthritis. *Arthritis Res Ther*, **12**(3), R107.

53. van Vollenhoven, R.F., Ernestam, S., Geborek, P., *et al*. (2009). Addition of infliximab compared with addition of sulfasalazine and hydroxychloroquine to methotrexate in patients with early rheumatoid arthritis (Swefot trial): 1-year results of a randomised trial. *Lancet,* **374**(9688), 459–466.

54. van Vollenhoven, R.F., Geborek, P., Forslind, K., *et al*. (2012). Conventional combination treatment versus biological treatment in methotrexate-refractory early rheumatoid arthritis: 2 year follow-up of the randomised, non-blinded, parallel-group Swefot trial. *Lancet,* **379**(9827), 1712–1720.

55. Goekoop-Ruiterman, Y.P., de Vries-Bouwstra, J.K., Allaart, C.F., *et al*. (2005). Clinical and radiographic outcomes of four different treatment strategies in patients with early rheumatoid arthritis (the BeSt study): A randomized, controlled trial. *Arthritis Rheum,* **52**(11), 3381–3390.

56. Moreland, L.W., O'Dell, J.R., Paulus, H.E., *et al*. (2012). A randomized comparative effectiveness study of oral triple therapy versus etanercept plus methotrexate in early aggressive rheumatoid arthritis: The treatment of Early Aggressive Rheumatoid Arthritis Trial. *Arthritis Rheum,* **64**(9), 2824–2835.

57. O'Dell, J.R., Mikuls, T.R., Taylor, T.H., *et al*. (2013). Therapies for active rheumatoid arthritis after methotrexate failure. *N Eng J Med,* **369**(4), 307–318.

58. van Vollenhoven, R.F., Chatzidionysiou, K. (2013). Rheumatoid arthritis. Triple therapy or etanercept after methotrexate failure in RA? *Nat Rev Rheumatol,* **9**(9), 510–512.

59. Hetland, M.L., Christensen, I.J., Tarp, U., *et al.* (2010). Direct comparison of treatment responses, remission rates, and drug adherence in patients with rheumatoid arthritis treated with adalimumab, etanercept, or infliximab: Results from eight years of surveillance of clinical practice in the nationwide Danish DANBIO registry. *Arthritis Rheum,* **62**(1), 22–32.

60. Hyrich, K.L., Lunt, M., Watson, K.D., *et al.* (2007). Outcomes after switching from one anti-tumor necrosis factor alpha agent to a second anti-tumor necrosis factor alpha agent in patients with rheumatoid arthritis: Results from a large UK national cohort study. *Arthritis Rheum,* **56**(1), 13–20.

61. Smolen, J.S., Kay, J., Doyle, M.K., *et al.* (2009). Golimumab in patients with active rheumatoid arthritis after treatment with tumour necrosis factor alpha inhibitors (GO-AFTER study): A multicentre, randomised, double-blind, placebo-controlled, phase III trial. *Lancet,* **374**(9685), 210–221.

62. Weinblatt, M.E., Fleischmann, R., Huizinga, T.W., *et al.* (2012). Efficacy and safety of certolizumab pegol in a broad population of patients with active rheumatoid arthritis: Results from the REALISTIC phase IIIb study. *Rheumatology,* **51**(12), 2204–2214.

63. Haraoui, B., Keystone, E.C., Thorne, J.C., *et al.* (2004). Clinical outcomes of patients with rheumatoid arthritis after switching from infliximab to etanercept. *J Rheumatol,* **31**(12), 2356–2359.

64. Bingham, C.O., 3rd, Ince, A., Haraoui, B., *et al.* (2009). Effectiveness and safety of etanercept in subjects with RA who have failed infliximab therapy: 16-week, open-label, observational study. *Curr Med Res Opin,* **25**(5), 1131–1142.

65. Buch, M.H., Bingham, S.J., Bejarano, V., *et al.* (2007). Therapy of patients with rheumatoid arthritis: Outcome of infliximab failures switched to etanercept. *Arthritis Rheum,* **57**(3), 448–453.

66. Furst, D.E., Gaylis, N., Bray, V., *et al.* (2007). Open-label, pilot protocol of patients with rheumatoid arthritis who switch to infliximab after an incomplete response to etanercept: The opposite study. *Ann Rheum Dis,* **66**(7), 893–899.

67. Bombardieri, S., Ruiz, A.A., Fardellone, P., *et al.* (2007). Effectiveness of adalimumab for rheumatoid arthritis in patients with a history of TNF-antagonist therapy in clinical practice. *Rheumatol,* **46**(7), 1191–1199.

68. Karlsson, J.A., Kristensen, L.E., Kapetanovic, M.C., *et al.* (2008). Treatment response to a second or third TNF-inhibitor in RA: Results from the South Swedish Arthritis Treatment Group Register. *Rheumatol,*47(4), 507–513.

69. Gomez-Reino, J.J., Carmona, L., Group, B. (2006). Switching TNF antagonists in patients with chronic arthritis: An observational study of 488 patients over a four-year period. *Arthritis Res Ther,* **8**(1), R29.

70. Chatzidionysiou, K., Askling, J., Eriksson, J., *et al.* (2014). Effectiveness of TNF inhibitor switch in RA: Results from the national Swedish register. *Ann Rheum Dis.*

71. Cohen, S.B., Emery, P., Greenwald, M.W., *et al.* (2006). Rituximab for rheumatoid arthritis refractory to anti-tumor necrosis factor therapy: Results of a multicenter, randomized, double-blind, placebo-controlled, phase III trial evaluating primary efficacy and safety at twenty-four weeks. *Arthritis Rheum,* **54**(9), 2793–2806.

72. Genovese, M.C., Schiff, M., Luggen, M., *et al.* (2008). Efficacy and safety of the selective co-stimulation modulator abatacept following 2 years of treatment in patients with rheumatoid arthritis and an inadequate response to anti-tumour necrosis factor therapy. *Ann Rheum Dis,* **67**(4), 547–554.

73. Finckh, A., Ciurea, A., Brulhart, L., *et al.* (2007). B cell depletion may be more effective than switching to an alternative anti-tumor necrosis factor agent in rheumatoid arthritis patients with inadequate response to anti-tumor necrosis factor agents. *Arthritis Rheum,* **56**(5), 1417–1423.

74. Finckh, A., Ciurea, A., Brulhart, L., *et al.* (2010). Which subgroup of patients with rheumatoid arthritis benefits from switching to rituximab versus alternative anti-tumour necrosis factor (TNF) agents after previous failure of an anti-TNF agent? *Ann Rheum Dis,* **69**(2), 387–393.

75. Soliman, M.M., Hyrich, K.L., Lunt, M., *et al.* (2012). Rituximab or a second anti-tumor necrosis factor therapy for rheumatoid arthritis patients who have failed their first anti-tumor necrosis factor therapy? Comparative analysis from the British Society for Rheumatology Biologics Register. *Arthritis Care Res,* **64**(8), 1108–1115.

76. Gomez-Reino, J.J., Maneiro, J.R., Ruiz, J., *et al.* (2012). Comparative effectiveness of switching to alternative tumour necrosis factor (TNF) antagonists versus switching to rituximab in patients with rheumatoid arthritis who failed previous TNF antagonists: The MIRAR Study. *Ann Rheum Dis,* **71**(11), 1861–1864.

77. Chatzidionysiou, K., van Vollenhoven, R.F. (2013). Rituximab versus anti-TNF in patients who previously failed one TNF inhibitor in an observational cohort. *Scand J Rheumatol,* **42**(3), 190–195.

78. Lipsky, P.E., van der Heijde, D.M., St Clair, E.W., *et al.* (2000). Infliximab and methotrexate in the treatment of rheumatoid arthritis. Anti-Tumor Necrosis Factor Trial in Rheumatoid Arthritis with Concomitant Therapy Study Group. *N Eng J Med,* **343**(22), 1594–1602.

79. Tanaka, Y., Takeuchi, T., Mimori, T., *et al.* (2010). Discontinuation of infliximab after attaining low disease activity in patients with rheumatoid arthritis:

RRR (remission induction by Remicade in RA) study. *Ann Rheum Dis,* **69**(7), 1286–1291.

80. van der Kooij, S.M., le Cessie, S., Goekoop-Ruiterman, Y.P., *et al.* (2009). Clinical and radiological efficacy of initial vs delayed treatment with infliximab plus methotrexate in patients with early rheumatoid arthritis. *Ann Rheum Dis,* **68**(7), 1153–1158.

81. van der Kooij, S.M., Goekoop-Ruiterman, Y.P., de Vries-Bouwstra, J.K., *et al.* (2009). Drug-free remission, functioning and radiographic damage after 4 years of response-driven treatment in patients with recent-onset rheumatoid arthritis. *Ann Rheum Dis,* **68**(6), 914–921.

82. Smolen, J.S., Emery, P., Fleischmann, R., *et al.* (2014). Adjustment of therapy in rheumatoid arthritis on the basis of achievement of stable low disease activity with adalimumab plus methotrexate or methotrexate alone: The randomised controlled OPTIMA trial. *Lancet,* **383**(9914), 321–332.

83. Tanaka, Y., Hirata, S., Kubo, S., *et al.* (2013). Discontinuation of adalimumab after achieving remission in patients with established rheumatoid arthritis: 1-year outcome of the HONOR study. *Ann Rheum Dis.*

84. O'Mahony, R., Richards, A., Deighton, C., *et al.* (2010). Withdrawal of disease-modifying antirheumatic drugs in patients with rheumatoid arthritis: A systematic review and meta-analysis. *Ann Rheum Dis,* **69**(10), 1823–1826.

85. Genovese, M.C., *et al.* (2015). Apremilast in patients with active rheumatoid arthritis: a phase II, multicenter, randomized, double-blind, placebo-controlled, parallel group study. *Arthritis Rheumatol,* doi: 10.1002/art. 39120. [Epub ahead of print].

86. Burmester, G.R., *et al.* (2013). Efficacy and safety of mavrilimumab in subjects with rheumatoid arthritis. *Ann Rheum Dis,* **72**(9), 1445–1452.

CHAPTER 6

ADVANCES IN THERAPIES FOR SPONDYLOARTHROPATHIES

Irene E. van der Horst-Bruinsma

Introduction

Spondyloarthritis (SpA) is a group of rheumatic diseases dominated by spinal symptoms, classified as axial SpA[1] or by peripheral arthritis, classified as peripheral SpA.[2] Axial SpA is subdivided in two types, ankylosing spondylitis (AS), which requires radiographic changes of the sacroiliac joints (according to the Modified New York Criteria[3]), and non-radiographic axial SpA, which is mainly based on a combination of clinical symptoms, the presence of the HLA-B27 antigen and signs of sacroiliitis by MRI. Non-radiographic axial SpA can progress towards AS within a couple of years. The clinical symptoms of axial SpA include inflammatory back pain during at least three months with an age at onset before 45 years and at least one of the other "SpA-features": arthritis, enthesitis (heel), uveitis, dactylitis, psoriasis, Crohn's disease/ulcerative colitis, good response to NSAIDs, family history of SpA and elevated CRP.[1,2] Peripheral SpA requires peripheral arthritis compatible with SpA (usually asymmetric and/ or predominant involvement of the lower limbs), enthesitis or dactylitis and at least one of the other SpA features, as mentioned before.[2]

Next to these articular symptoms, many patients with SpA also suffer from extra-articular manifestations (EAMs), such as anterior uveitis (25–30%), psoriasis (10–25%) or inflammatory bowel disease (IBD, 5–10%).[4]

Treatment of Spondyloarthritis

The majority of axial SpA patients respond very well to a combination of Non-Steroidal Anti-inflammatory drugs (NSAIDs) and exercise. Disease Modifying Anti-Rheumatic Drugs (DMARDs) have limited efficacy in this group of diseases and are mainly effective in case of peripheral SpA. Biologicals, however, especially the TNF blocking agents, have brought a dramatic improvement in patients who do not sufficiently respond to NSAIDs and exercise.[5]

Exercise and physical therapy are very important in SpA, in order to prevent restriction of spinal mobility and the development of disability, and to improve the symptoms of pain and stiffness. Effectiveness of these treatments is described in several studies[6–8] and patients should be referred to a physical therapist, who will teach the patient the exercises that should be performed regularly.

In one study, AS patients who were stable during anti-TNF (N=69) treatment had a significant increase in the Bath Ankylosing Spondylitis Metrology index (BASMI), range of motion and thoracic spine excursions after 12 sessions of physical therapy compared with controls.[6]

Moreover, physical exercise improves muscle strength and decreases the risk of cardiovascular disease.

Non-Steroidal Anti-Inflammatory Drugs (NSAIDs)

NSAIDs are regarded as the cornerstone of treatment in SpA and reduce pain and stiffness rapidly in 60% of the patients.[5,9] The most optimal combination is a slow release tablet taken in the evening (*e.g.*, diclofenac 100 mg), in combination with a fast-acting drug in the morning (*e.g.*, diclofenac 50 mg), which is effective in reducing pain at night and morning stiffness.

Several placebo-controlled trials with different NSAIDs, including cyclo-oxygenase-2 (Cox-2)-selective inhibitors, convincingly showed good efficacy compared with placebo treatment. The advantage of selective Cox-2 inhibitors (celecoxib, etoricoxib) is the lower risk of gastrointestinal side effects. Furthermore, a good response to NSAID treatment can be discriminative between chronic non-inflammatory back pain and inflammatory back pain due to SpA.

A few studies suggest that NSAIDs might delay radiological progression of the spine when given continuously over two years compared with an on-demand treatment schedule. Especially cases of SpA with a high risk of radiographic progression (*e.g.*, with raised CRP-levels and/or the presence of syndesmophytes) have been shown to benefit from continuous treatment with NSAIDs.[10–13]

Gastrointestinal side effects can be prevented by concomitant use of proton pump inhibitors (such as omeprazole) and the intake of NSAIDs during meals. Selective Cox-2 inhibitors can even further reduce the risk of gastrointestinal side effects compared with conventional NSAIDs.[14,15] Cardiovascular side effects occur in a minority of patients, especially in older patients with NYHA class III–IV heart failure.[16]

Similar efficacy can be expected in the treatment of non-radiographic axial SpA, although there are no studies in this area.

Disease Modifying AntiRheumatic Drugs (DMARDs)

The efficacy of most DMARDs in SpA is rather disappointing, especially in comparison to rheumatoid arthritis.[17] Sulfasalazine is effective in peripheral SpA and shows some efficacy on spinal symptoms as well but not on enthesitis.

Sulfasalazine (SSZ) has shown limited efficacy in SpA.[18–19] A pooled analysis showed that the difference between intervention groups was significant only in the case of a raised erythrocyte sedimentation rate and morning stiffness, favouring sulfasalazine over placebo, but not for any other variables. Only one trial investigating patients with a relatively short disease duration (<6 years) showed a benefit in primary outcome parameters, including back pain, spinal mobility and patient's well-being. However, several trials showed a higher efficacy of sulfasalazine compared with placebo in the presence of peripheral arthritis. Normally treatment at a dose of 2 × 1000 mg/day, which can be increased to 3 × 1000 mg/day, for a duration of up to four months is necessary before a treatment failure can be stated.

In a double-blind head to head comparison between sulfsasalazine and etanercept, sulfasalazine was very effective in reducing peripheral arthritis, but also decreased axial symptoms, as illustrated by a decrease of the ASAS 20 (Fig. 1).[19]

However, taking all results together SSZ is not recommended for the treatment of axial manifestations of AS but can be used in cases of peripheral arthritis in patients with AS.

Methotrexate, in contrast with the good results in rheumatoid arthritis, is not effective in axial SpA.[20–22] A 6-week open-label trial of methotrexate 20 mg subcutaneously once a week in AS patients did not show any effect on axial symptoms and only some improvement in peripheral symptoms. Therefore, methotrexate is not recommended for the axial manifestations of AS, though in some patients with predominantly peripheral arthritis a treatment trial might be justified.

Leflunomide was tested in AS in an open label study which showed efficacy only for the peripheral arthritis but not for the axial symptoms.[24]

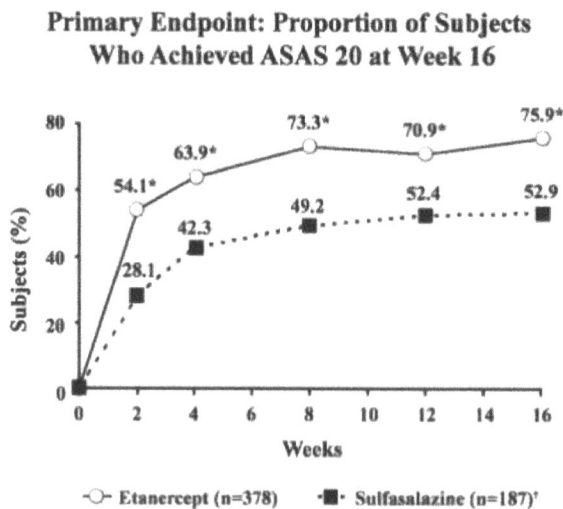

Primary Endpoint: Proportion of Subjects Who Achieved ASAS 20 at Week 16

Figure 1. Clinical efficacy and safety of etanercept versus sulfasalazine in patients with ankylosing spondylitis: a randomized, double-blind trial.[19]

This observation was confirmed by a randomized placebo controlled trial that did not show beneficial effects of leflunomide for the axial component of AS.[23]

Thalidomide has also been tested for the treatment of patients with AS in open uncontrolled trials with some beneficial effects, but is regarded as too toxic for widespread use.[25]

Other DMARDs such as cyclosporine, azathioprine, cyclophosphamide and mesalazine have not shown efficacy in axial SpA.[26]

Corticosteroids do not play a major part in the treatment of AS, in contrast to other inflammatory rheumatic diseases. Peripheral arthritis often improves if patients are treated with a moderate dose of prednisolone (20–30 mg/day) but axial manifestations improve only slightly, even if a relatively high dose of ≥50 mg/day of prednisolone is given. A few small studies describe good short-term efficacy of intravenous pulse methylprednisolone (1000 mg/day for three days) in patients with treatment refractory AS, but there is no evidence of a long-term effect of such treatment. Local corticosteroid injections are recommended for peripheral joint manifestations and are sometimes used for the treatment of enthesitis.

Contradictory results are described regarding the efficacy of intra-articular injections with corticosteroids into the sacroiliac joints. In a study with an injection of 40 mg of triamcinolone, the response rate was higher if the intra-articular position of the needle was guided by ultrasound, MRI or with X-rays.[27,28]

Bisphosphonates have been tested in AS in a 6-month randomized controlled trial; 60 mg of pamidronate given intravenously once a month was better than a small placebo-like dose of 10 mg pamidronate, with a significant improvement of function and pain. Such an effect only became evident after three months of treatment. A positive effect was not found in other open trials treating patients with AS with the same dosage over three months. Therefore, further studies are needed before this treatment can be recommended.[29,30]

Biologicals

TNF blocking agents give substantial improvement of SpA. Large placebo controlled trials have demonstrated the efficacy of infliximab, etanercept, adalimumab, golimumab and certolizumab pegol in 60–70% of SpA patients.[31–39] Anti-TNF therapy is indicated in case of persistently high disease activity (BASDAI $\geq$ 4) and insufficient response to NSAIDs or sulfasalazine in case of peripheral arthritis.[31] Patients with non-radiographic axial SpA also seem to benefit from treatment with TNF-blockers. Next to the improvement of axial symptoms in SpA patients, TNF blockers are very effective in the treatment of peripheral arthritis and enthesitis. Infliximab is given as an intravenous infusion at a dose of 5 mg/kg every 6–8 weeks, etanercept is given subcutaneously at a dose of 50 mg once a week, adalimumab at a dose of 40 mg subcutaneously every other week, golimumab at a monthly dose of 50 mg subcutaneously and certolizumab 200 mg every two weeks.

In nearly all AS studies *infliximab* was given intravenously at a dosage of 5 mg/kg body weight at weeks 0, 2, 6 and thereafter every 6–8 weeks.[32] In several open-label studies, an often dramatic improvement in signs and symptoms was seen beginning on the same day or in the days after the first infusion, which could subsequently be confirmed in placebo-controlled randomized controlled trials. In all these studies infliximab was given as monotherapy, without methotrexate. Normally, continuation of NSAID treatment was permitted. The crucial endpoint in all these studies was a 50% improvement in disease activity (BASDAI) or in a composite clinical score (ASAS percentage improvement). This endpoint was reached uniformly by about 50% of patients in the placebo-controlled trials with about $\leq$10% of the placebo group reaching this level of response, and in up to 60–70% in the open-label studies.

Long-term follow-up results from these studies have been published for up to eight years, showing good long-term efficacy if treatment is continued. In case of secondary non-response, patients can be tested for antibodies against infliximab which lower the serum trough levels and reduce efficacy of the drug.[33]

However, when infliximab was stopped after three years of treatment, almost all patients (97.6%) relapsed within one year. When treatment with infliximab was restarted, all but one patients improved similarly to the initial response and the drug was well-tolerated.

Several double-blind placebo-controlled trials with *etanercept* in AS demonstrated a very similar efficacy profile to that shown with infliximab and reduction of acute inflammation as shown by MRI.[34,35] In the first few studies, etanercept was given in a dose of 25 mg subcutaneously (SC) twice a week, but more recent studies showed that 50 mg SC given once a week has similar efficacy. Similarly to infliximab, a relapse occurred when treatment with etanercept was stopped and a comparable clinical response was seen when the drug was restarted. The long-term efficacy is good as well as the safety profile.[35]

Adalimumab is another TNF-blocking agent that has been shown to be effective for the treatment of AS in large randomized placebo-controlled studies.[36] In one study, which also included patients with total spinal ankylosis, a 50% response rate was observed. This underscores the fact that inflammation is still present in ankylosed patients and that they also benefit from treatment with TNF blocking agents. Long-term safety and efficacy are also shown in the majority of these patients. Secondary loss of response can also occur with adalimumab due to the development of antibodies against this drug.[37]

Golimumab has shown similar efficacy to the other three TNF blockers and is given in a dose of 50 mg SC once a month.[38] *Certolizumab* is administered subcutaneously at 200 mg every two weeks after a loading dose. This TNF blocker is also effective and safe in axial SpA.[39]

Other Biologicals (not Registered for Axial SpA)

Anakinra (an interleukin-1 receptor antagonist), *rituximab* and *abatacept* were only tested in small open label studies in AS. No relevant clinical responses were observed, especially in light of the fact that these trials were uncontrolled.[40–42,44,45] Treatment targeting the interleukin-6 pathway with *tocilizumab* was tested in formal randomized placebo-controlled studies, but failed to show a significant improvement over placebo.[43] In a large study with *sarilumab* (an IL6 receptor antagonist) in 250 patients also failed to show efficacy.[47] A small study with *apremilast* (a phosphodiesterase inhibitor) in 38 patients did not show a response.[49]

However, more recent studies targeting the interleukin-17 and 12/23 pathways showed more promising results. In a phase II trial with *secukinumab* (anti-IL17A) an ASAS20 response was seen in 13 out of 23 patients,[46] whereas *ustekinumab* (anti-IL12/23) showed an ASAS40 response in 13 out of 20 patients in an open label study.[48]

TNF Blockers in Patients with Non-Radiographic Axial SpA

In the case of insufficient response to NSAIDs, in combination with physical therapy and exercise, TNF blocking agents can be beneficial for a subgroup of severe cases of non radiographic axial SpA (Table 1).[50–53]

Recently several investigator-initiated placebo-controlled double-blind studies were performed in this group. In the first trial 46 patients with non-radiographic axial SpA were treated either with placebo or with 40 mg adalimumab given every second week over 12 weeks, followed by open-label treatment with adalimumab for altogether 48 weeks in all patients. The ASAS 40 response was significantly higher in the adalimumab group (36%) than in the placebo group (15%) at week 12. This response rate was similar at week 48 for the whole group.[51]

In another trial, patients with axial SpA with a symptom duration of ≤3 years had to be HLA-B27 positive and had to have a positive MRI showing active inflammation in the sacroiliac joint. In this trial, the ASAS 40 was reached after 16 weeks of infliximab treatment in 61% of the patients, compared with a placebo response of 19%.[50] Etanercept also appears to be as effective in nr-axSpA with bone marrow edema on MRI as in AS.[52] Recently, a phase III trial was published with certoluzimab in non-radiographic axial SpA which showed good efficacy after 24 weeks.[53]

Taken together, these data indicate that patients with nr-axSpA who do not respond to NSAIDs and physical therapy, and additionally have an increased CRP and/or inflammatory signs of the SI joints on MRI, respond well to TNF-blockers. However, the long-term effects of this early intervention have to be studied because the data so far are limited.

Table 1. Studies with TNF blockers in non-radiographic Axial Spondyloarthritis.

	Number of patients (N)	Duration (weeks)	ASAS 40% response (%)	Placebo response (%)
infliximab	20*	16	61	19
etanercept	40* (AS included)	48	70	31 on sulfasalazine
adalimumab	91	12	36	15
certolizumab	97*	12	47	17

* only patients with raised CRP and/or inflammation in the sacroiliac joints by MRI

Table 2. Efficacy of biologicals in Axial Spondyloarthritis.

	Target	AS	Non-radiographic
infliximab	TNF	+	+
etanercept		+	+
adalimumab		+	+
certolizumab		+	+
golimumab		+	?
anakinra	IL1 receptor	−	?
rituximab	B-cells	−	?
abatacept	T-cells	−	?
tocilizumab	IL6 receptor	−	?
sarilumab	IL6 receptor	−	?
apremilast	phosphodiesterase	−	?
secukinumab	IL17	+	?
ustekinumab	IL12/23	+	?

Legends table 2: + effective, — not effective, ? no data

TNF Blockers in Relation to Extra-articular Manifestations of SpA

Many patients with SpA suffer from extra-articular manifestations (EAMs), such as anterior uveitis, psoriasis or inflammatory bowel disease (Crohn's disease or ulcerative colitis), and this might be important in the choice of TNF blockers.[4]

Acute anterior uveitis is an acute attack with inflammation of the uvea and can be the first presenting symptom of the disease. In AS, the chance to develop uveitis is 25–30%.[54,55]

The attacks of uveitis are usually recurrent and unilateral and present with sudden ocular pain with redness and photophobia. Inflammation can lead to pupillary and lens dysfunction with blurring of vision. In some cases, glaucoma and severe visual impairment occur if adequate treatment is delayed. In case of suspicion of uveitis, it is recommended to refer the patient to the ophthalmologist as soon as possible. Most cases of acute uveitis can be treated successfully by the ophthalmologist with local corticosteroids and mydriatics. Sometimes, a high dosage of prednisone (up to 60 mg daily) or an intraocular injection with corticosteroids is necessary to suppress the inflammation. There is some evidence that the use of sulfasalazine reduces the recurrence rate of uveitis.[56] Other immunosuppressive drugs used by ophthalmologists to treat refractory uveitis, such as azathioprine and methotrexate, do not have much efficacy on the disease activity of SpA.

Overall, TNF-blocking agents can be useful for high disease activity in SpA as well as for refractory uveitis. Infliximab decreases the recurrence rate of uveitis and is effective in refractory uveitis.[57,58] In contrast to the usual treatment with infusions, intraocular injections with infliximab are toxic, inducing intraocular inflammation, and should be avoided.[59,60] There is much debate about the efficacy of etanercept for uveitis. Etanercept does not seem to prevent a relapse of uveitis and it was suggested that etanercept might even trigger attacks of uveitis.[61] However, a comparison of three randomised studies with etanercept in AS showed a lower number of cases with uveitis in the etanercept-treated patients compared with placebo indicating that etanercept does inhibit the recurrence of uveitis.[62] Reports on the efficacy of adalimumab for uveitis showed beneficial results in a retrospective analysis of placebo controlled trials: during treatment with adalimumab, the rate of acute uveitis flares was reduced by 51%.[63] In a prospective study, AS patients were treated with adalimumab because of their high disease activity and screened by an ophthalmologist for uveitis as well.[64] This study demonstrated a significant decrease (73%) of the recurrence rate of uveitis during adalimumab treatment.

Recent reports show that golimumab and certolizumab are also effective in refractory uveitis.[65]

It can be concluded that in most cases, attacks of anterior uveitis respond very well to (local) treatment by the ophthalmologist. In cases with refractory uveitis or a high uveitis recurrence rate, treatment with TNF blocking agents can be successful, especially if the treatment is indicated for high disease activity of SpA.

Psoriasis occurs in approximately 5–10% of the SpA patients, excluding those with psoriatic arthritis.[66] Skin manifestations of psoriasis respond to local corticosteroids or PUVA therapy. In case of psoriatic arthritis, NSAIDs, intra-articular injections with corticosteroids, and several DMARDs are effective, such as methotrexate and leflunomide.

Table 3. Efficacy of TNF blockers for extra-spinal manifestations of AS.

	Peripheral arthritis/ enthesitis	Uveitis	Ulcerative Colitis	Crohn's Disease	Psoriasis
infliximab	+	+	+	+	+
adalimumab	+	+	+	+	+
etanercept	+	+/−	−	−	+
golimumab	+	+	+	?	+
certolizumab	+	+	?	+	+

Legends: + effective, — not effective,? no data

TNF blockers, such as infliximab, etanercept, adalimumab, golimumab and certolizumab are efficacious for the skin and nail lesions of psoriasis in SpA.[66,67]

Inflammatory Bowel Disease (*IBD*) includes Crohn's disease and ulcerative colitis. Approximately 10% of the IBD patients develop SpA whereas the chance of SpA patients to develop IBD is 5–10%.[68–70] Treatment of IBD by the gastro-enterologist is based on immunosuppressive drugs and anti-TNF. NSAIDs can worsen colitis and their use is discouraged in SpA patients with IBD, except for celecoxib which does not seem to increase the risk of exacerbation of the IBD.[71] The use of sulfasalazine can be beneficial for both SpA as well as IBD. In contrast, other immunosuppressive drugs often used in IBD have in most cases not proven efficacious in SpA. The TNF blockers infliximab and adalimumab are effective in both SpA and IBD, whereas golimumab is effective in ulcerative colitis but has not yet been tested for Crohn's disease, and certolizumab has shown efficacy in Crohn's disease but has not been tested for ulcerative colitis.[72–77] Etanercept works well for spinal symptoms in SpA but not for IBD and new manifestations of IBD might even occur during etanercept treatment.[76] New onset manifestations of IBD are described for infliximab 0.2, etanercept 2.2 and adalimumab 2.3 per 100 patient years.[72]

Conclusions

NSAIDs and exercise remain the cornerstones of treatment in axial and peripheral SpA. DMARDs have limited efficacy, mainly in the case of peripheral arthritis, but probably some beneficial effects for spinal complaints can be attributed to sulfasalazine as well.

In the case of insufficient response to NSAIDs, TNF blockers are very effective in SpA, especially infliximab, etanercept, adalimumab, golimumab and certolizumab pegol. These drugs all work very well for the axial manifestations as well as for arthritis and enthesitis. Non-radiographic axial SpA with severe complaints and signs of inflammation also responds to TNF blockers, but long-term data are not yet available. Some new biologicals, such as secukinumab and ustekinumab show promising results in axial SpA.

Concerning the treatment of extra-spinal manifestations, anterior uveitis and psoriasis can be treated locally and also respond to all TNF blockers. In the case of IBD in SpA, the choice of anti-TNF therapy in SpA with IBD is in favor of infliximab and adalimumab rather than etanercept. Golimumab can be considered in cases of ulcerative colitis and certoluzimab in cases of Crohn's disease. Overall, it is important to realize that in SpA, extra-articular manifestations do occur frequently and should be taken into account in the choice of treatment.

Thus, TNF blockers are effective in case of insufficient response to conventional agents, and new biologicals show promising results in axial SpA.

References

1. Rudwaleit, M., *et al.* (2009). The development of Assessment of SpondyloArthritis international Society classification criteria for axial spondyloarthritis (part II): validation and final selection. *Ann Rheum Dis*, **68**, 777–783.
2. Rudwaleit, M., *et al.* (2011). The Assessment of SpondyloArthritis International Society classification criteria for peripheral spondyloarthritis and for spondyloarthritis in general. *Ann Rheum Dis*, **70**, 25–31.
3. Van der Linden, S., Valkenburg, H.A., Cats, A. (1984). Evaluation of the diagnostic criteria for ankylosing spondylitis; a proposal for the modification of the New York criteria. *Arthritis Rheum*, **27**, 361–368.
4. van der Horst-Bruinsma, I.E., Nurmohamed, M.T. (2012). Management and evaluation of extra-articular manifestations in spondyloarthritis. *Ther Adv Musculoskelet Dis*, **4**(6), 413–422.

5. Braun, J., vd Berg, R., Baraliakos, X., *et al.* (2011). 2010 update of the ASAS/EULAR recommendations for the management of ankylosing spondylitis. *Ann Rheum Dis*, **70**, 896–904.

6. Giannotti, E., Trainito, S., Arioli, G., Rucco, V., Masiero, S. (2014). Effects of physical therapy for the management of patients with ankylosing spondylitis in the biological era. *Clin Rheumatol*, **33**(9), 1217–1230.

7. Dagfinrud, H., Hagen, K.B., Kvien, T.K. (2008). Physiotherapy interventions for ankylosing spondylitis. *Cochrane Database Syst Rev*, (1):CD002822.

8. van den Berg, R., Baraliakos, X., Braun, J., van der Heijde, D. (2012). First update of the current evidence for the management of ankylosing spondylitis with non-pharmacological treatment and non-biologic drugs: a systematic literature review for the ASAS/EULAR management recommendations in ankylosing spondylitis. *Rheumatology*, **51**(8), 1388–1396.

9. Zochling, J., van der Heijde, D., Burgos-Vargas, R. *et al.* (2006). ASAS/EULAR recommendations for the management of ankylosing spondylitis. *Ann Rheumatic Dis*, **65**: 442–452.

10. Boersma, J.W. (1976). Retardation of ossification of the lumbar vertebral column in ankylosing spondylitis by means of phenylbutazone. *Scand J Rheumatol*, **5**, 60–64.

11. Wanders, A., Heijde, D., Landewe, R. *et al.* (2005). Nonsteroidal antiinflammatory drugs reduce radiographic progression in patients with ankylosing spondylitis: a randomized clinical trial. *Arthritis Rheum*, **52**: 1756–1765.

12. Kroon, F., Landewé, R., Dougados, M., van der Heijde, D. (2012). Continuous NSAID use reverts the effects of inflammation on radiographic progression in patients with ankylosing spondylitis, *Ann Rheum Dis*, **71**(10):1623–1629.

13. Poddubnyy, D., Rudwaleit, M., Haibel, H., Listing, J., Märker-Hermann, E., Zeidler, H., Braun, J., Sieper, J. (2012). Effect of non-steroidal anti-inflammatory drugs on radiographic spinal progression in patients with axial spondyloarthritis: results from the German Spondyloarthritis Inception Cohort. *Ann Rheum Dis*, **71**(10):1616–1622.

14. Sandborn, W.J., Stenson, W.F., Brynskov, J., Lorenz, R.G., Steidle, G.M., Robbins, J.L., Kent, J.D., Bloom, B.J. (2006). Safety of celecoxib in patients with ulcerative colitis in remission: a randomized, placebo-controlled, pilot study. *Clin Gastroenterol Hepatol*, **4**, 203–211.

15. Miedany, Y., Youssef, S., Ahmed, I., El Gaafary, M. (2006). The gastrointestinal safety and effect on disease activity of etoricoxib, a selective cox-2 inhibitor in inflammatory bowel diseases. *Am J Gastroenterol*, **101**, 311–317.

16. Nurmohamed, M.T., van der Horst-Bruinsma, I., Maksymowych, W.P. (2012). Cardiovascular and Cerebrovascular Diseases in Ankylosing Spondylitis: Current Insights. *Curr Rheumatol Rep*, **14**(5):415–421.

17. Horst-Bruinsma, I.E., van der Clegg, D.O., Dijkmans, B.A.C. (2002). Treatment of ankylosing spondylitis with disease modifying antirheumatic drugs. *Clin Exp Rheumatology*, **20**, S67–S70.

18. Amor, B., Kahan, A., Dougados, M., *et al.* (1984). Sulfasalazine and ankylosing spondylitis. *Ann Intern Med*, **101**, 878.

19. Braun, J., van der Horst-Bruinsma, I.E., Huang, F., Burgos-Vargas, R., Vlahos, B., Koenig, A.S., Freundlich, B. (2011). Clinical efficacy and safety of etanercept versus sulfasalazine in patients with ankylosing spondylitis: a randomized, double-blind trial. *Arthritis Rheum,* **63**(6), 1543–1551

20. Biasi, D., Carletto, A., Caramaschi, P., *et al.* (2000). Efficacy of methotrexate in the treatment of ankylosing spondylitis: a three-year open study. *Clin Rheumatol,* **19**, 114–117.

21. Gonzalez-Lopez, L., Garcia-Gonzalez, A., *et al.* (2004). Efficacy of methotrexate in ankylosing spondylitis: a randomized placebo-controled, double-blinded trial. *J Rheumatol,* **31**(8), 1568–1574

22. Chen, J., Veras, M.M., Liu, C., Lin, J. (2013). Methotrexate for ankylosing spondylitis. *Cochrane Database Syst Rev*, **2**, CD004524.

23. van Denderen, J.C., Van der Paardt, M., Nurmohamed, M.T., De Ryck, Y.M., Dijkmans, B.A., Van der Horst-Bruinsma, I.E. (2005). Double-blind, randomised, placebo-controlled study of leflunomide in the treatment of active ankylosing spondylitis. *Ann Rheum Dis*, **64**(12), 1761–1764.

24. Haibel, H., Rudwaleit, M., Braun, J., Sieper, J. (2005). Six months open label trial of leflunomide in active ankylosing spondylitis. *Ann Rheum Dis,* **64**(1), 124–126.

25. Lee, L., Lawford, R., McNeil, H.P. (2001). The efficacy of thalidomide in severe refractory spondylarthropathy: comment on the letter by Breban *et al.* [letter]. *Arthritis Rheum*, **44**: 2456–2457.

26. van Denderen, J.C., van der Horst-Bruinsma, I.E., Bezemer, P.D., Dijkmans, B.A.C. (2003). Efficacy and safety of mesalazine (Salofalk) in patients with ankylosing spondylitis: an open study in 20 patients. *J Rheumatol*, **30**(7), 1558–1560.

27. Hanly, J.G., *et al.* (2000). Efficacy of sacroiliac corticosteroid injections in patients with inflammatory spondylarthropathy: results of a 6 month controlled study. *J Rheumatol*, **27**, 719–722.

28. Fritz, *et al.* (2005). MRI –guided corticosteroid infliltration of the sacroiliac joints:Pain therapy of sacroiliitis in patients with ankylosing spondylitis. *RoFo*, **177**, 555–563.

29. Maksymowych, W.P., Jhangri, G.S., Fitzgerald, A.A., LeClercq, S., Chiu, P., Yan, A., Skeith, K.J., Aaron, S.L., Homik, J., Davis, P., Sholter, D., Russell, A.S. (2002). A six-month randomized, controlled, double-blind, dose response comparison of intravenous pamidronate (60 mg versus 10mg) in the treatment of nonsteroidal antiinflammatory drug-refractory ankylosing spondylitis: *Arthritis Rheum,* **46**(3), 766–773.

30. Grover, R., Shankar, S., Aneja, R., Marwaha, V., Gupta, R., Kumar, A. (2006). Treatment of ankylosing spondylitis with pamidronate: an open label study, *Ann Rheum Dis,* **65**, 688–689.

31. van der Heijde, D., Sieper, J., Maksymowych, W.P., *et al.* (2011). Assessment of SpondyloArthritis international Society. 2010 Update of the international ASAS recommendations for the use of anti-TNF agents in patients with axial spondyloarthritis. *Ann Rheum Dis,* **70**(6), 905–908.

32. van der Heijde, D., Dijkmans, B., Geusens, P., *et al.* (2005). Ankylosing Spondylitis Study for the Evaluation of Recombinant Infliximab Therapy Study Group. Efficacy and safety of infliximab in patients with ankylosing spondylitis: results of a randomized, placebo-controlled trial (ASSERT). *Arthritis Rheum,* **52**, 582–591.

33. de Vries, M.K., Wolbink, G.J., Stapel, S., de Vrieze, H., Van Denderen, J.C., Dijkmans, B.A., Aarden, L., van der Horst-Bruinsma, I.E. (2007). Decreased clinical response to infliximab in Ankylosing Spondylitis (AS) is correlated with anti-infliximab formation. *Ann Rheum Dis,* **66**(9), 1252–1254.

34. van der Heijde, D., Da Silva, J.C., Dougados, M., Pal, G., van der Horst-Bruinsma, I.E., Juanola, X., Olivieri, I., Raeman, F., Settas, L.D., Sieper, J., Szechinski, J., Walker, D., Boussuge, M.P., Wajdula, J.S., Paolozzi, L., Fatenejad, S. (2006). Once-weekly 50-mg dosing of Etanercept (Enbrel(R)) is as effective as 25-mg twice-weekly dosing in patients with ankylosing spondylitis. *Ann Rheum Dis,* **65**(12), 1572–1577.

35. Martín-Mola, E., Sieper, J., Leirisalo-Repo, M., Dijkmans, B.A., Vlahos, B., Pedersen, R., Koenig, A.S., Freundlich, B. (2010). Sustained efficacy and safety, including patient-reported outcomes, with etanercept treatment over 5 years in patients with ankylosing spondylitis. *Clin Exp Rheumatol,* **28**(2), 238–245.

36. Van der Heijde, D., Kivitz, A., Schiff, M.H., Sieper, J., Dijkmans, B.A.C., Braun, J., *et al.* (2006). Efficacy and safety of adalimumab in patients with ankylosing spondylitis. Results of a multicenter, randomized, double-blind, placebo-controlled trial. *Arthritis Rheum,* **54**, 2136–2146.

37. de Vries, M.K., Brouwer, E., van der Horst-Bruinsma, I.E., *et al.* (2009). Decreased clinical response to adalimumab in ankylosing spondylitis is associated with antibody formation. *Ann Rheum Dis,* **68**(11), 1787–1788.

38. Inman, R.D., Davis, J.C Jr, Heijde, D., Diekman, L., Sieper, J., Kim, S.I., Mack, M., Han, J., Visvanathan, S., Xu, Z., Hsu, B., Beutler, A., Braun, J. (2008). Efficacy and safety of golimumab in patients with ankylosing spondylitis: results of a randomized, double-blind, placebo-controlled, phase III trial. *Arthritis Rheum*, **58**, 3402–3412.

39. Landewé, R., Braun, J., Deodhar, A., Dougados, M., Maksymowych, W.P., Mease, P.J., Reveille, J.D., Rudwaleit, M., van der Heijde, D., Stach, C., Hoepken, B., Fichtner, A., Coteur, G., de Longueville, M., Sieper, J. (2014). Efficacy of certolizumab pegol on signs and symptoms of axial spondyloarthritis including ankylosing spondylitis: 24-week results of a double-blind randomised placebo-controlled Phase 3 study. *Ann Rheum Dis*, **73**(1), 39–47.

40. Haibel, H., Rudwaleit, M., Listing, J., Sieper, J. (2005). Open label trial of anakinra in active ankylosing spondylitis over 24 weeks. *Ann Rheum Dis*, **64**(2), 296–298.

41. Tan, A.L., Marzo-Ortega, H., O'Connor, P., *et al.* (2004). Efficacy of anakinra in active ankylosing spondylitis: a clinical and magnetic resonance imaging study. *Ann Rheum Dis*, **63**(9), 1041–1045.

42. Song, I.H., Heldmann, F., Rudwaleit, M., (2010). Different response to rituximab in tumor necrosis factor blocker-naive patients with active ankylosing spondylitis and in patients in whom tumor necrosis factor blockers have failed: a twenty-four-week clinical trial. *Arthritis Rheum*, **62**(5), 1290–1297.

43. Sieper, J., Porter-Brown, B., Thompson, L., Harari, O., Dougados, M. (2014). Assessment of short-term symptomatic efficacy of tocilizumab in ankylosing spondylitis: results of randomised, placebo-controlled trials. *Ann Rheum Dis*, **73**, 95–100.

44. Lekpa, F.K., Farrenq, V., Canouï-Poitrine, F., *et al.* (2012). Lack of efficacy of abatacept in axial spondylarthropathies refractory to tumor-necrosis-factor inhibition. *Joint Bone Spine*, **79**(1), 47–50.

45. Song, I.H., Heldmann, F., Rudwaleit, M., *et al.* (2011). Treatment of active ankylosing spondylitis with abatacept: an open-label, 24-week pilot study. *Ann Rheum Dis*, **70**(6), 1108–1110.

46. Baeten, D., Baraliakos, X., Braun, J., *et al.* (2013). Anti-interleukin-17A monoclonal antibody secukinumab in treatment of ankylosing spondylitis: a randomised, double-blind, placebo-controlled trial. *Lancet*, **382**(9906):1705–1713.

47. Sieper, J., Braun, J., Kay, J., Badalamenti, S., Radin, A.R., Jiao, L., Fiore, S., Momtahen, T., Yancopoulos, G.D., Stahl, N., Inman, R.D. (2014). Sarilumab for the treatment of ankylosing spondylitis: results of a Phase II, randomised, double-blind, placebo-controlled study (ALIGN). *Ann Rheum Dis,* doi: 10.1136/annrheumdis-2013-204963 [Epub ahead of print].

48. Poddubnyy, D., Hermann, K.G., Callhoff, J., Listing, J., Sieper, J. (2014). Ustekinumab for the treatment of patients with active ankylosing spondylitis: results of a 28-week, prospective, open-label, proof-of-concept study (TOPAS). *Ann Rheum Dis,* **73**(5), 817–823.

49. Pathan, E., Abraham, S., Van Rossen, E., Withrington, R., Keat, A., Charles, P.J., Paterson, E., Chowdhury, M., McClinton, C., Taylor, P.C. (2013). Efficacy and safety of apremilast, an oral phosphodiesterase 4 inhibitor, in ankylosing spondylitis. *Ann Rheum Dis,* **72**(9), 1475–1480.

50. Barkham, N., Keen, H.I., Coates, L.C., O'Connor, P., Hensor, E., Fraser, A.D., Cawkwell, L.S., Bennett, A., McGonagle, D., Emery, P. (2009). Clinical and imaging efficacy of infliximab in HLA-B27-Positive patients with magnetic resonance imaging-determined early sacroiliitis. *Arthritis Rheum,* **60**(4), 946–954. Erratum in: *Arthritis Rheum,* (2010) **62**(10), 3005.

51. Sieper, J., van der, H.D., Dougados, M., Mease, P.J., Maksymowych, W.P., Brown, M.A., *et al.* (2013). Efficacy and safety of adalimumab in patients with non-radiographic axial spondyloarthritis: results of a randomised placebo-controlled trial (ABILITY-1). *Ann Rheum Dis,* **72**(6), 815–822.

52. Song, I.H., Hermann, K., Haibel, H., Althoff, C.E., Listing, J., Burmester, G., *et al.* (2011). Effects of etanercept versus sulfasalazine in early axial spondyloarthritis on active inflammatory lesions as detected by whole-body MRI (ESTHER): a 48-week randomised controlled trial. *Ann Rheum Dis,* **70**(4), 590–596.

53. Landewe, R., Braun, J., Deodhar, A., Dougados, M., Maksymowych, W.P., Mease, P.J., *et al.* (2014). Efficacy of certolizumab pegol on signs and symptoms of axial spondyloarthritis including ankylosing spondylitis: 24-week results of a double-blind randomised placebo-controlled Phase 3 study. *Ann Rheum Dis,* **73**(1):39–47.

54. Linder, R., Hoffmann, A., Brunner, R. (2004). Prevalence of the spondyloarthritides in patients with uveitis. *J Rheumatol,* **31**(11), 2226–2229.

55. Linssen, A., Rothova, A., Valkenburg, H.A., Dekker-Saeys, A.J., *et al.* (1991). The lifetime cumulative incidence of acute anterior uveitis in a normal population and its relation to ankylosing spondylitis and histocompatibility antigen HLA-B27. *Invest Ophthalmol Vis Sci,* **32**(9), 2568–2578.

56. Munoz-Fernandez, S., Hidalgo, V., Fernandez-Melon, J., *et al.* (2003). Sulfasalazine reduces the number of flares of acute anterior uveitis over a one-year period. *J Rheumatol,* **30**(6), 1277–1279.

57. El-Shabrawi, Y., Hermann, J. (2002). Anti-tumor necrosis factor-alpha therapy with infliximab as an alternative to corticosteroids in the treatment of

human leukocyte antigen B27-associated acute anterior uveitis. *Ophthalmology*, **109**(12), 2342–2346.

58. Braun, J., Baraliakos, X., Listing, J., Sieper, J. (2005). Decreased incidence of anterior uveitis in patients with ankylosing spondylitis treated with the anti-tumor necrosis factor agents infliximab and etanercept. *Arthritis Rheum,* **52**(8), 2447–2451.

59. Giganti, M., Beer, P.M., Lemanski, N., Hartman, C., Schartman, J., Falk, N. (2010). Adverse events after intravitreal infliximab (Remicade). *Retina,* **30**(1), 71–80.

60. Wu, L., Hernandez-Bogantes, E., Roca, J.A., Arevalo, J.F., Barraza, K., Lasave, A.F. (2011). Intravitreal tumor necrosis factor inhibitors in the treatment of refractory diabetic macular edema: a pilot study from the Pan-American Collaborative Retina Study Group. *Retina,* **31**(2), 298–303.

61. Rosenbaum, J.T. (2004). Effect of etanercept on iritis in patients with ankylosing spondylitis. *Arthritis Rheum,* **50**(11), 3736–3737.

62. Sieper, J., Koenig, A., Baumgartner, S., Wishneski, C., Foehl, J., Vlahos, B., Freundlich, B. (2010). Analysis of uveitis rates across all etanercept ankylosing spondylitis clinical trials. *Ann Rheum Dis,* **69**(1), 226–229.

63. Rudwaleit, M., Rødevand, E., Holck, P., Vanhoof, J., Kron, M., Kary, S., Kupper, H. (2009). Adalimumab effectively reduces the rate of anterior uveitis flares in patients with active ankylosing spondylitis: results of a prospective open-label study. *Ann Rheum Dis,* **68**(5), 696–701.

64. van Denderen, J.C., Visman, I.M., Nurmohamed, M.T., Suttorp-Schulten M.S., van der Horst-Bruinsma, I.E. (2014). Adalimumab significantly reduces the recurrence rate of anterior uveitis in patients ankylosing spondylitis. *J Rheumatol,* **41**(9), 1843–1848.

65. Cordero-Coma, M., Calvo-Río, V., Adán, A., Blanco, R., Alvarez-Castro, C., Mesquida, M., Calleja, S., González-Gay, M.A., Ruíz de Morales, J.G. (2014). Golimumab as rescue therapy for refractory immune-mediated uveitis: a three-center experience. *Mediators Inflamm,* **2014**, 717598.

66. Gossec, L., Smolen, J.S., Gaujoux-Viala, C., Ash, Z., Marzo-Ortega, H., van der Heijde, D., FitzGerald, O., Aletaha, D., Balint, P., Boumpas, D., Braun, J., Breedveld, F.C., Burmester, G., Cañete, J.D., de Wit, M., Dagfinrud, H., de Vlam, K., Dougados, M., Helliwell, P., Kavanaugh, A., Kvien, T.K., Landewé, R., Luger, T., Maccarone, M., McGonagle, D., McHugh, N., McInnes, I.B., Ritchlin, C., Sieper, J., Tak, P.P., Valesini, G., Vencovsky, J., Winthrop, K.L., Zink, A., Emery, P. (2012). European League Against Rheumatism. European League Against Rheumatism recommendations for the management of psoriatic arthritis with pharmacological therapies. *Ann Rheum Dis,* **71**(1), 4–12.

67. Reich, K., Ortonne, J.P., Gottlieb, A.B., Terpstra, I.J., Coteur, G., Tasset, C., Mease, P. (2012). Successful treatment of moderate to severe plaque psoriasis with the PEGylated Fab' certolizumab pegol: results of a phase II randomized, placebo-controlled trial with a re-treatment extension. *Br J Dermatol*, **167**(1), 180–190.

68. Mielants, H., Veys, E.M., Cuvelier, C., De Vos, M. (1988). Ileocolonoscopy and spondarthritis.Br *J Rheumatol*, **27**(2), 163–164.

69. Mielants, H., Veys, E.M., Goemaere, S., Goethals, K., Cuvelier, C., De Vos, M. (1991). Gut inflammation in the spondyloarthropathies: clinical, radiologic, biologic, and genetic features in relation to the type of histology. A prospective study. *J Rheumatol*, **18**(10), 1542–1551.

70. de Vries, M., van der Horst-Bruinsma, I., van Hoogstraten, I., van Bodegraven, A., von Blomberg, B.M., Ratnawati, H., Dijkmans, B. (2010). pANCA, ASCA, and OmpC antibodies in patients with ankylosing spondylitis without inflammatory bowel disease. *J Rheumatol*, **37**(11), 2340–2344.

71. Sandborn, W.J., Stenson, W.F., Brynskov, J., Lorenz, R.G., Steidle, G.M., Robbins, J.L., Kent, J.D., Bloom, B.J. (2006). Safety of celecoxib in patients with ulcerative colitis in remission: a randomized, placebo-controlled, pilot study. *Clin Gastroenterol Hepatol*, **4**(2), 203–211.

72. Braun, J., Baraliakos, X., Listing, J., Davis, J., van der Heijde, D., Haibel, H., Rudwaleit, M., Sieper, J. (2007). Differences in the incidence of flares or new onset of inflammatory bowel diseases in patients with ankylosing spondylitis exposed to therapy with anti-tumor necrosis factor alpha agents. *Arthritis Rheum*, **57**(4), 639–647.

73. Hanauer, S.B., Feagan, B.G., Lichtenstein, G.R., Mayer, L.F., Schreiber, S., Colombel, J.F., Rachmilewitz, D., Wolf, D.C., Olson, A., Bao, W., Rutgeerts, P. (2002). ACCENT I Study Group. Maintenance infliximab for Crohn's disease: the ACCENT I randomised trial. *Lancet*, **359**(9317), 1541–1549.

74. Rutgeerts, P., Sandborn, W.J., Feagan, B.G., Reinisch, W., Olson, A., Johanns, J., Travers, S., Rachmilewitz, D., Hanauer, S.B., Lichtenstein, G.R., de Villiers, W.J., Present, D., Sands, B.E., Colombel, J.F. (2005). Infliximab for induction and maintenance therapy for ulcerative colitis. *N Engl J Med*, **353**(23), 2462–2476. Erratum in: *N Engl J Med*, (2006), **354**(20), 2200.

75. Sandborn, W.J., Rutgeerts, P., Enns, R., Hanauer, S.B., Colombel, J.F., Panaccione, R., D'Haens, G., Li, J., Rosenfeld, M.R., Kent, J.D., Pollack, P.F. (2007). Adalimumab induction therapy for Crohn disease previously treated with infliximab: a randomized trial. *Ann Intern Med*, **146**(12), 829–838.

76. Sandborn, W.J., Hanauer, S.B., Katz, S., Safdi, M., Wolf, D.G., Baerg, R.D., Tremaine, W.J., Johnson, T., Diehl, N.N., Zinsmeister, A.R. (2001). Etanercept

for active Crohn's disease: a randomized, double-blind, placebo-controlled trial. *Gastroenterology,* **121**(5), 1088–1094.

77. Schreiber, S., Rutgeerts, P., Fedorak, R.N., Khaliq-Kareemi, M., Kamm, M.A., Boivin, M., *et al.* (2004). A randomized, placebo-controlled trial of certolizumab pegol (CDP870) for treatment of Crohn's disease. *Gastroenterology,* **129**(3), 807–818.

CHAPTER 7

ADVANCES IN THERAPIES FOR SYSTEMIC LUPUS ERYTHEMATOSUS

Noémi Győri, Chiara Tani, and Marta Mosca

Introduction

Systemic lupus erythematosus (SLE) is a multi-systemic inflammatory disease with a broad spectrum of clinical manifestations. This chronic autoimmune condition is characterized by a flaring nature and can vary from mild to potentially life-threatening. The word "lupus" in Latin means *wolf*, and "erythro" is derived from the Greek terminology indicating "*redness*" or "*blush*". The above appellation originates with the reddish, butterfly-shaped malar rash that the disease classically exhibits across the nose and cheeks. The dermatological manifestation of the disease was first documented in the Middle Ages. The discovery of the lupus erythematosus (LE) cell in the mid-1900s significantly contributed to further understanding of the pathophysiology and clinical-laboratory features of the disease, which provided a basis for advances in therapy.

Epidemiology

SLE can develop in people of all ages, gender, and ethnicities; however, it is more prevalent in females at proportions that are nine times that of males, with the disease onset peaking between 20–30 years of age. There are also regional disparities in both incidence and prevalence of SLE with the highest in people of Afro-American, Afro-Caribbean, and Hispanic American descents, making ethnicity an important factor to consider regarding lupus development. The current incidence is reported to be 1 to 25/100,000 in North America, South America, Europe and Asia.

Etiology and Pathogenesis

A great deal of evidence indicates that both susceptible genetic profiles and environmental factors are responsible for triggering the onset of SLE and disease flares. Although SLE is not completely understood, it is multifactorial in etiology.

Genetics

The genetic association of SLE has been well documented, with many family studies revealing the concordance rate in monozygotic twins as 24–35%, compared to 2–5% in dizygotic twins. Furthermore, 10–12% of patients with lupus are reported to have first- or second-degree family members also affected with the disease.[1,2] A large number of SLE susceptibility loci have been identified over the last decade, indicating genes responsible for immune functions such as immune complex clearance (complement and phagocytosis), lymphocyte signaling (T and B cell signaling) and the innate immune response (interferon and NFκB signaling). The major histocompatibility complex (MHC) was the first region identified to be associated with SLE. It contains the classical human leukocyte antigen (HLA) class I, II and III regions that encode the genes involved in antigen presentation, as well as genes coding for cytokines, and early complement factors. The class II alleles HLA-DR2 (DRB1*1501) and HLA-DR3 (DRB1*0301) are apparently the most consistently associated genetic risk factors for lupus. Interestingly, HLA-DQ and –DR alleles show a strong association with SLE autoantibodies.[3,4] A strong relationship has also been documented between deficiencies of early classical pathway complement components (C1q, C2, and C4) and the development of SLE. The plasma and cell-surface proteins of the complement system mediate the inflammatory responses to the immune complexes which assist in the clearance of pathogens.[5] Also documented in the literature is the gender disparity associated with SLE, in keeping with the hypothesis that sex hormones and genetic variation on chromosome X might contribute to a higher risk of lupus.

Environmental factors

A number of environmental agents, such as ultraviolet radiation, exposure to cigarette smoke, hormonal factors, infectious or endogenous viruses (such as Epstein-Barr Virus, Varicella Zoster Virus and cytomegalovirus) have been demonstrated to be associated with the occurrence of SLE. Research suggests that a variety of environmental contributors induce oxidative stress, which subsequently reduces DNA methylation in CD4+ T-cells and enhances autoimmunity. Ultraviolet-B (UV-B) exposure promotes pro-inflammatory apoptosis, extensive release of autoantigens and pro-inflammatory cytokines. Tobacco smoke has been reported to activate alveolar macrophages, induce myeloperoxidase activity and production of free radicals. Certain drugs and chemical agents (such as hydralazine, procainamide, TNF-inhibitors) have also been identified as possible contributors to the development of lupus-like disease. The role of certain environmental triggers in the development of SLE in susceptible individuals has been established but none of these factors have been identified as a direct cause of the disease.[6]

Immunopathogenesis

Both innate and adaptive immune mechanisms are implicated in the pathogenesis of SLE. The aforementioned genetic predisposition and specific environmental factors contribute to a systemic malfunction that is mediated by a global loss of self-tolerance with the subsequent development of a pathological immune response. The defective clearance of apoptotic cells, increased antigenic load, loss of immune tolerance, excessive T cell activation, impaired B cell suppression, and the shifting of Th1 to Th2 immune responses lead to B cell hyperactivity and the production of pathogenic autoantibodies. The central immunological failure in patients with SLE is characterized by the presence of autoantibodies to widespread endogenous nuclear self-antigens (such as antinuclear antibodies and anti-double stranded DNA antibodies) and extensive deposition of immune complexes in affected tissues. These immune complexes potently activate the classical complement pathway resulting in hypocomplementemia and deposition of complement at sites of tissue damage. Excessive production of cytokines (such as IFN-α, IL-6, IL-10, IL23 and TNF) also contributes to the inflammatory process through stimulating immune response and organ damage in SLE.

Clinical and Serological Features of SLE

SLE is characterized by protean manifestations and a heterogeneous clinical picture among patients as almost any organ system can be affected by the disease with an extremely wide range of severity.

Major clinical manifestations

Constitutional symptoms include generalized manifestations of the disease process such as fever, malaise, fatigue, anorexia and weight loss. These nonspecific complaints are common, especially at disease onset, being reported in up to 95% in inception cohorts. Malaise and fatigue are the most common constitutional symptoms associated with SLE; fatigue in SLE is reported by up to 95% of patients, with fatigue being persistent, unpredictable and typically not resolved by rest.

Other than disease activity, fatigue in SLE can be due to anemia, medications, hormonal disturbances, concomitant fibromyalgia or affective disorders.[7]

Fever reflecting disease activity is described in up to 90% of the patients; infections, malignancies and drug reactions have to be ruled out.[8]

Musculoskeletal involvement in SLE is common, and is reported in up to 90% of patients during the disease course. Arthritis in SLE is a frequent manifestation and it is often one of the first symptoms of the disease. Most patients with SLE have a non-erosive polyarthritis, characterized by soft tissue swelling and tenderness in joints, most commonly in the hands,

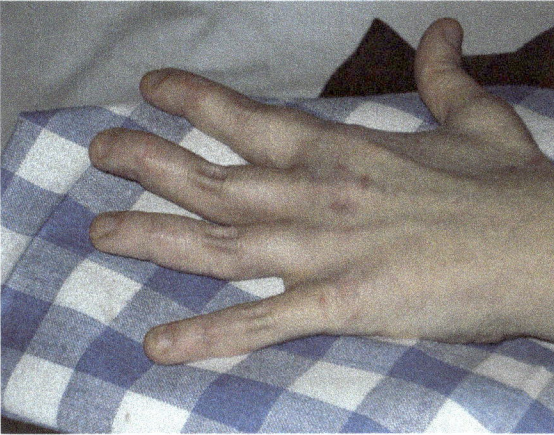

Figure 1. Jaccoud's arthropathy.

wrists and knees. While for decades joint involvement in SLE has been considered mild and non-erosive, many studies have recently showed that patients with SLE develop joint deformities and, in up to 10% of the cases, an erosive deforming arthritis. From the patient's perspective, musculo-skeletal involvement is one of the most commonly reported symptoms with a major impact on quality of life, employment and social life.

In 10–35% of patients Jaccoud's syndrome is described (Fig. 1); it is a severely deforming variant of joint involvement which mainly affects hands and feet with multiple non-erosive subluxations, mild aching and little or no evidence of synovitis.[9]

Cutaneous manifestations are present in 70–85% of patients and often represent the first sign of the disease. Mucocutaneous lesions have been classified into LE-specific and LE-nonspecific. The LE-specific cutane-ous findings cover three subtypes of cutaneous lupus erythematosus (CLE): acute CLE (ACLE), subacute CLE (SCLE), and chronic CLE (CCLE) (Table 1) (Figs. 2 and 3). Cutaneous lupus is discussed further in Chapter 11 of this book.

LE-nonspecific lesions include Raynaud's phenomenon, oral ulcers, livedo reticularis, thrombophlebitis, leukocytoclastic vasculitis, and non-scarring alopecia as the most frequent manifestations[10] (Fig. 4).

Table 1.   Subtypes of cutaneous lupus erythematosus (CLE).

Acute cutaneous lupus erythematosus (ACLE)	• Localized form (malar rash) • Generalized form
Subacute cutaneous lupus erythematosus (SCLE)	• Annular form • Papulosquamous form

Chronic cutaneous lupus erythematosus (CCLE)	• Discoid lupus erythematosus (DLE)
	  Localized form
	  Disseminated form
	• Lupus erythematosus profundus (LEP; LE panniculitis)
	• Chilblain lupus erythematosus (CHLE)

Intermittent cutaneous lupus erythematosus (ICLE)	• Lupus erythematosus tumidus (LET)

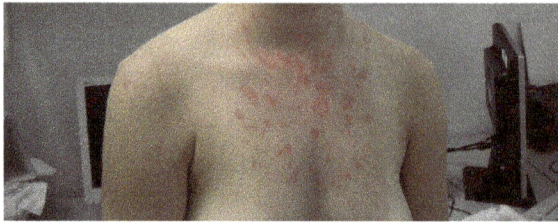

Figure 2.   Subacute cutaneous lupus. Annular variant.

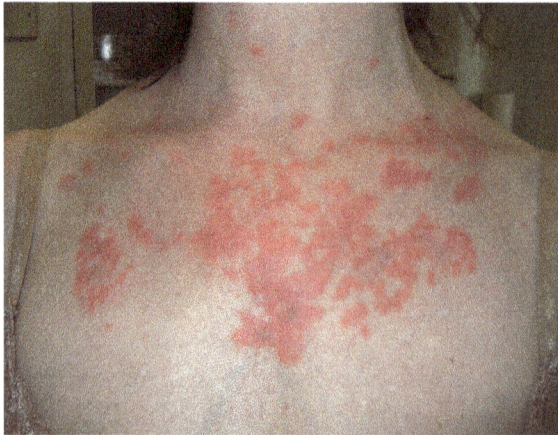

Figure 3.   Subacute cutaneous lupus. Papulosquamous variant.

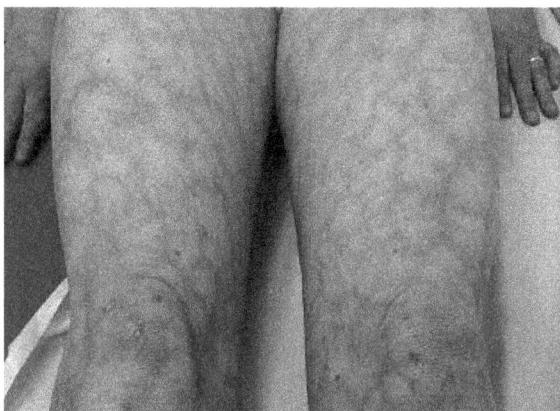

Figure 4.   Livedo reticularis in SLE.

Involvement of the kidney in the course of the disease is present in a majority of patients (50–70%) and recent findings suggest a higher incidence, since a considerable proportion of patients with SLE have silent lupus nephritis (LN). An abnormal urinalysis with or without an elevated plasma creatinine concentration is present in a large proportion of patients at the time of diagnosis of LN, and the most frequently observed abnormality in patients with LN is proteinuria.

From a histopathological perspective, renal biopsy findings are classified according to the current classification of lupus nephritis [International Society of Nephrology (ISN)/Renal Pathology Society, 2003] into six (I–VI) classes[11] (Table 2).

The heart is frequently involved in SLE; depending on methods of assessment, sensitive imaging techniques demonstrated cardiovascular involvement in more than 50% of the patients. All three layers of the heart (pericardium, myocardium and endocardium) can be affected in SLE. Pericarditis is the most common cardiovascular manifestation of SLE as isolated or recurrent episodes; symptomatic pericarditis is estimated to occur in 25% of SLE patients during the disease course, while asymptomatic pericardial effusion is more common and recorded in about 40% of patients. Rarely, cardiac tamponade, constrictive pericarditis and purulent pericarditis can complicate pericarditis in SLE. Myocarditis can

Table 2. International Society of Nephrology (ISN)/Renal Pathology Society classification of lupus nephritis.

Class	Description	Histological findings
Class I	Minimal mesangial lupus nephritis	Normal glomeruli by light microscopy, but mesangial immune deposits by immunofluorescence
Class II	Mesangial proliferative lupus nephritis	Purely mesangial hypercellularity of any degree or mesangial matrix expansion by light microscopy, with mesangial immune deposits
Class III	Focal lupus nephritis	Active or inactive focal, segmental or global endo- or extracapillary glomerulonephritis involving 50% of all glomeruli, typically with focal subendothelial immune deposits, with or without mesangial alterations
Class III (A/C)	focal proliferative and sclerosing lupus nephritis	Active and chronic lesions
Class III (A)	focal proliferative lupus nephritis	Active lesions
Class III (C)	focal sclerosing lupus nephritis	Chronic inactive lesions with glomerular scars
Class IV	Diffuse lupus nephritis	Active or inactive diffuse, segmental or global endo- or extracapillary glomerulonephritis involving >50% of all glomeruli, typically with diffuse subendothelial immune deposits, with or without mesangial alterations. This class is divided into diffuse segmental (IV-S) lupus nephritis when >50% of the involved glomeruli have segmental lesions, and diffuse global (IV-G) lupus nephritis when >50% of the involved glomeruli have global lesions. Segmental is defined as a glomerular lesion that involves less than half of the glomerular tuft. This class includes cases with diffuse wire loop deposits but with little or no glomerular proliferation

(Continued)

Table 2.   (*Continued*)

Class	Description	Histological findings
Class IV-(A)	diffuse segmental proliferative lupus nephritis	Active lesions
Class IV- (A/C)	diffuse proliferative and sclerosing lupus nephritis	Active and chronic lesions
Class IV-(C)	diffuse sclerosing lupus nephritis	Chronic inactive lesions with scars
Class V	Membranous lupus nephritis	Global or segmental subepithelial immune deposits or their morphologic sequelae by light microscopy and by immunofluorescence or electron microscopy, with or without mesangial alterations
Class VI	Advanced sclerosis lupus nephritis	90% of glomeruli globally sclerosed without residual activity

be clinically detected in 3–15% of SLE patients although it appears to be much more prevalent in autopsy studies suggesting the largely subclinical nature of lupus-associated myocarditis. Anatomical and functional valvular abnormalities are prevalent in SLE (50–60% in studies with transesophageal echocardiography), mainly affecting mitral and aortic valves. Libman–Sacks endocarditis (a non-bacterial verrucous variant) is the most specific finding while valvular thickening and regurgitation are more frequently observed. Verrucous endocarditis is generally asymptomatic and the verrucae usually are near the edge of the valves thus leading to hemodynamically significant impairment in only 3–4% of SLE patients. Infectious endocarditis, stroke or peripheral embolism, and chorda tendinea rupture are possible complications. Cardiovascular complications are an emerging issue in SLE patients, being one of the major causes of morbidity and mortality. Coronary artery disease (CAD), including myocardial infarction, angina and sudden death, is described with a prevalence ranging from 6% to 10% with a risk of developing CAD in SLE patients 4–8 times higher than in the general population. In young women with SLE, the risk of myocardial infarction is increased 50-fold. Different mechanisms are involved in its pathogenesis including accelerated atherosclerosis, coronary arteritis, thrombotic events or embolization of valvular material, vasospasm and hypertension.[12]

The pattern of lung involvement in SLE includes pleural, parenchymal, vascular and airway disease manifestations. Infections and drug toxicities should also be considered (Table 3).

Approximately 30–50% of patients with SLE develop symptomatic pleural inflammation in the form of pleurisy manifesting as sharp chest pain aggravated on deep breathing and/or shortness of breath. Pleural effusion is usually bilateral and the pleural fluid is exudative in nature. Although acute lupus pneumonitis is uncommon, seen in 1–12% of patients, it is one of the most serious complications of the disease. Chronic interstitial lung disease (ILD) or interstitial pneumonitis is described in 3–13% of patients of SLE with long-standing disease. Shrinking lung syndrome (SLS) is defined as unexplained dyspnea, small lung volumes, and restrictive lung physiology typically with mono- or bilateral elevation of the diaphragmatic domes on chest radiographs.[13]

Many SLE patients develop neurological or psychiatric symptoms (NPSLE) during the course of the disease, with a reported cumulative prevalence of NPSLE of 30–40%. Most NPSLE events occur at disease onset or within the first years of the disease, usually in the presence of generalized disease activity. Risk factors significantly associated with NPSLE events include general SLE activity or damage, previous events and antiphospholipid antibodies.

In 40% of cases, NPSLE is secondary to other causes such as metabolic derangement based on SLE damage to organs other than the brain or due to side effects of drug treatment. In the remaining 60% of the cases, NP symptoms are primarily attributed to the disease process. Primary NPSLE can be divided into focal and diffuse disease. The focal disease includes the occurrence of thrombo-embolic events and seizures as the most frequent manifestations (5–10% and 7–10% respectively). Diffuse primary NPSLE is a group of neurological, psychiatric, and cognitive symptoms comprising a wide range of conditions with headache and cognitive dysfunction being the most frequently observed (10–60% and 10–80% respectively). Often, no abnormalities are found on conventional neuro-imaging techniques in this group.[14]

Laboratory abnormalities

Hematological disorders are reported in over 80% of patients with SLE at some point in the disease course; the major manifestations are anemia, leukopenia and thrombocytopenia.

Anemia is a common hematological abnormality in SLE and can result from different pathogenetic mechanisms. The most frequent form (60–80%) is the anemia of chronic disease which results from suppressed erythropoiesis secondary to chronic inflammation. Autoimmune hemolytic anemia is reported in up to 10% of the patients.

Leukopenia is common in SLE both at disease onset and during follow-up; a white blood cell count of less than 4500/μL has been noted in approximately 50% of patients, especially during active phases of the disease, while more severe forms are reported to occur in 15–20% of patients. It is usually secondary to lymphopenia, neutropenia or a combination of both and it generally reflects disease activity. However, ongoing therapies with immunosuppressive drugs, especially azathioprine and cyclophosphamide, should be considered in the differential diagnosis as possible causes of leukopenia in SLE. The prevalence of lymphopenia (lymphocytes less than 1500/μL) in SLE ranges from 20–81%; both T and B lymphocytes are reduced, while natural killer cells can be increased. Neutropenia has a prevalence of 40–50% in SLE and may be mediated by anti-neutrophil antibodies. Mild thrombocytopenia (platelet counts between 100,000/μL and 150,000/μL) is observed in 25–50% of patients, while a platelet count under 50,000/μL is less frequent.[15]

Autoantibodies

SLE is characterized by the aberrant production of a broad and heterogeneous group of autoantibodies; more than one hundred autoantibodies have been described in SLE patients; among these autoantibodies, those that are directed to nuclear (ANA), cytoplasmatic, and cellular membrane antigens are considered the serological hallmark of the disease.

Anti-DNA antibodies constitute a subgroup of ANA that bind to either single-stranded or double stranded DNA; both subtypes of DNA-binding antibodies may be found in SLE but because of their higher specificity, anti-dsDNA antibodies are used in routine clinical practice for diagnostic as well as monitoring purposes. Moreover, it is generally accepted that anti-dsDNA antibodies, in particular of the IgG isotype, have an important pathogenetic role in SLE. Overall, anti-dsDNA are present in around 70% of SLE patients, and the serum levels of anti-dsDNA are significantly associated with renal involvement and disease activity.

Patterns of disease course

Three main patterns of SLE activity have been described: relapsing-remitting (RR), chronic active (CA), and long quiescent (LQ). The CA pattern is the most frequent, characterizing more than half of SLE patients; the least common pattern is LQ (described in up to 25% of the patients) while the RR pattern is intermediate in frequency (up to 35%).[16]

Late manifestations, damage

It has been suggested that the spectrum of clinical manifestations and the causes of death in SLE patients differ depending on the time of evolution of the disease. Indeed, long-term observational studies seem to support the idea that most of the SLE inflammatory manifestations tend to be less common after a long-term evolution of the disease, probably reflecting the effect of therapy as well as the gradual remission of the disease in many patients.

Conversely, other medical problems are prevalent in patients with long disease duration and may cause morbidity in SLE patients including cardiovascular diseases, infections, hypertension, osteoporosis and fractures, joint deformities, drug-induced cytopenias and neoplasms. In particular, athero-thrombotic events as the result of an accelerated atherosclerotic process have a prominent role, significantly affecting both morbidity and mortality in SLE.

The accrual of organ damage as a result of disease activity or drug side effects is the dominant issue in long-term disease; male gender, older age, longer disease duration, Afro-Caribbean and Indo-Asian ethnicity are considered risk factors for damage as well as persistent disease activity. Renal or neuropsychiatric involvement also predicts damage accrual. Glucocorticoids and immunosuppressants showed an association with damage accrual.[17]

Instruments for measuring clinical disease activity and damage (*SLEDAI, ECLAM, BILAG*)

The assessment of disease activity in SLE is a pivotal issue in every day care as well as in clinical trials and research. Over the past years, many indices have been developed to objectively measure lupus disease activity and several of these have been validated.

The most widely used indices are the British Isles Lupus Assessment Group (BILAG) index, the European Consensus Lupus Activity Measurement (ECLAM), the Systemic Lupus Activity Measure (SLAM), the Systemic Lupus Erythematosus Disease Activity Index (SLEDAI) and the Lupus Activity Index (LAI). The ECLAM, SLAM, SLEDAI and LAI, provide a single summary score for activity, while the BILAG provides assessment scales for individual organs and systems.

Although each of these composite indices has been developed with the same aim to assess disease activity in SLE, each includes different items to evaluate organ systems and different laboratory measures. All the composite measures have a greater or lesser degree of validation, and none has been accepted as the preferred or standard measure of choice.

The Systemic Lupus International Collaborating Clinics/American College of Rheumatology-Damage Index: SLICC/ACR-DI (SDI) has been validated for damage assessment in SLE; it is an organ-based system, detecting damage in patients regardless of its cause, which may have resulted from disease activity, treatment or comorbidities.[18]

Prognosis

Because of better knowledge of the pathogenetic mechanisms and prognostic factors as well as more effective and aggressive treatment, the prognosis for SLE has improved markedly over the past decades. Recent studies have shown that 5-year survival is now near 90–95% and that 70–85% of patients survive at 10 years after disease onset. However, SLE patients have poor long-term prognosis and increased mortality compared to the general population. Renal injury is the most important predictor of mortality in patients with SLE. Overall, common causes of death are infections, while disease activity contributes to about a third of early deaths but less commonly to late deaths. Cardiovascular events are more common causes of death in longstanding disease.[19,20]

Therapy

General concepts on SLE management and treat-to-target recommendations

The clinical picture in SLE is extremely variable, due to the interplay of features of disease activity, alternating phases of remission and flares, disease and drug-induced damage, comorbidities, and drug toxicities: all these aspects need to be considered in the management of SLE patients.

Recently, Treat-to-target (T2T) Recommendations have been published to guide physicians in the treatment of SLE. According to T2T Recommendations, "Treatment of SLE should aim at ensuring long-term survival, preventing organ damage, and optimizing health-related quality-of-life, by controlling disease activity and minimizing comorbidities and drug toxicity."[21]

From the T2T Recommendations, some important concepts might be extrapolated:

- In a chronic and potentially invalidating disease such as SLE, the patient must be central in the decision-making process.
- The health care providers must be aware of the multifaceted nature of SLE, possibly implying that care be delivered by more than one type of specialist.
- SLE can cause severe dysfunctions at various organ levels that might be underdiagnosed until the development of life-threatening conditions; for this reason patients should be monitored regularly, with adjustment of therapy at reasonable time intervals.
- A low level of disease activity or remission predicts better long-term patient outcome; this implies not only that these conditions represent the main treatment targets, but also that at least one validated disease activity measure should be regularly assessed in the routine evaluation of SLE.
- It is well-known that flares affect long-term patient outcomes, thus representing the third therapeutic goal in SLE.

- Damage has been shown to predict further damage and to seriously increase the risks of morbidity and mortality. It is associated with disease activity, disease flares and drug toxicity. Therefore, it appears mandatory to control these factors for avoiding the development of damage and to regularly measure irreversible damage by a validated index [Systemic Lupus International Collaborating Clinics/American College of Rheumatology SLICC Damage Index (SDI)].
- From the patients' point of view, the ultimate goal in their disease is "to survive and to survive well." Accordingly, rheumatologists should aim at optimizing patients' HRQoL, trying to ensure their social functioning.
- Considering the damage accrual associated with chronic therapy with GC (of which a "safe dose" in SLE does not seem to exist), their use should be carefully minimized, aiming at complete withdrawal when possible.

In an attempt to summarize these concept, we can identify different goals of SLE treatment: (1) induction of remission: aimed at rapidly controlling disease activity for prolonged periods; (2) maintenance of remission and flare prevention; (3) treatment of comorbidities; and (4) maintaining a good quality of life. These aspects make the treatment of SLE complex and dependent on the use of combinations of drugs.

In the following paragraphs, we will review the available information on old and new therapies for SLE.

Treatment of SLE: Traditional Therapeutic Agents

Glucocorticoids

The introduction of glucocorticoids (GC) in the early 1950s has changed the history of SLE and contributed greatly to the improvement of patient survival. GC are still the first choice treatment of acute SLE, but are also used in the maintenance of remission and are often continued long-term.[22,24]

The most commonly used GC in the treatment of SLE are prednisone/prednisolone (PDN) and methylprednisolone (MP). Low dose GC (0.1–0.2 mg/kg/day) are generally used as maintenance treatment; low to medium (0.2–0.5 mg/kg/day) doses are used in the treatment of mild disease activity, particularly cutaneous, musculoskeletal, haematological and constitutional manifestations. In patients with mild to moderate SLE flares, GC might be administered either as an increase in daily oral dose, followed by rapid tapering, or as an intramuscular (i.m.) [triamcinolone] injection [(100 mg)]. Pulse GC have been used since the 1970s to obtain rapid control of activity in severe disease while minimizing toxicity. Intravenous methylprednisolone (MP) (500 mg to 1000 mg) appears more immunosuppressive than oral MP, as it has a more prolonged duration of action and induces more profound or sustained changes in neutrophils, lymphocytes, and humoral immunity.

Cumulative dose of glucocorticoids, irrespective of the route of administration, is predictive of osteoporotic fractures, coronary artery disease, and cataracts. In addition, the risk of avascular necrosis and stroke increases in association with high-dose prednisone treatment.

Assessment and correction of comorbidities and/or side-effects (especially diabetes, osteoporosis, peptic ulcer, glaucoma, cataract) should be performed before and during treatment. Adherence to guidelines on the prevention of glucocorticoid-induced osteoporosis is strongly recommended. Patients receiving chronic therapy who undergo surgery are at risk to develop adrenal insufficiency, and therefore should receive glucocorticoid replacement therapies. Before starting GC therapy, assessment for the presence of chronic infections (tuberculosis, hepatitis B and C viruses) is advised in endemic areas.[23]

Although there is general agreement on the toxicity of GC and the need to avoid long-term administration of these drugs, up to 80% of patients are chronically treated with these drugs in the majority of published cohorts. In addition, no agreement exists on tapering schedules for GC which are based primarily on the physician's experience and clinical judgment. Therefore, it is important to define not only when and how GC should be used in SLE treatment but also if, when and how these drugs should be discontinued. Discontinuation should be very gradual and monitoring should be very strict.

Antimalarial agents

Hydroxychloroquine (HCQ) is the most widely used antimalarial agent, at doses ranging from 200 mg to 400 mg per day. Other antimalarials are chloroquine (250 mg/day) and quinacrine (100 mg/day). Mucocutaneous and articular manifestations were the original indications for the use of antimalarials in SLE. Data show, however, that these drugs may have benefit in a wider variety of disease manifestations and that withdrawal of antimalarials is associated with an increased risk of SLE flares. In addition, therapy with HCQ appears associated with a reduced risk of irreversible damage, cardiovascular events, and death.

Ocular toxicity represents the major side effect of chloroquine and hydroxychloroquine.

Taken together, these data suggest that antimalarials have a long-term protective effect against disease flares in SLE and act as disease-modifying agents and could be viewed as a (long-term) background therapy for SLE and should be continued long-term, whenever tolerated.[25,26]

Cyclophosphamide

Cyclophosphamide (CYC), an alkylating agent, is considered the standard treatment for severe organ involvement in SLE. In fact, although controlled studies are mainly available on the treatment of lupus nephritis (LN), CYC has been successfully used for treating patients with myocarditis, systemic or gastrointestinal vasculitis and extensive skin involvement.[27–29]

Two different intravenous protocols have been used. The first published intravenous CYC protocol (the so-called NIH protocol), consisted of monthly pulses of CYC (750 mg/m^2) followed by quarterly pulses of a similar dose for two additional years. Subsequently, a lower dose protocol (Eurolupus protocol) was developed consisting of the administration of six fortnightly CYC pulses at 500 mg each followed by maintenance therapy with azathioprine (AZA) at a dose of 2 mg/kg/day.[30] This low dose protocol appears associated with a lower incidence of side effects and similar efficacy. Oral CYC is rarely used, due to the incidence of side effects mainly associated with a high cumulative dose.

Short-term toxic effects of CYC are dominated by risk of infections, nausea and vomiting, hemorrhagic cystitis, leukopenia and liver toxicity. Long-term toxicity of CYC is mainly represented by gonadal toxicity and increased risk of cancer. Ovarian toxicity is related to cumulative doses of CYC and increasing age; in women aged >32 years, an average cumulative dose of 8 g will result in ovarian failure in 50% of the patients.[31]

A positive relationship between cumulative CYC dose and cervical intraepithelial neoplasia (CIN) was observed; in particular each 1 g in cumulative CYC exposure corresponded to a 13% increase in risk of CIN.[32]

In conclusion, side effects appear mostly related to the cumulative dose of the drug, and low dose protocols appear effective in controlling disease activity and inducing remission. Therefore, short-term protocols with a cumulative CYC dose ranging between 6 g and 9 g followed by maintenance therapy with other immunosuppressive drugs have received increasing support.

Mycophenolate mofetil

Mycophenolate mofetil (MMF) has gradually been introduced into the therapeutic armamentarium for SLE. Initially the indication to start MMF therapy has been disease that was resistant to other immunosuppressive drugs, with doses ranging from 1500 mg to 2000 mg daily. Many studies are now available showing that MMF is effective in the induction and maintenance of remission of lupus nephritis.[33,34]

Compared to CYC, MMF may have the advantage of improved safety, especially the absence of ovarian toxicity. MMF side effects are generally few and not severe, consisting of gastrointestinal manifestations (nausea, vomiting), haematological abnormalities and infections. Ethnic differences have been reported in the effectiveness of MMF which appears to be more effective in Afro-American patients.[33,34]

MMF represents a valid alternative to CYC in the treatment of LN. In addition, data from the MAINTAIN trial have shown the equivalence of MMF and Azathioprine in maintaining remission after the Eurolupus protocol in LN patients.

Mycophenolate sodium is also available on the market; this formulation seems to have better gastrointestinal tolerability.

Other immunosuppressive drugs

Other immunosuppressive drugs more commonly used in the treatment of SLE are azathioprine (AZA), methotrexate (MTX), and cyclosporine A (CsA).[35,36]

AZA is used for the treatment of skin, serositis, haematological manifestations, as a steroid sparing agent and in the maintenance phase of severe
SLE and lupus nephritis. Azathioprine is generally administered at a daily
dose of 1–2 mg/kg, but doses up to 2.5 mg/kg/day have also been used.

MTX at doses up to 15–25 mg/week seems to be very effective not
only in the treatment of articular manifestations refractory to steroids and
antimalarials, but also for serositis, and cutaneous manifestations.

CsA, at doses ranging from 2 mg/kg/day to 4 mg/kg/day, has been
used to treat a variety of clinical manifestations, such as pleural effusions
and haematologic manifestations.

Therapeutic protocols

Therapy of active SLE is mainly related to the type and severity of each
single manifestation and is guided by the most severe manifestations. The
majority of the available data on SLE therapy derive from observational
studies, and few controlled studies are available mainly for the treatment
of lupus nephritis. Therefore a trial-and-error approach is commonly
adopted. In Table 3, a summary of the main indications and dosages for
traditional drugs is reported.

Treatment of mild SLE is based on the administration of low doses of
glucocorticoids (0.1–0.2 mg/kg/day) and antimalarial drugs (mainly
hydroxychloroquine 200 mg/day). While the suspension of glucocorticoids should be considered, data suggest that antimalarials should be
continued long-term.

Moderate SLE is generally treated with medium doses of glucocorticoids (0.2–0.5 mg/kg/day) in association with immunosuppressive drugs
such as azathioprine, cyclosporine or methotrexate. As discussed earlier,
the choice of one drug over another is based on major clinical expression
of the disease (*e.g.* methotrexate for arthritis, cyclosporine for haematological problems, and azathioprine for serositis, haematological and cutaneous involvement).

Severe manifestations are treated with combined glucocorticoids
(pulse or high dose ~1 mg/kg/day) and cyclophosphamide, and subsequently remission is maintained with other immunosuppressive drugs.

Table 3. Traditional drugs in the treatment of disease manifestations.

Drug	Manifestations	Dose
Cyclophosphamide	Lupus nephritis Neurological manifestations Severe disease	500 mg every 2 weeks for 3 months (Eurolupus) 0.75 g/m2 monthly for 6 months (NIH)
Mycophenolate mofetil	Lupus nephritis (induction and maintenance) Other manifestations of severe disease	2–3 g/day
Azathioprine	Lupus nephritis maintenance Serositis Hematological manifestations	100–150 mg/day
Methotrexate	Cutaneous manifestations Articular manifestations Serositis Lupus nephritis maintenance	10–25 mg/week
Cyclosporin-A	Hematological manifestations Serositis Articular manifestations Lupus nephritis maintenance	Up to 3.5_mg/kg/day

What's New in the Treatment of SLE

Over the last decades, the introduction of glucocorticoids and immuno-suppressive drugs and the optimization of therapeutic protocols have played an important role in the improvement of patient outcomes.

However, with currently available protocols, complete remission of disease activity is relatively rare. On the contrary, the majority of patients experience either chronically active disease or disease flares. Similarly, damage accrual remains and, despite the correlation between the cumulative GC dose and damage accrual, GC are still used in the long-term treatment of SLE patients. Finally, patients' quality of life is often poor.

These data highlight limits of existing therapeutic options used to control SLE. In this scenario, a number of new drugs targeting different pathways of the immune response are under development, and some are already available in clinical practice.

Belimumab and SLE

Belimumab is a fully human monoclonal antibody against soluble B-lymphocyte stimulator (BLyS). Based on two large phase III trials results, belimumab has been approved for the treatment of SLE patients with active disease.[37,38]

A pooled analysis of two phase III trials, BLISS-52 and BLISS-76 has shown that factors associated with a better response were higher disease activity, anti-dsDNA positivity, low complement and glucocorticoid therapy.[39] BLISS studies were not designed to define which type of organ involvement would benefit most from this therapy. However, analyses suggest a significant effect for the musculoskeletal and mucocutaneous domains of both BILAG and SELENA SLEDAI indices. Based on these data, belimumab has been the first drug approved for treatment of SLE after 50 years. The drug is administered at a dose of 10 mg/kg every two weeks for the first month and every 28 days thereafter.[40]

"Real life" data from registries suggest that clinical improvement is observed in the first six months of treatment. No prospective steroid-sparing studies have been conducted so far but post-hoc data from clinical trials as well as registry data suggest that a reduction of GC dose is obtained in more patients treated with belimumab.[41–43]

We may summarize that available data support the use of belimumab in patients with high disease activity, positive autoantibodies and low complement. However, treatment with belimumab might also be considered (1) when disease activity is controlled but the patient is receiving a GC dose >7.5 mg/day prednisone or equivalent; (2) when the use of traditional immunosuppressive drugs is limited by the risk of interaction with additional therapies (*e.g.*, anticoagulants and antiepileptic drugs; (3) in patients with intolerance to traditional immunosuppressive drugs.[37]

Although clinical trials excluded patients with severe active kidney and neurological involvement, a post hoc analysis of the phase III trials suggests that belimumab may be beneficial for renal outcomes such as renal flares, renal remission, renal organ disease improvement, and proteinuria reduction. Interestingly, better results were obtained in patients receiving concomitant mycophenolate mofetil.[44] Finally, no data are available to suggest the optimal duration of treatment in responsive patients and a possible tapering strategy.

Rituximab and SLE

The first reports concerning the use of rituximab (RTX) in the treatment of SLE were case reports and small series in which the drug had been used for the treatment of patients with severe organ involvement refractory to traditional drugs. Over the past 10 years, clinical evidence has accumulated supporting the efficacy of RTX in the treatment of SLE.[45,46]

RTX is most commonly administered in two 1000 mg doses two weeks apart; usually B cell depletion occurs within two weeks after the first infusion and B cell repopulation after 3 to 40 months. Flares of disease activity have been reported in about 40% of the treated patients, occurring simultaneously or after B cell reconstitution. Retreatment with RTX was effective and safe.

Two large randomized studies aimed at assessing the efficacy of RTX in the treatment of moderate-severe SLE and lupus nephritis failed to reach their primary endpoint.

At present, from the existing literature, RTX is generally considered as a rescue therapy for severe cases.[45]

Two new studies are underway to assess the efficacy of RTX in treating lupus nephritis. In the RING protocol, RTX is used to treat those patients who have failed to achieve renal remission after initial induction therapy with the Eurolupus protocol or with MMF. In the second study, RTX is used in a protocol aimed at treating lupus nephritis without chronic glucocorticoid therapy (the "RITUXILUP" protocol). In an open-label study, at least partial renal responses were seen in most patients and about half achieved a complete renal response.[47]

Epratuzumab and SLE

CD22 is a transmembrane sialoglycoprotein expressed on most mature B-cells which acts as a regulator of B-cell activation and migration. Epratuzumab is a humanized monoclonal antibody targeting CD22.

Two international, randomized, controlled trials (ALLEVIATE-1 and -2) and an open-label extension study (SL0006) have been conducted to assess the effects of epratuzumab in patients with moderately-to-severely active SLE. Both trials were discontinued because of lack of drug supply.[48,49]

Exploratory analyses showed a response at 12 weeks in 44.1% and 30.0% for epratuzumab 360 mg/m^2 and 720 mg/m^2, respectively, versus 20.0% for placebo and no safety signals.

In addition epratuzumab treatment produced improvements in physician global assessment, patient global assessment and health-related quality of life.

Subsequently a phase IIb, multicentre, randomised controlled study (EMBLEM) was conducted in patients with moderate-severe SLE to identify the appropriate drug regimen for phase III trials.[50]

Clinical improvements were observed with epratuzumab 600 mg weekly, 1200 mg every other week, and in the 2400 mg total dose. Treatment was well-tolerated and beneficial effects of the 2400 mg dose were observed as early as eight weeks. At present, phase III studies have concluded enrollment and are ongoing.[50]

Novel Biologics Currently in Development

The critical role of B cells in autoantibody formation, antigen presentation and T cell interactions has been highlighted by advanced research in deducing the complex pathogenesis of SLE. Numerous novel biological agents have also shown treatment efficacy in lupus (Table 4).

A phase II clinical trial (PEARL-SC) recently evaluated *Blisibimod,* a human "peptibody", an immunoglobulin-like molecule that has been synthetically produced to selectively target BLyS. The study suggests that the use of high dose blisibimod (200 mg weekly) is associated with a sustained significant decrease in SLEDAI and anti-ds DNA, and an increase in C3 and C4 in patients with SLE.[51] *Tabalumab* is a monoclonal antibody that antagonises BLyS in both membrane and soluble forms (unlike belimumab, which is thought to target soluble BLyS only).

Tabalumab has been studied in two phase III trials, ILLUMINATE 1 and 2. While ILLUMINATE 1 narrowly failed to meet the endpoint of a significant reduction of disease activity measured with the SRI-5, in ILLUMINATE 2 the higher Tabalumab dose was effective in meeting the endpoint. No increased incidence of side effects was observed in Tabalumab treated patients. In spite of these positive results, Lilly has decided to stop the development of this drug. Additional data from these trials are expected.[52]

Table 4. New biological agents in the treatment of SLE.

Target	Agent	Mechanism of action	Key clinical trials	Key results
B cells	Rituximab	Chimeric monoclonal anti CD-20 antibody	Phase III (EXPLORER) Phase III (LUNAR)	While patients in uncontrolled studies showed improvements, these two controlled trials did not meet their primary endpoints.
B cells	Belimumab	BLyS inhibitor	Phase III (RING) Phase III (BLISS 52) Phase III (BLISS 76) Phase III (BLISS-LN) Phase III/IV (EMBRACE)	ONGOING Both these trials achieved their primary endpoints
B cells	Atacicept	Blys and APRIL inhibitor	Phase II/III (APRIL-LN) Phase II/III (APRIL-SLE)	Patient with moderate SLE show clinical improvement compared to placebo
B cells	Blisibimod	Selective BLyS inhibitor	Phase II (PEARL-SC)	Promising results with high dose blisibimod (200 mg weekly)
B cells	Tabalumab	Both membrane and soluble BLyS antagonist	Phase III (ILLUMINATE 1 Phase III (ILLUMINATE 2)	NEGATIVE clinically significant improvement with high dose tabalumab

B cells	Epratuzumab	Humanized monoclonal anti CD-22 antibody	Phase II (EMBLEM) Phase III (EMBODY)	Positive results for 2400 mg/total dose ONGOING
T cells	Abatacept	T-cell costimulation blockade	Phase IIb Phase II/III Phase II (ACCESS), Phase III	Negative results ONGOING
Cytokines	Sifalimumab	IFN-α inhibitor	Phase I Phase II	Improvement
Cytokines	Rontalizumab	IFN-α inhibitor	Phase I Phase II	Clinical improvement compared to placebo
Cytokines	Tocilizumab	Humanized monoclonal antibody against IL-6 receptor	Phase I	Clinical and serological improvement in mild to moderate SLE

Atacicept is a recombinant fusion protein containing both human IgG and the extracellular section of the B cell surface receptor TACI. This biologic agent is able to inhibit TACI receptor activation by both APRIL and BLyS. Atacicept has been reported to be associated with a 45–60% attenuation in mature B cells, associated with significant dose dependent decreases in autoantibody levels.[53,54] *Laquinimod* is an oral medication that has been shown to be effective in the treatment of relapsing-remitting multiple sclerosis.[55] Laquinimod exerts immunomodulating effects on antigen presenting cells that direct T cells toward an anti-inflammatory cascade. Preliminary results of a phase IIa randomized placebo-controlled study, indicated that a combination of laquinimod (0.5 mg and 1.0 mg/day), mycophenolate mofetil and glucocorticoids had an additive effect in improving renal function and proteinuria in patients with lupus nephritis.[56] Serum levels of IL-6 are elevated in patients with active SLE and correlated with disease activity and anti-dsDNA levels. *Tocilizumab* has been shown to improve both disease activity and serum anti-dsDNA levels in an open-label phase I study with patients with mild to moderate lupus. Laboratory analysis revealed that activated T and B cells, plasmablasts, and post-switched memory B cells were decreased with tocilizumab treatment, while antigen-inexperienced IgD+CD27- B cells and mature naive B cells increased significantly.[57,58] *Sirukumab* is another anti-IL-6 monoclonal antibody and was tested in a phase I placebo-controlled study in patients with either SLE or cutaneous lupus. Sirukumab has been reported to be associated with a dose-independent reduction in total white blood cell, absolute neutrophil and platelet counts and minor elevations in total cholesterol levels.[59] An increased expression of type I interferon (IFN) regulated genes (an IFN signature) has been reported in blood and tissue cells from patients with SLE and other autoimmune diseases as well. *Sifalimumab* (MEDI-545) is a fully humanized anti-IFN-α monoclonal antibody that binds specifically to most IFN-α subtypes and prevents signaling through the type I IFN receptor. A phase Ia placebo-controlled study suggests that sifalimumab has some potential in inhibiting type I IFN-induced mRNAs in SLE patients with moderate disease activity.[60] Another phase I randomized study in patients with moderate-to-severe disease activity showed sustained inhibition of IFN gene signature after sifalimumab treatment.[61] *Rontalizumab* is another human IgG1 monoclonal antibody that neutralizes all known isoforms of human IFN-α. A phase I double-blind placebo-controlled trial of rontalizumab in SLE patients established safety of this agent and its efficacy in reducing the expression of IFN-regulated genes. In a phase II trial, SLE patients with moderate to severe disease activity were randomized to receive either rontalizumab or placebo. The study suggested that the proportion of IFN signature-negative patients achieving improvement (as measured by the SLE Responder Index and frequency of flares) was significantly higher in the rontalizumab group compared to the placebo group.[62,63]

Treatment of Comorbidities

Long-term survival and follow-up of patients with SLE have demonstrated the emergence of comorbid conditions that impact on prognosis and survival. Patients with SLE appear at increased risk for cardiovascular disease, hypertension, diabetes, osteoporosis and some types of cancer.[64]

Cardiovascular disease and SLE: treatment of traditional and SLE related risk factors

Premature atherosclerosis and increased incidence of cardiovascular disease (CVD) among patients with SLE are well established. Data from the literature have shown that this increased incidence cannot be fully explained by traditional CVD risk factors. On this basis, SLE could be included in the group of conditions in which the use of predictive charts is insufficient.

For this reason, some authors have proposed that SLE should be considered as a coronary heart disease high-risk state (much like diabetes mellitus) and have suggested different targets for risk factor modification specifically tailored to SLE patients.

The reported prevalence of hypertension among SLE patients ranges from 14% to 52%, with half of the examined studies reporting a prevalence ≥40%. Published data on lipid profiles agree on a high prevalence (ranging from 11.5% to 75%) of dyslipidemia (most frequently assessing cholesterol levels) in SLE patients. Current prednisone dose and cumulative prednisone dose have been correlated with total cholesterol levels in different studies. Fewer data are available on whether the prevalence of diabetes (prevalence ranging from 0.9% to 11.2%) or obesity is increased. It might be expected that SLE patients have a more sedentary lifestyle;

indeed one study reported a 70% prevalence of sedentary lifestyle according to the American Heart Association Guidelines.

EULAR Recommendations suggest that at baseline and during follow-up at least once a year, patients are assessed for traditional CV risk factors with patient history, patient examination (blood pressure and body mass index) and laboratory exams (*i.e.* blood cholesterol and blood glucose). Patients should receive counselling to control modifiable CV risk factors such as smoking, obesity and a sedentary lifestyle.[64,65]

No SLE specific data are yet available to define the optimal targets for cardiovascular risk factors, however ideal target values for classic risk factors and indications for additional interventions in SLE patients according to recent preliminary guidelines are suggested in Table 5.

Osteoporosis

The prevalence of osteoporosis among SLE patients varies from 4% to 24% (spine 7–23%, femur 3–23%). When only premenopausal patients are evaluated, the prevalence of osteoporosis ranges between 10–20%. Vertebral fractures have a prevalence ranging between 7.6% and 37% and are more commonly observed in post-menopausal women.

Sub-optimal vitamin D status is common in patients with SLE, related to the limitation of sun exposure, glucocorticoid exposure and renal function. This deficiency has an impact on bone mass and remodelling and may be correlated with disease activity as well.[66]

Adequate supplementation of vitamin D is advised and correction of vitamin D insufficiency or deficiency with the administration of high doses is mandatory.

Osteoporosis is a well-established side effect of chronic glucocorticoid use; although the incidence of osteoporosis is time and dose dependent,

Table 5.   Ideal target values for classic risk factors in SLE.

Risk factor	"Ideal" target values
Blood pressure	<130 mmHg systolic and diastolic <80 mmHg
LDL cholesterol	<2.6 mmol/l
Diabetes mellitus	Fasting blood glucose <7.0 mmol/l
Obesity	Body mass index < 25 kg/m^2

there is no consensus about a "safe" dose. According to the EULAR-based recommendations on the management of systemic glucocorticoid therapy in rheumatic diseases, if a patient is started on prednisone >7.5 mg daily and continues on prednisone for more than three months, calcium and vitamin D supplementation should be prescribed.

Bisphosphonates are recommended in post-menopausal women with a history of fractures, with a T score of −2.5 or below and fractures or at high risk.

No data are available on the use of bisphosphonates in premenopausal women if pregnancy is planned. In these cases, the decision should be based on the patient risk profile for fractures.[23]

Cancer screening

SLE patients appear at high risk of developing cervical dysplasia due to an increased incidence of human papilloma virus (HPV) infection.

It has been recommended that patients with SLE undergo cancer screening according to the guidelines for the general population. However, as far as cervical intraepithelial neoplasm is concerned, Pap smears should be performed according to guidelines for immunosuppressed patients; HPV DNA testing may improve the specificity of the diagnosis and therefore should be considered.[64]

Adherence to therapy

Adherence to therapy could be defined as the extent to which a patient follows the prescriptions of physicians. Non-adherence to therapy is a generalized problem in the treatment of patients with chronic diseases, including rheumatic diseases. Different studies have shown non-adherence to therapy in up to 50% of patients, and has been reported particularly for hydroxychloroquine, calcium, vitamin D, and bisphosphonates.

Non-adherence to therapy may impact on the control of disease activity and the development of damage and therefore needs to be considered in our routine patient assessment: the failure of a drug to control disease activity could be due to the patients' non-adherence rather than the drug's ineffectiveness.

Conclusions

Over the past 50 years, the management and treatment of SLE has greatly changed regarding optimization and development of traditional immuno-suppressive drug protocols leading to increased patient survival. Nonetheless, SLE patients still present with flares, chronically active disease, and accrued damage. Also due to the side effects of drug therapy, the need for improved treatment strategies is required. Patient management based on a Treat-to-Target approach and the availability of new biotechnological drugs will inform future strategies to improve patient outcomes.

References

1. Block, S.R. (2006). A brief history of twins. *Lupus*, **15**, 61–64.
2. Ramos, P.S., Brown, E.E., Kimberly, R.P., Langefeld, C.D. (2010). Genetic factors predisposing to systemic lupus erythematosus and lupus nephritis. *Semin Nephrol*, **30**, 164–176.
3. Fernando, M.M., Stevens, C.R., Sabeti, P.C., Walsh, E.C., McWhinnie, A.J., Shah, A. *et al.* (2007). Identification of two independent risk factors for lupus within the MHC in United Kingdom families. *PLoS Genet*, **3**, 192.
4. Graham, R.R., Ortmann, W., Rodine, P., Espe, K., Langefeld, C., Lange, E. *et al.* (2007). Specific combinations of HLA-DR2 and DR3 class II haplo-types contribute graded risk for disease susceptibility and autoantibodies in human SLE. *Eur J Hum Genet*, **15**, 823–830.
5. Pickering, M.C., Botto, M., Taylor, P.R., Lachmann, P.J., Walport, M.J. (2000). Systemic lupus erythematosus, complement deficiency, and apopto-sis. *Adv Immunol*, **76**, 227–324.
6. Mak, A., Tay, S.H. (2014). Environmental factors, toxicants and systemic Lupus Erythematosus. *Int J Mol Sci.* **15**, 16043–16056.
7. Cleanthous, S., Tyagi, M., Isenberg, D.A., Newman, S.P. (2012). What do we know about self-reported fatigue in systemic lupus erythematosus? *Lupus*, **21**, 465–476.
8. Rovin, B.H., Tang, Y., Sun, J., Nagaraja, H.N., Hackshaw, K.V., Gray, L., *et al.* (2005). Clinical significance of fever in the systemic lupus erythema-tosus patient receiving steroid therapy. *Kidney Int*, **68**, 747–759.
9. Fernández, A., Quintana, G., Matteson, E.L., Restrepo, J.F., Rondón, F., Sánchez, A., Iglesias, A. (2004). Lupus arthropathy: historical evolution from deforming arthritis to rhupus. *Clin Rheumatol*, **23**, 523–526.

10. Kuhn, A., Landmann, A. (2014). The classification and diagnosis of cutaneous lupus erythematosus. *J Autoimmun*, 48–49, 14–19.
11. Weening, J.J., D'Agati, V.D., Schwartz, M.M., Seshan, S.V., Alpers, C.E., Appel, G.B., *et al.* (2004). The classification of glomerulonephritis in systemic lupus erythematosus revisited. *J Am Soc Nephrol*, **15**, 241–250.
12. Doria, A., Iaccarino, L., Sarzi-Puttini, P., Atzeni, F., Turriel, M., Petri, M. (2005). Cardiac involvement in systemic lupus erythematosus. *Lupus*, **14**, 683–686.
13. Carmier, D., Marchand-Adam, S., Diot, P., Diot, E. (2010). Respiratory involvement in systemic lupus erythematosus. *Rev Mal Respir*, **27**, e66–78.
14. Muscal, E., Brey, R.L. (2010). Neurologic manifestations of systemic lupus erythematosus in children and adults. *Neurol Clin*, **28**, 61–73.
15. Newman, K., Owlia, M.B., El-Hemaidi, I., Akhtari, M. (2013). Management of immune cytopenias in patients with systemic lupus erythematosus -old and new. *Autoimmun Rev*, **12**, 784–791.
16. Barr, S.G., Zonana-Nacach, A., Magder, L. S,, Petri, M. (1999). Patterns of disease activity in systemic lupus erythematosus. *Arthritis Rheum*, **42**, 2682–2688.
17. Gordon, C. (2002). Long-term complications of systemic lupus erythematosus. *Rheumatology*, **41**, 1095–1100.
18. Griffiths, B., Mosca, M., Gordon, C. (2005). Assessment of patients with systemic lupus erythematosus and the use of lupus disease activity indices. *Best Pract Res Clin Rheumatol*, **19**, 685–708.
19. Urowitz, M.B., Gladman, D.D., Tom, B.D., Ibañez, D., Farewell, V.T. (2008). Changing patterns in mortality and disease outcomes for patients with systemic lupus erythematosus. *J Rheumatol*, **35**, 2152–2158.
20. Ippolito, A., Petri, M. (2008). An update on mortality in systemic lupus erythematosus. *Clin Exp Rheumatol*, **26**, S72–79.
21. van Vollenhoven, R.F., Mosca, M., Bertsias, G., Isenberg, D., Kuhn, A., Lerstrøm, K. *et al.* (2014). Treat-to-target in systemic lupus erythematosus: recommendations from an international task force. *Ann Rheum Dis*, **73**, 958–967.
22. Badsha, H., Kong, K.O., Lian, T.Y., Chan, S.P., Edwards, C.J., Chng, H.H. (2002). Low-dose pulse methylprednisolone for systemic lupus erythematosus flares is efficacious and has a decreased risk of infectious complications. *Lupus*, **8**, 508–513.
23. Hoes, J.N., Jacobs, J.W.G., Boers, M., Boumpas, D., Buttgereit, F., Caeyers, N., *et al.* (2007). EULAR evidence based recommendations on the management of systemic glucocorticoid therapy in rheumatic diseases. *Ann Rheum Dis*, **66**, 1560–1567.

24. van Vollenhoven, R.F. (1998). Corticosteroids in rheumatic disease. Understanding their effects is key to their use. *Postgrad Med*, **103**(2), 137–142.
25. The Canadian hydroxychloroquine study group. (1998). A long-term study of hydroxychloroquine withdrawal on exacerbations in systemic lupus erythematosus. *Lupus*, **7**, 80–85.
26. Ruiz-Irastorza, G., Egurbide, M.-V., Pijoan, J.-I., Garmendia, M., Villar, I., Martinez-Berriotxoa, A., *et al.* (2006). Effect of antimalarials on thrombosis and survival in patients with systemic lupus erythematosus. *Lupus*, **15**, 577–583.
27. Austin II, H.A., Klippel, J.H., Balow, J.E., le Richie, N.G., Steinberg, A.D., Plotz, P.H. *et al.* (1986). Therapy of lupus nephritis. Controlled trial of prednisone and cytotoxic drugs. *N Eng J Med*, **314**, 614–619.
28. Boumpas, D.T., Austin, H.A. 3rd, Vaughn, E.M., Klippel, J.H., Steinberg, A.D., Yarboro, C.H. *et al.* (1992). Controlled trial of pulse methylprednisolone versus two regimens of pulse cyclophosphamide in severe lupus nephritis. *Lancet*, **340**, 741–745.
29. Illei, G.G., Austin III, H.A., Crane, M., Collins, L., Gourley, M.F., Yarboro, C.H. *et al.* (2001). Combination therapy with pulse cyclophosphamide plus pulse methylprednisolone improves long-term renal outcome without adding toxicity in patients with lupus nephritis. *Ann Int Med*, **135**, 248–257.
30. Houssiau, F.A., Vasconcelos, C., D'Cruz, D., Sebastiani, G.D., de Ramon Garrido, E., Danieli, M.G. *et al.* (2002). Immunosuppressive therapy in lupus nephritis the euro-lupus nephritis trial, a randomized trial of low-dose versus high-dose intravenous cyclophosphamide. *Arthritis Rheum*, **46**, 2121–2131.
31. Ioannidis, J.P., Katsifis, G.E., Tzioufas, A.G., Moutsopoulos, H.M. (2002). Predictors of sustained amenorrhea from pulsed intravenous cyclophosphamide in premenopausal women with systemic lupus erythematosus. *J Rheumatol*, **29**, 2129–2135.
32. Ognenovski, V., Marder, W., Somers, E.C., Johnston, C.M., Ferrehi, J.G., Selvaggi, S.M. *et al.* (2004). Increased incidence of cervical intraepithelial neoplasia in women with systemic lupus erythematosus treated with intravenous cyclophosphamide. *J Rheumatol*, **31**, 1763–1767.
33. Touma, Z., Gladman, D.D., Urowitz, M.B., Beyene, J., Uleryk, E.M., Shah, P.S. (2011). Mycophenolate mofetil for induction treatment of lupus nephritis: a systematic review and metaanalysis. *J Rheumatol*, **38**, 69–78.
34. Maneiro, J.R., Lopez-Canoa, N., Salgado, E., Gomez-Reino, J.J. (2014). Maintenance therapy of lupus nephritis with mycophenolate or azathioprine: systematic review and meta-analysis. *Rheumatology*, **53**, 834–838.
35. Callen, J.P., Spencer, L.V., Burruss, J.B., Holtman, J. (2001). Azathioprine: an effective, corticosterois sparing therapy for patients with recalcitrant cuta-

neous lupus erythematosus or with recalcitrant cutaneous leukocytoclastic vasculitis. *Arch Dermatol*, **127**, 515–522.

36. Sakthiswary, R., Suresh, E. (2014). Methotrexate in systemic lupus erythematosus: a systematic review of its efficacy. *Lupus*, **23**, 225–235.
37. Navarra, S.V., Guzman, R.M., Gallacher, A.E., Hall, S., Levy, R.A., Jimenez, R.E. *et al.* (2011). Efficacy and safety of belimumab in patients with active systemic lupus erythematosus: a randomised, placebo-controlled, phase 3 trial. *Lancet*, **377**, 721–731.
38. Furie, R., Petri, M., Zamani, O., Cervera, R., Wallace, D.J., Tegzová, D. (2011). A phase III, randomized, placebo-controlled study of belimumab, a monoclonal antibody that inhibits B lymphocyte stimulator, in patients with systemic lupus erythematosus. *Arthritis Rheum*, **63**, 3918–3930.
39. van Vollenhoven, R.F., Petri, M.A., Cervera, R., Roth, D.A., Ji, B.N., Kleoudis, C.S., *et al.* (2012). Belimumab in the treatment of systemic lupus erythematosus: high disease activity predictors of response. *Ann Rheum Dis*, **71**, 1343–1349.
40. Manzi, S., Sanchez-Guerrero, J., Merrill, J.T., Furie, R., Gladman, D., *et al.* (2012). Effects of belimumab, a B lymphocyte stimulator-specific inhibitor, on disease activity across multiple organ domains in patients with systemic lupus erythematosus: combined results from two phase III trials. *Ann Rheum Dis*, **71**, 1833–1838.
41. Ginzler, E.M., Wallace, D.J., Merrill, J.T., Furie, R.A., Stohl, W., Chatham, W.W. *et al.* (2014). Disease control and safety of belimumab plus standard therapy over 7 years in patients with systemic lupus erythematosus. *J Rheumatol*, **41**, 300–309.
42. Strand, V., Levy, R.A., Cervera, R., Petri, M.A., Birch, H., Freimuth, W.W., *et al.* (2014). Improvements in health-related quality of life with belimumab, a B-lymphocyte stimulator-specific inhibitor, in patients with autoantibody-positive systemic lupus erythematosus from the randomised controlled BLISS trials. *Ann Rheum Dis*, **73**, 838–844.
43. Parodis, I., Svenungsson, E., Axelsson, M. and Gunnarsson, I. (2014). Decreased disease activity and corticosteroid usage and no renal flares during belimumab treatment in patients with systemic lupus erythematosus. *Arthritis and Rheum*, **66**, 11 (Supplement).
44. Dooley, M.A., Houssiau, F., Aranow, C., D'Cruz, D.P., Askanase, A., Roth, D.A., *et al.* (2013). Effect of belimumab treatment on renal outcomes: results from the phase 3 belimumab clinical trials in patients with SLE. *Lupus*, **22**, 63–72.

45. Ekö, S.L., van Vollenhoven, R.F. (2014). Rituximab and lupus-a promising pair? *Curr Rheumatol Rep*, **16**, 444.
46. Gunnarsson, I., Sundelin, B., Jónsdóttir, T., Jacobson, S.H., Henriksson, E.W., van Vollenhoven, R.F. (2007). Histopathologic and clinical outcome of rituximab treatment in patients with cyclophosphamide-resistant proliferative lupus nephritis. *Arthritis Rheum*, **56**, 1263–1272.
47. Condon, M.B., Ashby, D., Pepper, R.J., Cook, H.T., Levy, J.B., Griffith, M., *et al.* (2013). Prospective observational single-centre cohort study to evaluate the effectiveness of treating lupus nephritis with rituximab and mycophenolate mofetil but no oral steroids. *Ann Rheum Dis*, **72**, 1280–1286.
48. Wallace, D.J., Gordon, C., Strand, V., Hobbs, K., Petri, M., Kalunian, K., *et al.* (2013). Efficacy and safety of epratuzumab in patients with moderate/severe flaring systemic lupus erythematosus: results from two randomized, double-blind, placebo-controlled, multicentre studies (ALLEVIATE) and follow-up. *Rheumatology*, **52**, 1313–1322.
49. Strand, V., Petri, M., Kalunian, K., Gordon, C., Wallace, D.J., Hobbs, K., *et al.* (2014). Epratuzumab for patients with moderate to severe flaring SLE: health-related quality of life outcomes and corticosteroid use in the randomized controlled ALLEVIATE trials and extension study SL0006. *Rheumatology*, **53**, 502–511.
50. Wallace, D.J., Kalunian, K., Petri, M.A., Strand, V., Houssiau, F.A., Pike, M. *et al.* (2014). Efficacy and safety of epratuzumab in patients with moderate/severe active systemic lupus erythematosus: results from EMBLEM, a phase IIb, randomised, double-blind, placebo-controlled, multicentre study. *Ann Rheum Dis*, **73**, 183–190.
51. Furie, R.A., Leon, G., Thomas, M., Petri, M.A., Chu, A.D., Hislop, C., *et al.* (2014). A phase 2, randomised, placebo-controlled clinical trial of blisibimod, an inhibitor of B cell activating factor, in patients with moderate-to-severe systemic lupus erythematosus, the PEARL-SC study. *Ann Rheum Dis*.
52. https://investor.lilly.com/releasedetail.cfm?ReleaseID=874281
53. Ginzler, E.M., Wax, S., Rajeswaran, A., Copt, S., Hillson, J., Ramos, E. *et al.* (2012). Atacicept in combination with MMF and corticosteroids in lupus nephritis: results of a prematurely terminated trial. *Arthritis Res Ther*, **14**(1):R33.
54. Wofsy, D., Isenberg, D., Licu, D. (2013). Efficacy and safety of atacicept for prevention of flares in subjects with moderate to severe systemic lupus erythematosus (SLE) [abstract]. *Arthritis Rheum*, **65**(Suppl 10), 1591.
55. Kieseier, B.C. (2014). Defining a role for laquinimod in multiple sclerosis. *Ther Adv Neurol Disord*, **7**(4), 195–205.

56. Jayne, D., Appel, G., Chan, T.M., Barkay, H., Weiss, R., Wofsy, D. (2013). A randomized controlled study of laquinimod in active lupus nephritis patients in combination with standard of care. *Ann Rheum Dis*, **72**, 164.
57. Illei, G.G., Shirota, Y., Yarboro, C.H., Daruwalla, J., Tackey, E., Takada, K., *et al.* (2010). Tocilizumab in systemic lupus erythematosus: data on safety, preliminary efficacy, and impact on circulating plasma cells from an openlabel phase I dosage-escalation study. *Arthritis Rheum*, **62**, 542.
58. Shirota, Y., Yarboro, C., Fischer, R., Pham, T.H., Lipsky, P., Illei, G.G., *et al.* (2013). Impact of anti-interleukin-6 receptor blockade on circulating T and B cell subsets in patients with systemic lupus erythematosus. *Ann Rheum Dis*, **72**, 118–128.
59. Szepietowski, J.C., Nilganuwong, S., Wozniacka, A., Kuhn, A., Nyberg, F., van Vollenhoven, R.F., *et al.* (2013). Phase I, randomized, double-blind, placebo-controlled, multiple intravenous, dose-ascending study of sirukumab in cutaneous or systemic lupus erythematosus. *Arthritis Rheum*, **65**, 2661–2671.
60. Merrill, J.T., Wallace, D.J., Petri, M., Kirou, K.A., Yao, Y., White, W.I., *et al.* (2011). Lupus Interferon Skin Activity (LISA) Study Investigators. Safety profile and clinical activity of sifalimumab, a fully human anti-interferon a monoclonal antibody, in systemic lupus erythematosus: a phase I, multicentre, double-blind randomised study. *Ann Rheum Dis*, **70**, 1905–1913.
61. Petri, M., Wallace, D.J., Spindler, A., Chindalore, V., Kalunian, K., Mysler, E., *et al.* (2013). Sifalimumab, a human anti-interferon-a monoclonal antibody, in systemic lupus erythematosus: a phase I randomized, controlled, dose-escalation study. *Arthritis Rheum*, **65**, 1011–1021.
62. McBride, J.M., Jiang, J., Abbas, A.R., Morimoto, A., Li, J., Maciuca, R., *et al.* (2012). Safety and pharmacodynamics of rontalizumab in patients with systemic lupus erythematosus: results of a phase I, placebo-controlled, double-blind, dose-escalation study. *Arthritis Rheum*, **64**(11), 3666–3676.
63. Kalunian, K., Merrill, J.T., Maciuca, R. (2012). Efficacy and safety of rontalizumab (anti-interferon alpha) in SLE subjects with restricted immunosuppressant use: results of a randomized, double-blind, placebo-controlled phase 2 study [abstract]. *Arthritis Rheum*, **64**(Suppl 10), 2622.
64. Mosca, M., Tani, C., Aringer, M., Bombardieri, S., Boumpas, D., Brey, R., *et al.* (2010). European League Against Rheumatism recommendations for monitoring patients with systemic lupus erythematosus in clinical practice and in observational studies. *Ann Rheum Dis*, **69**, 1269–1274.

65. Bruce, I.N. (2005). Cardiovascular disease in lupus patients: Should all patients be treated with statins and aspirin? *Best Pract Res Clin Rheumatol*, **19**, 823–838.
66. Toloza, S.M., Cole, D.E., Gladman, D.D., Ibañez, D., Urowitz, M.B. (2010). Vitamin D insufficiency in a large female SLE cohort. *Lupus*. **19**, 13–19.

CHAPTER 8

ADVANCES IN THERAPIES FOR SYSTEMIC SCLEROSIS

Vanessa Smith and Filip De Keyser

Introduction

Systemic sclerosis (SSc) is a rare multisystem connective tissue disease characterised by microvascular damage, fibrosis of the skin and internal organs and specific immunologic abnormalities. The clinical expression and course of the disease are very heterogeneous and may be coupled with serious morbidity and mortality. As yet, no treatment has been proven through randomised controlled trials to halt the natural progression of the "clinically recognizable" disease.

This chapter offers a general overview of the disease and its treatment and hints at future perspectives.

Epidemiology

Epidemiological studies in SSc have been hampered by the rarity of this condition, the imprecise estimation of date of onset and referral bias.[1] Incidence and prevalence of SSc vary according to the population studied. The prevalence in the United States has been described as 276 cases per million adults, in Europe as 8–15 cases per million.[2,3] Several recent series estimate a prevalence of about 1/10.000, with incidence rates of about

1/100.000.[4] The incidence increases with age and peaks between 45 and 64 years in both sexes.[2, 5, 6] Females are disproportionally affected, with a female to male ratio between 4:1 and 7:1.[2] Blacks are at higher risk than whites.[2, 5]

Pathogenesis

The pathogenesis of SSc is very complex and largely unknown.[7] Relevant data on pathogenic mechanisms are limited and difficult to interpret since most of the available information is derived from cross-sectional studies and from patients in various stages of the disease, often after treatment. Moreover, there are no satisfactory animal models of scleroderma.[8] It is generally accepted that there is an interaction between the main presentations of this disease: vascular damage, excessive collagen deposition (fibrosis) and autoimmunity.[8]

The hierarchy and relevance of cells and soluble mediators in the pathogenesis are not clear. In addition, the primary triggering event in SSc is unknown. Environmental factors may trigger, while various events and genetics also play a role.

Environmental factors

Several environmental stimuli have been postulated as triggering events. Among these are:

- Viral triggers, such as cytomegalovirus and parvovirus B19, through mechanisms of molecular mimicry.[9,10]
- Chemical components: *e.g.*, silica, solvents.[11]

Genetic predisposition and (epi)genetics

Studies of twins have failed to show a significant genetic component.[12] Nevertheless, there is support for an indirect genetic predisposition:

- Offspring of patients with SSc have a small but definite risk (<1%) of developing the disorder themselves.[13]

- Choctaw Americans have a higher prevalence of developing the disease than the rest of the population of the USA.[14]
- A multitude of genetic studies, ranging from candidate-gene studies to genome-wide association studies, have identified a large number of genetic susceptibility factors for SSc.[15] In this way the altered expression of >2500 genes involved in different biological functions, such as cell proliferation, antigen presentation and chemokine production have been described.[16–21] Attention has also been drawn to the role of epigenetic phenomena in SSc such as DNA methylation patterns, histone modifications and microRNAs.[15]

Immune activation/inflammation

Both humoral and cellular immune system alterations play a role in the pathogenesis of SSc. The activation of humoral immunity is witnessed by the presence of SSc-specific antibodies: anti-topoisomerase I/Scl-70 (anti-topo I), anti-centromere (ACA), anti-PM/Scl, anti-fibrillarin, anti-RNA polymerase I/III antibodies and anti-Th/To.[22]

Recently, autoantibodies against non-nuclear antigens have been described; among these are anti-fibrillin-1, anti-metalloproteinase (MMP)-1 and -3, anti-platelet derived growth factor receptor (PDGFR), anti-endothelial cells, anti-fibroblast, anti-angiotensin II type I receptor and anti-endothelin-1 type A receptor.[23–25]

The activation of cellular immunity is demonstrated among other things by the presence of mononuclear cell infiltrates that are found in the skin and lungs of patients with SSc.[26] The lesions consist mostly of T cells, B cells, dendritic cells, mast-cells and macrophages.[26] T cells in skin lesions are predominantly CD4+ cells, display markers of activation, exhibit oligoclonal expansion (suggesting activation in response to an unknown autoantigen) and are predominantly type 2 helper T (Th2)-cells, which produce profibrotic cytokines such as IL-4 and IL-13. In addition to the abnormal activation of T cells, disturbances in B cell homeostasis appear to be involved in the process of fibrosis and autoantibody production in SSc.[27] For example, one study showed that CD19 expression on B cells is increased in SSc patients to a level that leads to the production of autoantibodies in a mouse model. In addition, upregulated expression of CD80 and CD86 on memory B cells of SSc patients suggests that these cells are chronically activated.[27] Immune and resident cells cross-talk through cytokines and chemokines (non-exhaustive list: IL-1, 4, 6, 13, CXCL-8, 12, CCL-2, 5).[17]

Vascular damage

Vascular changes are ubiquitous in the small (capillaries and arterioles) and medium-sized vessels of patients with SSc. A vascular, inflammatory phase is believed to be the initial event in SSc.[8] The lesions are marked by loss of endothelial cells, proliferating pericytes, smooth-muscle cells and immune inflammatory events in the perivascular space.[28]

Endothelial damage

An unknown trigger causes progressive endothelial cell activation and endothelial damage resulting in apoptosis which results in capillary break-down.[29–31] The progressive loss of capillaries is not compensated as both angiogenesis and vasculogenesis are impaired in SSc.[29–31] The ensuing reduction of blood flow subsequently leads to hypoxia and oxidative stress which also play a role in the orchestration of vascular damage and fibrosis.[32]

Secondarily to endothelial dysfunction, platelets attach to the denuded endothelial surface and release TGF-β and connective tissue growth factor (CTGF), which in turn promote proliferation of smooth muscle cells in the wall of the vessel and surrounding fibroblasts.[29] Platelet aggregation causes *in situ* thrombosis.

Intimal fibrosis and periadventitial fibrosis

Activated smooth muscle cells are believed to migrate into the intimal layer, where they differentiate into myofibroblasts.[31] These then secrete collagen and other extracellular matrix proteins, causing intimal prolifera-tion that progressively narrows the lumen of the affected vessels, with subsequent reduction of the blood flow and hypoxia. Pericytes and vascular smooth muscle cells of the vascular wall proliferate vigorously, resulting in increased vascular wall thickness.[8]

Perivascular mononuclear cell infiltration

The activated endothelial cells express adhesion molecules which promote perivascular inflammatory infiltrates by enabling the transmigration of inflammatory cells through the endothelium.[26] The resulting endothelial cell disease is believed to result in the overproduction of contributors to vasoconstriction and fibrosis (such as endothelin [ET], angiotensin and serotonin), and eventually, an underproduction of vasodilators (prostacyclin, nitric oxide [NO]). This is phenotypically reflected in vascular hyperreactivity to cold, best exemplified by Raynaud's phenomenon (RP). All the above described structural changes (lumen narrowing, intimal and periadventitial fibrosis, capillary loss) result in an obliterative disease.[28] This occlusive, vasoconstrictive vasculopathy leads to the subsequent clinical manifestation of, for example, trophic lesions such as digital ulcers. Of note, the above described "vasoconstrictors and vasodilators" are targets in current and future therapies (see further).

Fibrosis

Fibrosis is also ubiquitous in SSc. There is fibrosis of the skin, which is disabling and disfiguring, and fibrosis of internal organs, contributing to morbidity and mortality. Histologic examination of lesional skin demonstrates a marked increase in thickness of the dermis. Normal dermal architecture is replaced by the dense accumulation of thickened and tightly packed collagen fibres. Except in the earliest stages of the disease, the dermis is usually devoid of inflammatory cells and fibroblasts are reduced.[33]

The role of fibroblasts in normal wound healing versus SSc

Normal wound healing

In normal wound healing, initial dermal injury is followed by an influx of macrophages and lymphocytes and 3 to 5 days later by the influx of fibroblasts. These turn into myofibroblasts, which are characterized among others things by smooth muscle actin.

Myofibroblasts are responsible for producing an extracellular matrix, contracting collagen fibers and closing the wound.[34] Profibrotic signaling competes with negative feedback from the matrix to produce an adequate fibrotic response, adequate scar formation, remodeling and termination. By two weeks following tissue injury, myofibroblasts undergo apoptosis which continues until the repaired tissue is almost acellular.[34]

Pathological wound healing in SSc

In SSc, wound healing is not correctly terminated and remodeled because of the persistence of profibrotic "on" signals, or the failure to generate "off" signals. In addition (myo)fibroblasts are prevented from undergoing apoptosis. Subsequently there is persistent activation of collagen genes (which differentiates SSc from normal response to injury), which is responsible for uncontrolled production of collagen, fibronectin and other extracellular-matrix components.[26]

Several factors in the activation of the fibroblasts have been identified. Among these are interleukins, chemokines (CXCL-4 and CCL-2), cytokines (TGF-β [key-profibrotic cytokine], CTGF, PDGF and ET), thrombin, ROS, activating antibodies, pericytes, direct cell-cell contact and tissue hypoxia.[8,26] Other mediators with important roles include the Wnt-β-catenin signaling pathway and lipid mediators (lysophosphatidic acid and sphingosine-1-phosphate).[35] Of note, some of these mediators are targeted by (novel) therapies.

Classification, Clinical Manifestations and Prognosis

Classification criteria

The former, but still frequently used, American College of Rheumatology (ACR) criteria for SSc were intended to allow classifying patients with definite disease.[36] The major criterion for definite SSc was skin thickening proximal to the metacarpophalangeal joints (Fig. 1a). The minor criteria were sclerodactyly (skin thickening of the fingers), digital pitting scars or loss of substance from the finger pad (depressed areas at the tips of the fingers or loss of digital pad tissue due to ischemia) (Fig. 1b–c) and bibasilar pulmonary fibrosis. When a patient meets the one major criterion

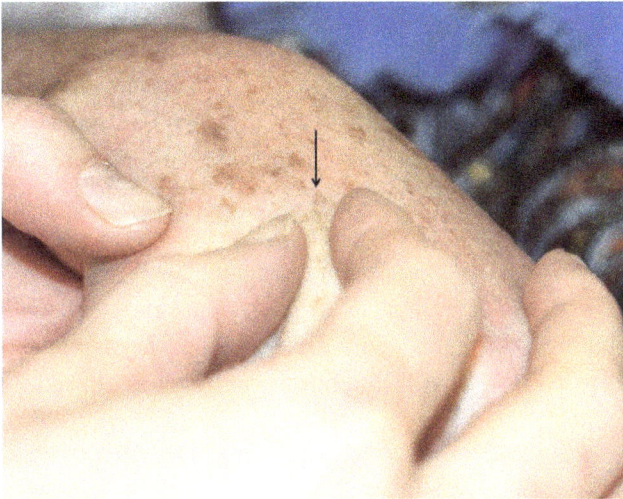

(a)

Figure 1a.   Major ACR criterion for SSc.

Skin thickening proximal to metacarpophalangeal joints. Note that the skin cannot be pinched. ($\leftarrow$)

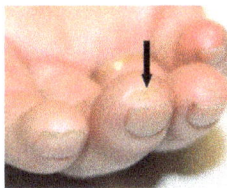

(b)

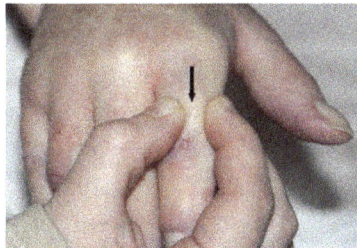

(c)

Figure 1b–c.   Minor ACR criteria for SSc.

Pitting scars (b) ($\leftarrow$); sclerodactyly (c) ($\leftarrow$)

or two of the minor criteria, the sensitivity and specificity to classify the patient correctly are 97% and 98%. The value of these criteria lies in the fact that they clearly point out that skin thickening is distinctive for SSc, occurring rarely in control patients.

A drawback of these criteria is that they are biased towards the fibrotic component of the disease. Consequently these criteria lack sensitivity for patients who predominantly have vascular manifestations of the disease, such as early SSc (see below) or limited cutaneous SSc.

Hence, new ACR/ European league against rheumatism (EULAR) criteria including vascular, immunologic and fibrotic manifestations have recently been published with the aim to encompass a broader spectrum of SSc.[37]

Clinical manifestations

The clinical manifestations of SSc are characterized by heterogeneity, varying from patients having almost no detectable skin involvement to patients with widespread skin involvement. In recent years, a descriptive sub-classification of diffuse cutaneous disease (DcSSc) versus limited cutaneous disease (LcSSc) has become widely accepted and used in clinical practice.[38] The value of this sub-classification lies in the fact that it is indicative both of the stage at which certain organ involvements may occur and also of mortality.

Subgroups based on skin involvement

LeRoy and Medsger proposed in 1988 two major clinical subsets based on the extension of the skin involvement.[38] A patient is defined as having DcSSc when the affected skin is proximal to elbow and knees (*i.e.* affecting upper arms, thighs, or trunk) (Fig. 2). When these changes remain distal to the elbows and knees, the patient is defined as having LcSSc. The skin involvement occurs, in most cases of patients with DcSSc, progressively during the first years of the "clinically recognisable" disease until a plateau is reached. In many cases, there are little or no further changes after this stage.[39]

The percentage of patients with the former subtype varies considerably across studies, for example between 17.0–44.6%.[2,6,40–42]

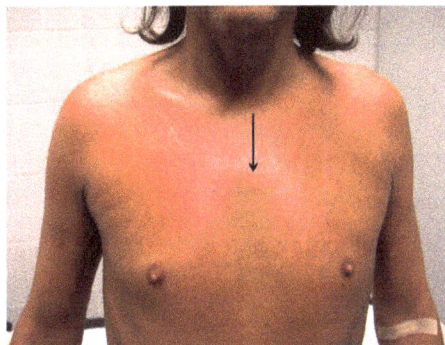

Figure 2. Patient with DcSSc.

This patient has skin involvement proximal to elbows and knees, more especially involving the thorax, where the taut and shiny may be noted. (←)

Organ involvement

Patients with DcSSc and LcSSc differ in the prevalence of organ manifestations. The most recent study on this was published in 2011 by the EULAR Scleroderma Trials and Research group (EUSTAR) (Table 1). In this study, prevalences of organ manifestations paralleled those of earlier published studies.[2,6,41] The time interval between the onset of Raynaud's phenomenon and skin and internal organ involvement varied significantly between disease subsets, being shorter for DcSSc and longer for LcSSc. Prominent clinical symptoms, such as digital ulcers, skin involvement, joint contractures, synovitis, tendon friction rubs, muscle weakness and/ or atrophy and organ involvement more specifically lung fibrosis, gastrointestinal tract, cardiovascular involvement and kidney involvement occured mostly in DcSSc whilst pulmonary arterial hypertension (PAH) occurred in equal frequencies in both subsets.[42]

Natural history of the disease

Patients with LcSSc nearly always have RP for years (even decades) before other clinical manifestations of SSc appear. The presence of skin thickening is typically restricted to the distal extremities (fingers, hands, distal forearms) and face.

Table 1. Organ involvement in patients with SSc according to subgroup.

	LcSSc	DcSSc	P value
ACR criteria fulfilled (%)	100	100	
Peripheral vascular involvement			
Raynaud's Phenomenon (%)	96.6	96.1	NS
Time from onset RP to onset first non-RP symptoms (years)	5.1	1.8	<0.001
Digital ulcers (%)	32.7	42.4	<0.001
ANA positive (%)	93.7	93.5	NS
ACA positive (%)	48.2	7.2	<0.001
Scl70 positive (%)	23.2	59.8	<0.001
RNA polymerase III positive (%)	1.2	4.7	<0.01
Musculoskeletal involvement			
Joint synovitis (%)	12.7	20.0	<0.001
Tendon friction rubs (%)	5.1	18.4	<0.001
Lung involvement			
Pulmonary arterial hypertension (%)	20.7	22.1	NS
Lung fibrosis (on HRCT) (%)	43.5	64.1	<0.001
Restrictive defect (lung function test) (%)	23.3	45.9	<0.001
Gastrointestinal involvement			
Esophageal symptoms (%)	66.4	69.5	<0.01
Stomach symptoms (%)	22.4	27.1	<0.001
Intestinal symptoms (%)	23.2	24.1	NS
Heart involvement			
Conduction blocks (%)	10.1	12.2	<0.01
Diastolic function abnormal (%)	17.2	18.0	NS
Pericardial effusion (%)	6.4	11.9	<0.001
Kidney involvement			
Renal crisis (%)	1.0	4.0	<0.001

ACA: anticentromere antibodies; ACR: American College of Rheumatology;[36] ANA: antinuclear antibodies; DcSSc: diffuse cutaneous systemic sclerosis; HRCT: high-resolution CT; LcSSc: limited cutaneous systemic sclerosis; NS: not significant; RNA: ribonucleic acid; RP: Raynaud's phenomenon; Scl70: anti-topoisomerase I antibodies. After Meier *et al.*[42]

Late and serious internal organ involvements are malabsorption and PAH.[43, 44] The mean survival in patients with PAH is 1.5–2 years.[45]

DcSSc characteristically has a prodromal phase of fatigue, arthralgias (or overt polyarthritis), carpal tunnel syndrome, puffy fingers, swollen legs and feet before the development of RP or skin thickening. The skin thickening typically evolves fast, in the first months or years. Severe internal organ involvement (gastrointestinal [GI], lung, heart, kidney) most often occurs during the first three years and carries a poor prognosis (see below).[46] After several years (> 5) and after skin involvement has reached its peak, it is unusual for new internal organ involvement to occur. Complications in this stage result from progression of fibrosis of the internal organs.

Severe organ involvement occurs in 31% of patients with DcSSc and portends poor survival. A large, single centre study with consecutive follow-up of patients with DcSSc (n = 953) showed that the 9-year cumulative survival rate in patients with severe organ involvement was 38%, while in patients without severe organ involvement it was 72%.

The most frequent severe organ involvement is severe skin involvement (defined as a mRSS >40 of a maximum possible score of 51) followed by severe renal, pulmonary, cardiac and severe GI involvement (Fig. 3).[46]

Subgroups based on SSc-selective autoantibodies

Another way to handle the extreme heterogeneity in clinical features and prognoses in SSc is to group patients by antibody profiles. This sub-grouping also has clinical and prognostic value, but is not used as often as that based on skin involvement because in most SSc centres, not all SSc-specific antibodies are detected routinely.

One representative feature of the immunological abnormalities in SSc patients is the presence of antinuclear antibodies (ANA), which are present in more than 90% of SSc patients.[47] ACA and anti-topo I antibodies are the classic ANA found in SSc. In addition to these ANA, anti-nucleolar antibodies (ANoA) are found less frequently in SSc subjects and comprise clinically distinct subsets. ANoA produce nucleolar staining patterns by indirect immunofluorescence staining (IIF) on human epithelioma type 2 (HEp-2) cells. ANoA are directed against different nucleolar proteins such as RNA polymerase (RNAP), small nuclear ribonucleoproteins (snRNP, Th/To) and

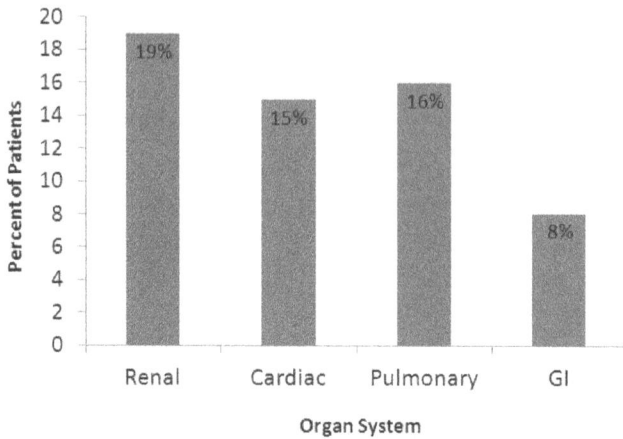

Figure 3.   Frequency of severe organ system involvement in 953 patients with systemic sclerosis and diffuse cutaneous involvement.

Renal: malignant arterial hypertension and/or rapidly progressive renal failure and/or microangiopathic hemolytic anemia (MAH). Patients with new-onset hypertension without increases in serum creatinine levels or MAH were not included, even if they were successfully treated with an angiotensin-converting enzyme (ACE) inhibitor. **Cardiac:** cardiomyopathy with a decrease in left ventricular ejection fraction and symptoms of congestive heart failure, symptomatic pericarditis that included pericardial pain or cardiac decompensation from effusion, or an arrhythmia attributable to scleroderma heart disease requiring treatment. Patients who had an asymptomatic decrease in the ejection fraction, an asymptomatic pericardial effusion or asymptomatic arrhythmias were not considered to have severe heart involvement. Non-scleroderma-related heart problems and non-specific asymptomatic changes on echocardiogram, electrocardiogram or Holter monitor were also not considered severe involvement. **Pulmonary:** pulmonary fibrosis (PF) on chest radiograph, with a forced vital capacity <55% of predicted. **GI tract:** malabsorption syndrome, repeated episodes of intestinal pseudo-obstruction or severe GI problems requiring hyperalimentation. Diarrhea responsive to antibiotics without malnutrition, bloating after meals, and esophageal stricture are evidence of significant GI involvement but were not classified as severe unless they were associated with a 10% weight loss or hospitalization. **After Steen *et al.*[46]**

fibrillarin components (U3RNP).[48] Among them, anti-RNAP frequently do not produce nucleolar staining with IIF but yield instead a speckled nucleolar pattern. They are specific for SSc and are rarely found in other diseases or in healthy individuals.[49] Screening for ANA is usually performed by IIF using HEp-2 cells, which is very sensitive.[50] Except for ACA, it is difficult to identify the specific ANA by IIF. Therefore additional techniques such as enzyme-linked immunosorbent assay (ELISA), immunodiffusion, immuno-precipitation and immuno assay are required to confirm ANA in a patient's serum.[51–55]

Mortality

Standardized mortality ratio, age adjusted mortality versus the general population and causes of death

SSc is associated with a significant reduction in survival compared with the general population. Standardised mortality ratios range, in different cohorts, from 1.5 to 7.2.[41] Causes of death are attributed to SSc in 55% of cases and comprise pulmonary fibrosis (35%), pulmonary arterial hypertension (26%), cardiac causes, mainly heart failure and arrhytmias (26%). Of the non-SSc related causes of death, infections (33%) and malignancies (31%) are followed by cardiovascular causes (29%).[56]

Predictors of mortality

Studies investigating predictors of mortality in SSc show diverging results, depending on sample sizes, determinants investigated, patient demographics (*e.g.*, different ethnicities), clinical subsets (different proportions of patients with DcSSc and LcSSc) and organ involvement and are thus difficult to compare.[1] In addition, different definitions of onset, such as the first symptom, the first physician diagnosis or the first centre visit, have been used. Consequently, several variables have been brought forward by various studies as predictive factors. Two illustrative examples follow. First, one single-centre prospective study proposed a prediction of five-year survival following presentation with SSc, with inclusion of incident cases (n = 280 [restricted to those subjects who both contracted the disease and also were referred after the starting year of the study]). Disease onset was defined as date of first self-reported skin change. All patients fulfilled the ACR criteria. This study showed that the combination of proteinuria, elevated ESR and low carbon monoxide diffusing capacity (DLCO) had an accuracy of >80% in predicting mortality within five years in new SSc patients, at first presentation in a SSc clinic. This study has been recently externally validated in a large EUSTAR cohort.[57] Second, a recent meta-analysis addressed incident cases (n = 1645) within six months of SSc diagnosis. SSc onset was defined from onset of first systemic sclerosis related symptom. Standardized definitions were used for disease subtype and organ involvement (renal, pulmonary, cardiac, and esophageal). In multivariate analyses adjusted for age and sex, renal (hazard ratio [HR]: 1.9; 95%-confidence interval [CI]: 1.4–2.5), cardiac (HR: 2.8; 95%-CI: 2.1–3.8), pulmonary (HR: 1.6; 95%-CI: 1.3–2.2) and anti-topo I antibodies (HR: 1.3; 95%-CI: 1.0–1.6) independently increased the risk of death.

A common denominator throughout the studies is that DcSSc and severe involvement of the heart, lungs and kidney adversely affected survival.[58–60]

Therapy

There is no approved "disease modifying anti-rheumatic drug" (DMARD) based on randomized controlled trials (RCT) that stops the natural evolution of the disease in SSc. At this very moment, clinical trials in SSc have focused on treating organ-specific manifestations. Some organ specific treatments are based on evidence resulting from RCT, others are based on expert opinion and some are mainly based on extrapolation from other diseases (such as the treatment of PAH and gastro-esophageal reflux [GER] disease). Most trials show only modest to moderate effects. Consequently, there is a need for continuous search for more appropriate therapies.

On a more positive note, recent prospective RCTs have shown beneficial effects on mortality in the treatment of PAH and early DcSSc.[61, 62]

Current therapies

Raynaud's phenomenon and digital ulcers

Based on expert opinion, analgesics are used to manage severe pain due to ischemia and ulceration. Adjunctive therapy such as warm clothing, gloves and paraffin baths may be prescribed in the treatment of RP.[63] There is evidence from RCTs that treatment with calcium channel blockers (CCB), prostanoids, fluoxetine, endothelin receptor antagonists (ERA), phosphodiesterase type 5 inhibitors (PDE-5-I), statins and topical nitro-glycerine application modulates peripheral vascular involvement in SSc.[64–82]

A meta-analysis of six placebo-controlled trials with calcium antago-nists in RP secondary to SSc showed a moderate reduction in number and severity of attacks.[64] The results of two RCT suggest a comparable effect of CCB and intravenous (IV) prostanoids on digital ulcer healing.[65, 66] A meta-analysis of treatments with prostanoids, including the results of five RCT with IV iloprost, one RCT with oral iloprost and one RCT with oral cisaprost, showed that both IV and oral prostanoids are effective in the treatment of SSc-RP, the former much more so than the latter.[67–77] Two RCTs indicate that IV prostanoids improved digital ulcer healing.[71,72] One small RCT describes fluoxetine to be superior to calcium channel blockers (nifedipine) in the treatment of SSc-related RP.[78] ERA (bosentan) have been shown to prevent the number of new digital ulcer formation in two RCT (especially in DcSSc patients) but neither trial indicated effectiveness in healing digital ulcers. One RCT showed the benefit of an angiotensin receptor antagonist (Losartan) in reducing the frequency and severity of RP attacks, and a recent meta-analysis of six RCT showed a significant but moderate benefit of PDE-5 inhibitors for the same purpose.[79, 80] In addition, PDE-5 inhibitors were suggested to have a healing effect on digital ulcers. An open-controlled trial comparing statins to placebo demonstrated a 50% relative reduction in the risk of developing new digital ulcers.[81] Next to oral therapy, topical therapy in the form of nitroglycerine application has also shown efficacy in alleviating RP symptoms based on a recent RCT.[82]

SSc-related PAH

PAH occurs in both subsets and within five years of disease duration in half of the cases, and is associated with high mortality rates. PAH is often advanced by the time of diagnosis with the majority of patients being in New York Heart Association (NYHA) functional class III or IV.[83] Early therapeutic intervention (NYHA functional class II) is associated with better survival. In this way, for example three-year survival in patients differed along their NYHA functional class: survival in NYHA functional class II was 80% whereas in NYHA functional class III, it was 72% and in NYHA functional class IV, 30% ($p = 0.006$).[83] As early treatment favors survival, it makes sense to screen patients based on validated screening algorithms.[83–86]

Treatment of SSc-related PAH follows the recently published recommendations of the Task Force for Diagnosis and Treatment of Pulmonary Hypertension of the European Society of Cardiology (ESC) and European Respiratory Society (ERS).[87] Evidence, based on RCT/meta-analyses, exists for treatment of NYHA functional class II, III and IV. More specifically, patients in NYHA class II should be treated with ERA (bosentan, ambrisentan, macitentan) or the PDE-5 inhibitors (sildenafil, tadalafil and riociguat) which have proven efficacy on either haemodynamics and morbidity, or a survival benefit versus historical controls.[61, 87–97] Notably, as the first drug in this field macitentan showed a reduction of both morbidity and mortality in a prospective event-driven study.[61] Also, based on EULAR recommendations, prostanoid therapy with epoprostenol (IV [flolan or veletri]), treprostinil (IV, subcutaneous or inhaled) or iloprost (inhaled) is to be used in NYHA class III or IV or when monotherapy with ERA or a PDE-5 inhibitor fails.[98–103]

Simultaneous use of more than one PAH-specific class of drugs is recommended by the Task Force of ESC and ERS for PAH patients responding inadequately to initial monotherapy and this recommendation may be followed in the treatment of SSc-PAH as well.[87,104]

SSc-related skin involvement

Diffuse skin involvement is a harbinger of severe morbidity/mortality. Only recently did RCTs demonstrate beneficial effects of therapies for this subset of SSc patients. Thus, haemopoietic stem cell transplantation (HSCT) was shown to be beneficial in two RCTs.[62,105] The first small randomised trial allocated 19 DcSSc patients to non-myeloablative HSCT or monthly pulses of cyclophosphamide (standard of care [=controls]). All patients who received HSCT achieved the primary endpoint, a decrease of modified Rodnan skin score (mRSS) by > 25% or an increase in forced vital capacity (FVC) by more than 10% at month 12, versus none of the controls. In the second randomised clinical trial, 156 early DcSSc patients were randomly allocated to HSCT or cyclophosphamide.[62] The trial showed that HSCT was superior in the primary outcome, survival and event-free survival, and also showed that the mRSS, one of the secondary endpoints, diminished significantly: −19.9 versus −8.8 in the control group, $p<0.001$.

The ability of other therapeutic compounds to modulate skin involvement in SSc, such as methotrexate (MTX), prostanoids, steroids and cyclophoshamide has been tested in small RCT or in RCTs for patients with organ involvement other than skin involvement as the primary outcome. Due to modest efficacy or detrimental side-effects (steroids), these agents are not believed to be top candidates to stop expanding skin involvement in SSc.

Concerning MTX, two RCT have shown a moderate effect of MTX on skin disease.[100] The first RCT included both LcSSc and DcSSc and both "early" and "non-early" patients. A significantly larger proportion of patients on MTX 15 mg/week reached predefined response criteria at 24 weeks than the placebo group. In addition, a trend towards improvement of skin score in the study population ($p = 0.06$) was demonstrated at week 24. The other RCT studied patients with "early" (disease duration <3 years from first non-RP SSc-related manifestation) SSc and treated with MTX for 12 months. mRSS dropped significantly (-4.3 points in the MTX treated group versus +1.8 in the placebo group [$p < 0.009$]) in an intent-to-treat-analysis.[106, 107] Bayesian analysis showed that the probability of a better outcome than placebo was 94% for the mRSS, 96% for the University of California, Los Angeles (UCLA) skin score and 88% for physician global assessment.[108] One RCT with pulse therapy with IV prostanoids found beneficial effects on skin score, as did also an RCT with IV pulse therapy with corticosteroids (dexamethasone).[66,109] Nevertheless, steroids are being used with caution as it is generally accepted that prednisolone ≥15 mg/day may trigger scleroderma renal crisis (see below). The impact of steroid use on the development of scleroderma renal crisis was evaluated in four retrospective studies, involving 544 patients, all suggesting an association between steroid treatment and the occurrence of scleroderma renal crisis.[110–113] A case-control analysis showed that 36% of patients with scleroderma renal crisis had received prednisone at a dose of 15 mg/day or more within six months preceding the onset of the crisis, compared to 12% matched controls (odds ratio 4.4; 95% — CI 2.1 to 9.4; $p < 0.001$).[111]

Lastly, skin score was affected beneficially (evaluated as secondary outcome measure) in a multi-centre large RCT with daily oral cyclophosphamide for 12 months versus placebo designed to evaluate the efficacy of cyclophosphamide in SSc-related interstitial lung disease (ILD) (see below [the Scleroderma Lung Study]). In this study cyclophosphamide had a beneficial effect on skin score throughout the 12 months of treatment, but the effects were not sustained following treatment cessation.[114, 15]

SSc-related renal crisis

There has been no RCT concerning the treatment of SSc-related renal crisis. Moreover, due to the rarity of this condition and its high mortality, it is unlikely that any will be conducted in the future. Based on an impressive survival benefit since its adoption, ACE-inhibition is now considered the treatment of choice for SSc-renal crisis. A prospective analysis of 108 patients with SSc-renal crisis showed that those treated with ACE-inhibition had 1-year and 5-year survival rates of 76% and 66% respectively, whereas the survival rates in the same time frames of those not treated this way were 15% and 10% respectively ($p < 0.001$).[116, 117] In addition, since the adoption of ACE-inhibition, 61% of patients with renal crisis have had a good outcome, as defined by the absence of requirement for sustained dialysis. As to whether ACE-inhibition may prevent future development of renal crisis, the reply is inconclusive as well-designed prospective studies are lacking.[118]

SSc-related gastrointestinal disease

In the absence of large long-term RCT, proton pump inhibitors are recommended for GER on the basis of expert opinion in combination with one small RCT describing a beneficial effect on GER symptoms.[119]

For motility disturbances, metoclopramide, octreotide and erythromycine are being used based on expert opinion.[120–123] When malabsorption caused by bacterial overgrowth occurs, empirical courses of broad-spectrum antibiotics such as quinolones or amoxicillin-clavulanic acid may be given, based on expert opinion.[124]

SSc-related interstitial lung disease

Immunosuppressive therapy is indicated in patients with moderate to severe ILD with a duration of less than four years or worsening lung function.[125]

Nevertheless, therapeutic options are limited. To date, only cyclophosphamide and stem cell transplantation have evidence through RCT for favorable effects on lung function.[62, 105, 114] In this way, strong immunosupression for one year with daily oral cyclophosphamide has been shown, in a large multi-centre RCT (the Scleroderma Lung Study I) with lung outcome as primary aim, to have modest beneficial effects on SSc-ILD lung function and dyspnea. Following cessation of treatment at 12 months, patients were followed up for a second year to see if the benefits of cyclophosphamide persisted. Pulmonary function and health status continued to improve until 18 months but the former deteriorated thereafter.[114, 115] At 24 months, only the beneficial effect on dyspnea had not waned. In an explanatory subanalysis, the differences observed between the treatment groups in FVC at 12 and 18 months were much greater in subjects who exhibited more severe restrictive lung disease at baseline, suggesting that the overall treatment effect may have been driven primarily by this subset.[115] Another randomised controlled study used IV cyclophosphamide in combination with oral corticosteroids followed by maintenance immunosuppression with azathioprine. This study reported an improvement in FVC at one year but failed to achieve statistical significance. Given the complications of long-term cyclophosphamide use (malignant disease, and haemorrhagic cystitis), consideration will be given to strategies that minimize cyclophosphamide exposure.[126]

HSCT has shown efficacy for lung function through two RCT (see above). The first had lung function, more specifically amelioration of FVC of at least 10% at one year after transplantation (and/or skin involvement) as primary outcome.[105] The second evaluated lung involvement as secondary outcome but equally to it suggested beneficial effects on lung involvement.[62] Nevertheless, due to iatrogenic transplant related mortality, these procedures are reserved for specialised centres.

Future treatments in systemic sclerosis

Treatment of SSc remains a challenge. To date, no treatment for skin or organ disease has proved unequivocally effective.[127] Potential future candidates are directed towards the three main components of the disease: inflammatory, vascular and fibrotic.[128,129] Future candidate therapies that are being assessed in a randomized setting are depicted in Table 2. In addition, some small trials are underway that are mainly directed at the fibrotic component of the disease. Thus, the TGF-β (key profibrotic cytokine) axis, which includes a large number of ligands, receptors and accessory molecules, is being targeted[125] and several small studies are under way that target fibroblast recruitment, fibrocyte differentiation and integrin signalling.[125]

Early Systemic Sclerosis

SSc is a heterogeneous autoimmune disorder characterised by vasculopathy, as well as progressive fibrosis of the skin and internal organs. When patients meet the ACR criteria, they already have "clinically recognizable" scleroderma (skin involvement) that can be classified as belonging to either the limited cutaneous (LcSSc) or the diffuse cutaneous subset (DcSSc).[38, 131] Patients with "clinically recognizable" SSc undergo morbidity and mortality. As yet, no treatment has been proven, through randomized controlled trial, to halt the natural progression of the "clinically recognizable" disease. Consequently, efforts are being made to study the disease "early", before the "clinically recognizable" disease has set in and irreversible damage has occurred, as this may create a window of opportunity for treatment.[132] With this aim in mind, LeRoy and Medsger in 2001 proposed criteria for the "early" diagnosis of SSc, with RP as the single major criterion. These criteria incorporate SSc-specific autoimmune antibodies and microvascular techniques, more specifically the "scleroderma-type" changes on capillaroscopy (a tool to evaluate the microcirculation at the nailfold and with diagnostic and biomarker characteristics).[22,133,134] Like the ACR criteria, the LeRoy and Medsger criteria include patients with "clinically recognizable" SSc (with skin involvement), LcSSc and DcSSc. But in addition to that, they also allow patients to be included "earlier", before skin involvement has occurred. This third group of patients is classified as having limited systemic sclerosis (LSSc), identified by the presence of RP plus the presence of SSc-specific autoimmune antibodies and/or typical "scleroderma-type" abnormalities on capillaroscopy.[135] The third group is referred to as "prescleroderma", as there is no skin involvement, and subsequently as "early" systemic sclerosis. Interestingly, these LeRoy's criteria have recently been validated.[136]

Table 2. Candidate future therapies that are currently being assessed in a RCT setting.

		Mode of action/Target	Clinical Trials.gov Identifier:	Indication	Primary clinical outcome measure
Inflammatory	Immunoglobulin IV	Anti-inflammatory	NCT01785056	Diffuse skin involvement	mRSS
	Belimumab	B-cell (BLyS)	NCT01670565	Diffuse skin involvement	mRSS
	Rituximab	B-cell (CD20)	NCT01748084	Active polyarthritis	Number of tender and swollen joints
	Mycophenolate Mofetil	T-cell	NCT00883129	Interstitial lung disease	FVC
	Pomalidomide	Anti-inflammatory	NCT01559129	Interstitial lung disease	FVC
	Abatacept	T-cell (CTLA4)	NCT00442611	Diffuse skin involvement	mRSS
	AIMSPRO	Anti-inflammatory	NCT00769028	Diffuse skin involvement	mRSS
	Tocilizumab	IL-6R	NCT01532869	Diffuse skin involvement	mRSS
	Rilonacept	IL-1	NCT01538719	Diffuse skin involvement	mRSS
Fibrotic	P144	TGF-β1	NCT00574613	Diffuse and limited skin involvement	Skin hardness
Vascular	Selexipag	Prostacyclin agonist	NCT02260557	SSc-RP	Number of RP attacks per week
	Zibotentan	ETA receptor	NCT02047708	Acute and chronic renal insufficiency	Soluble Vascular Cell Adhesion Molecule
	Macitentan	ETA/ETB receptor	NCT01474109	Digital Ulcers	Number of digital ulcers

mRSS: modified Rodnan skin score; BLyS = Soluble human B-lymphocyte stimulator; CD20: cluster of differentiation 20; FVC: forced vital capacity; CTLA4: cytotoxic T-lymphocyte antigen; AIMSPRO: Anti-inflammatory IMmuno-Suppressive PROduct: caprine immunglobulins and various small molecular weights species including cytokines;[130] IL-6R: interleukin 6 receptor; TGF: transforming growth factor; RP: Raynaud's phenomenon; ET: endothelin

Of note, recently additional criteria for the very early diagnosis of systemic sclerosis (VEDOSS) have been proposed which run in line with the LeRoy's criteria[137]

Conclusions

SSc is a devastating orphan disease characterised by systemic immunological, vascular and fibrotic abnormalities. Clinical manifestations are heterogeneous and associated with serious morbidity and mortality. No approved disease modifying treatment is available. There is a high unmet need to stop the natural course of the disease with progressive vasculopathy and fibrotic remodelling. New targets are aimed at tackling the three main components of the disease. Future therapies may be aimed at targeting the disease "early", before clinically overt disease and complications have set in.

References

1. Kernéis, S., Boëlle, P., Grais, R., Pavillon, G., Jougla, E., Flahault, A., *et al.* (2010). Mortality trends in systemic sclerosis in France and USA, 1980–1998: An age-period-cohort analysis. *Eur J Epidemiol*, **25**(1), 55–61.
2. Mayes, M.D., Lacey, J.V., Jr., Beebe-Dimmer, J., Gillespie, B.W., Cooper, B., Laing, T.J., *et al.* (2003). Prevalence, incidence, survival, and disease characteristics of systemic sclerosis in a large US population. *Arthritis Rheum*, **48**(8), 2246–2255.
3. Alamanos, Y., Voulgari, P.V., Drosos, A.A. (2004). Epidemiology of rheumatic diseases in Greece. *J Rheumatol*, **31**(8), 1669–1670; author reply 70–71.
4. Matucci Cerinic, M., Miniati, I., Denton, C. Eular On-line Course on Rheumatic Diseases — module n°20 — Systemic Sclerosis-Epidemiology. [cited 2007–2009; Available from: http://www.eular-onlinecourse.org]
5. Medsger, T.A., Jr., Masi, A.T. (1978). The epidemiology of systemic sclerosis (scleroderma) among male U.S. veterans. *J Chronic Dis*, **31**(2), 73–85.
6. Walker, U.A., Tyndall, A., Czirjak, L., Denton, C., Farge-Bancel, D., Kowal-Bielecka, O., *et al.* (2007). Clinical risk assessment of organ manifestations in systemic sclerosis: a report from the EULAR Scleroderma Trials And Research group database. *Ann Rheum Dis*, **66**(6), 754–763.
7. Derk, C.T., Jimenez, S.A. (2003). Systemic sclerosis: Current views of its pathogenesis. *Autoimmun Rev*, **2**(4), 181–191.

8. Gabrielli, A., Avvedimento, E.V., Krieg, T. (2009). Mechanisms of disease: scleroderma. *N Eng J Med*, **360**(19), 1989–2003.

9. Hamamdzic, D., Harley, R.A., Hazen-Martin, D., LeRoy, E.C. (2001). MCMV induces neointima in IFN-gammaR-/- mice: intimal cell apoptosis and persistent proliferation of myofibroblasts. *BMC Musculoskelet Disord*, **2**(3), 1–12.

10. Ohtsuka, T., Yamazaki, S. (2004). Increased prevalence of human parvovirus B19 DNA in systemic sclerosis skin. *J Dermatol*, **150**(6), 1091–1095.

11. Diot, E., Lesire, V., Guilmot, J.L., Metzger, M.D., Pilore, R., Rogier, S., *et al.* (2002). Systemic sclerosis and occupational risk factors: a case-control study. *Occup Environ Med*, **59**(8), 545–549.

12. Feghali-Bostwick, C., Medsger, T.A., Jr., Wright, T.M. (2003). Analysis of systemic sclerosis in twins reveals low concordance for disease and high concordance for the presence of antinuclear antibodies. *Arthritis Rheum*, **48**(7), 1956–1963.

13. Arnett, F.C., Cho, M., Chatterjee, S., Aguilar, M.B., Reveille, J.D., Mayes, M.D. (2001). Familial occurrence frequencies and relative risks for systemic sclerosis (scleroderma) in three United States cohorts. *Arthritis Rheum*, **44**(6), 1359–1362.

14. Arnett, F.C., Howard, R.F., Tan, F., Moulds, J.M., Bias, W.B., Durban, E., *et al.* (1996). Increased prevalence of systemic sclerosis in a Native American tribe in Oklahoma. Association with an Amerindian HLA haplotype. *Arthritis Rheum*, **39**(8), 1362–1370.

15. Broen, J., Radstake, T., Rossato, M. (2014). The role of genetics and epigenetics in the pathogenesis of systemic sclerosis. *Nat Rev Rheumatol*, **10**(11), 671–681.

16. Whitfield, M.L., Finlay, D.R., Murray, J.I., Troyanskaya, O.G., Chi, J.T., Pergamenschikov, A., *et al.* (2003). Systemic and cell type-specific gene expression patterns in scleroderma skin. *Proc Nat Acad Sci USA*, **100**(21), 12319–12324.

17. Katsumoto, T., Whitfield, M., Connolly, M. (2011). The pathogenesis of systemic sclerosis. *Annu Rev Pathol*, **6**: 509–537.

18. Milano, A., Pendergrass, S., Sargent, J., George, L., McCalmont, T., Connolly, M., *et al.* (2008). Molecular subsets in the gene expression signatures of scleroderma skin. *PLoS One*, **3**(7), e2696.

19. Johnson, R.W., Tew, M.B., Arnett, F.C. (2002). The genetics of systemic sclerosis. *Curr Rheumatol Rep*, **4**(2), 99–107.

20. Radstake, T., Gorlova, O., Rueda, B., Martin, J.E., Alizadeh, B., Palomino-Morales, R., *et al.* (2010). Genome-wide association study in systemic sclerosis identifies CD247 as a new susceptibility locus. *Nat Genet*, **42**: 426–429.

21. Arnett, F.C., Gourh, P., Shete, S., Ahn, C.W., Honey, R., Agarwal, S.K., *et al.* (2010). Major Histocompatibility Complex (MHC) class II alleles, haplotypes, and epitopes which confer susceptibility or protection in the fibrosing autoimmune disease systemic sclerosis: Analyses in 1300 Caucasian, African-American and Hispanic cases and 1000 controls. *Ann Rheum Dis*, **69**(5), 822–827.

22. LeRoy, E.C., Medsger, T.A., Jr. (2001). Criteria for the classification of early systemic sclerosis. *J Rheumatol*, **28**(7), 1573–1576.

23. Mihai, C., Tervaert, J. (2010). Anti-endothelial cell antibodies in systemic sclerosis. *Ann Rheum Dis*, **69**(2), 319–324.

24. Hénault, J., Robitaille, G., Senécal, J., Raymond, Y. (2006). DNA topoisomerase I binding to fibroblasts induces monocyte adhesion and activation in the presence of anti-topoisomerase I autoantibodies from systemic sclerosis patients. *Arthritis Rheum*, **54**(3), 963–973.

25. Riemekasten, G., Philippe, A., Näther, M., Slowinski, T., Müller, D., Heidecke, H., *et al.* (2011). Involvement of functional autoantibodies against vascular receptors in systemic sclerosis. *Ann Rheum Dis*, **70**(3), 530–536.

26. Codullo, V., Distler, O., Montecucco, C. Pathophysiology of systemic sclerosis. In: Cutolo, M., Smith, V., editors. *Novel Insights into Systemic Sclerosis Management*. London: Future Medicine Ltd; (2013). p. 23–35.

27. Sato, S., Fujimoto, M., Hasegawa, M., Takehara, K. (2004). Altered blood B lymphocyte homeostasis in systemic sclerosis: Expanded naive B cells and diminished but activated memory B cells. *Arthritis Rheum*, **50**(6), 1918–1927.

28. Wigley, F., Hummers, L. Management: Holistic approach to systemic sclerosis. In: Clements, P., Furst, D., editors. *Systemic Sclerosis*. Philadelphia: Lippincot Williams and Wilkins; (2004). p. 371–384.

29. Kuwana, M., Okazaki, Y., Yasuoka, H., Kawakami, Y., Ikeda, Y. (2004). Defective vasculogenesis in systemic sclerosis. *Lancet*, **364**(9434), 603–610.

30. Distler, O., Distler, J., Scheid, A., Acker, T., Hirth, A., Rethage, J., *et al.* (2004). Uncontrolled expression of vascular endothelial growth factor and its receptors leads to insufficient skin angiogenesis in patients with systemic sclerosis. *Circ Res*, **95**(1), 109–116.

31. Hummers, L.K., Wigley, F.M. (2003). Management of Raynaud's phenomenon and digital ischemic lesions in scleroderma. *Rheum Dis Clin North Am*, **29**(2), 293–313.

32. Gabrielli, A., Svegliati, S., Moroncini, G., Pomponio, G., Santillo, M., Avvedimento, E. (2008). Oxidative stress and the pathogenesis of scleroderma: The Murrell's hypothesis revisited. *Semin Immunopathol*, **30**(3), 329–337.

33. Varga, J., Korn, J.H. Pathogenesis: Emphasis on human data. In: Clements P., furst, D., editors. *Systemic Sclerosis*. Philadelphia: Lippincott Williams and Wilkins; (2004). p. 63–97.

34. Kissin, E.Y., Korn, J.H. (2003). Fibrosis in scleroderma. *Rheum Dis Clin North Am*, **29**(2), 351–369.

35. Beyer, C., Distler, O., Distler, J.H. (2012). Innovative antifibrotic therapies in systemic sclerosis. *Curr Opin in Rheumatol*, **24**(3), 274–280.

36. Preliminary criteria for the classification of systemic-sclerosis (sclero-derma). (1980). Subcommittee for scleroderma criteria of the American Rheumatism Association Diagnostic and Therapeutic Criteria Committee. *Arthritis Rheum*, **23**(5), 581–590.

37. van den Hoogen, F., Khanna, D., Fransen, J., Johnson, S.R., Baron, M., Tyndall, A., *et al*. (2013). 2013 classification criteria for systemic sclerosis: An American college of rheumatology/European league against rheuma-tism collaborative initiative. *Ann Rheum Dis*, **72**(11), 1747–1755.

38. LeRoy, E.C., Black, C., Fleischmajer, R., Jablonska, S., Krieg, T., Medsger, T.A., *et al*. (1988). Scleroderma (systemic-sclerosis) — Classification, subsets and pathogenesis. *J Rheumatol*, **15**(2), 202–205.

39. Black, C., Dieppe, P., Huskisson, T., Hart, F. (1986). Regressive systemic sclerosis. *Ann Rheum Dis*, **45**(5), 384–388.

40. Giordano, M., Valentini, G., Migliaresi, S., Picillo, U., Vatti, M. (1986). Different antibody patterns and different prognoses in patients with sclero-derma with various extent of skin sclerosis. *J Rheumatol*, **13**(5), 911–916.

41. Ioannidis, J.P., Vlachoyiannopoulos, P.G., Haidich, A.B., Medsger, T.A., Jr., Lucas, M., Michet, C.J., *et al*. (2005). Mortality in systemic sclerosis: An international meta-analysis of individual patient data. *Am J Med*, **118**(1), 2–10.

42. Meier, F., Frommer, K., Dinser, R., Walker, U., Czirjak, L., Denton, C., *et al*. (2012). Update on the profile of the EUSTAR cohort: An analysis of the EULAR Scleroderma Trials and Research group database. *Ann Rheum Dis*, **71**(8), 1355–1360.

43. Hachulla, E., de Groote, P., Gressin, V., Sibilia, J., Diot, E., Carpentier, P., *et al*. (2009). The three-year incidence of pulmonary arterial hypertension associated with systemic sclerosis in a multicenter nationwide longitudinal study in France. *Arthritis Rheum*, **60**(6), 1831–1839.

44. Marie, I., Ducrotte, P., Denis, P., Menard, J.F., Levesque, H. (2009). Small intestinal bacterial overgrowth in systemic sclerosis. *Rheumatology (Oxford)*, **48**(10), 1314–1319.

45. Kawut, S.M., Taichman, D.B., Archer-Chicko, C.L., Palevsky, H.I., Kimmel, S.E. (2003). Hemodynamics and survival in patients with pulmonary arterial hypertension related to systemic sclerosis. *Chest*, **123**(2), 344–350.

46. Steen, V.D., Medsger, T.A., Jr. (2000). Severe organ involvement in systemic sclerosis with diffuse scleroderma. *Arthritis Rheum*, **43**(11), 2437–2444.

47. Tan, E.M. (1989). Antinuclear antibodies: Diagnostic markers for autoimmune diseases and probes for cell biology. *Adv Immunol*, **44**, 93–151.

48. Lischwe, M.A., Ochs, R.L., Reddy, R., Cook, R.G., Yeoman, L.C., Tan, E.M., *et al.* (1985). Purification and partial characterization of a nucleolar scleroderma antigen (Mr = 34,000; pI, 8.5) rich in NG,NG-dimethylarginine. *J Biol Chem*, **260**(26), 14304–14310.

49. Harvey, G., Black, C., Maddison, P., McHugh, N. (1997). Characterization of antinucleolar antibody reactivity in patients with systemic sclerosis and their relatives. *J Rheumatol*, **24**(3), 477–484.

50. Ho, K.T., Reveille, J.D. (2003). The clinical relevance of autoantibodies in scleroderma. *Arthritis Res Ther*, **5**(2), 80–93.

51. Van Praet, J., Van Steendam, K., Smith, V., De Bruyne, G., Mimori, T., Bonroy, C., *et al.* (2011). Specific anti-nuclear antibodies in systemic sclerosis patients with and without skin involvement: An extend methodological approach. *Rheumatology (Oxford)*, **50**(7), 1302–1309.

52. Hamaguchi, Y. (2010). Autoantibody profiles in systemic sclerosis: Predictive value for clinical evaluation and prognosis. *J Dermatol*, **37**(1), 42–53.

53. Bonroy, C., Verfaillie, C., Smith, V., Persijn, L., De Witte, E., De Keyser, F., *et al.* (2013). Automated indirect immunofluorescence antinuclear antibody analysis is a standardized alternative for visual microscope interpretation. *Clin Chem Lab Med*, **51**(9), 1771–1779.

54. Bonroy, C., Smith, V., Van Steendam, K., Van Praet, J., Deforce, D., Devreese, K., *et al.* (2012). Fluoroenzymeimmunoassay to detect systemic sclerosis-associated antobodies: Diagnostic performance and correlation with conventional techniques. *Clin Exp Rheumatol*, **30**(5), 748–755.

55. Bonroy, C., Van Praet, J., Smith, V., Van Steendam, K., Mimori,, T., Deschepper, E., *et al.* (2012). Optimization and diagnostic performance of a single multiparameter lineblot in the serological workup of systemic sclerosis. *J Immunol Methods*, **379**(1–2), 53–60.

56. Tyndall, A., Bannert, B., Vonk, M., Airò, P., Cozzi, F., Carreira, P., *et al.* (2010). Causes and risk factors for death in systemic sclerosis: A study from the EULAR Scleroderma Trials and Research (EUSTAR) database. *Ann Rheum Dis*, **69**(10), 1809–1815.

57. Fransen, J., Popa-Diaconu, D., Hesselstrand, R., Carreira, P., Valentini, G., Beretta, L., *et al.* (2011). Clinical prediction of 5-year survival in systemic

sclerosis: Validation of a simple prognostic model in EUSTAR centres. *Ann Rheum Dis*, **70**(10), 1788–1792.

58. Jacobsen, S., Halberg, P., Ullman, S. (1998). Mortality and causes of death of 344 Danish patients with systemic sclerosis (scleroderma). *Brit J Rheumatol*, **37**(7), 750–755.

59. Bryan, C., Howard, Y., Brennan, P., Black, C., Silman, A. (1996). Survival following the onset of scleroderma: results from a retrospective inception cohort study of the UK patient population. *Brit J Rheumatol*, **35**(11), 1122–1126.

60. Hesselstrand, R., Scheja, A., Akesson, A. (1998). Mortality and causes of death in a Swedish series of systemic sclerosis patients. *Ann Rheum Dis*, **57**(11), 682–686.

61. Pulido, T., Adzerikho, I., Channick, R., Delcroix, M., Galiè, N., Ghofrani, H., *et al.* (2013) Macitentan and morbidity and mortality in pulmonary arterial hypertension. *New Engl J Med*, **369**(9), 809–818.

62. van Laar, J., Farge, D., Sont, J., Naraghi, K., Marjanovic, Z., Larghero, J., *et al.* (2014). Autologous hematopoietic stem cell transplantation vs intravenous pulse cyclophosphamide in diffuse cutaneous systemic sclerosis: A randomized clinical trial. *JAMA*, **311**(24), 2490–2498.

63. Wigley, F., Cutolo, M. Raynaud's phenomenon. In: Hachulla E, Czirják L, editors. *EULAR Textbook on Systemic Sclerosis*. 1st ed. London: BMJ Publishing Group Ltd; (2013). p. 115–128.

64. Thompson, A.E., Shea, B., Welch, V., Fenlon, D., Pope, J.E. (2001). Calcium-channel blockers for Raynaud's phenomenon in systemic sclerosis. *Arthritis Rheum*, **44**(8), 1841–1847.

65. Rademaker, M., Cooke, E.D., Almond, N.E., Beacham, J.A., Smith, R.E., Mant, T.G., *et al.* (1989). Comparison of intravenous infusions of iloprost and oral nifedipine in treatment of Raynaud's phenomenon in patients with systemic sclerosis: A double blind randomised study. *Bmj*, **298**(6673), 561–564.

66. Scorza, R., Caronni, M., Mascagni, B., Berruti, V., Bazzi, S., Micallef, E., *et al.* (2001). Effects of long-term cyclic iloprost therapy in systemic sclerosis with Raynaud's phenomenon. A randomized, controlled study. *Clin Exp Rheumatol*, **19**(5), 503–508.

67. Belch, J.J., Capell, H.A., Cooke, E.D., Kirby, J.D., Lau, C.S., Madhok, R., *et al.* (1995). Oral iloprost as a treatment for Raynaud's syndrome: A double blind multicentre placebo controlled study. *Ann Rheum Dis*, **54**(3), 197–200.

68. Kyle, M.V., Belcher, G., Hazleman, B.L. (1992). Placebo controlled study showing therapeutic benefit of iloprost in the treatment of Raynaud's phenomenon. *J Rheumatol*, **19**(9), 1403–1406.

69. Lau, C., Belch, J., Madhok, R., Cappell, H., Herrick, A., Jayson, M., *et al.* (1993). A randomised, double-blind study of cicaprost, an oral prostacyclin analogue, in the treatment of Raynaud's phenomenon secondary to systemic sclerosis. *Clin Exp Rheumatol*, **11**(1), 35–40.

70. McHugh, N.J., Csuka, M., Watson, H., Belcher, G., Amadi, A., Ring, E.F., *et al.* (1988). Infusion of iloprost, a prostacyclin analogue, for treatment of Raynaud's phenomenon in systemic sclerosis. *Ann Rheum Dis*, **47**(1), 43–47.

71. Wigley, F.M., Seibold, J.R., Wise, R.A., McCloskey, D.A., Dole, W.P. (1992). Intravenous iloprost treatment of Raynaud's phenomenon and ischemic ulcers secondary to systemic sclerosis. *J Rheumatol*, **19**(9), 1407–1414.

72. Wigley, F.M., Wise, R.A., Seibold, J.R., McCloskey, D.A., Kujala, G., Medsger, T.A., Jr., *et al.* (1994). Intravenous iloprost infusion in patients with Raynaud phenomenon secondary to systemic sclerosis. A multicenter, placebo-controlled, double-blind study. *Ann Intern Med*, **120**(3), 199–206.

73. Yardumian, D.A., Isenberg, D.A., Rustin, M., Belcher, G., Snaith, M.L., Dowd P.M., *et al.* (1998). Successful treatment of Raynaud's syndrome with Iloprost, a chemically stable prostacyclin analogue. *Brit J Rheumatol*, **27**(3), 220–226.

74. Pope, J., Fenlon, D., Thompson, A.E., Shea, B., Furst, D., Wells, G. (1998). Iloprost and cisaprost for Raynaud's phenomenon in progressive systemic sclerosis. *Cochrane Database Syst Rev*, **2**: CD000953.

75. Wigley, F.M., Korn, J.H., Csuka, M.E., Medsger, T.A., Jr., Rothfield, N.F., Ellman, M., *et al.* (1998). Oral iloprost treatment in patients with Raynaud's phenomenon secondary to systemic sclerosis: A multicenter, placebo-controlled, double-blind study. *Arthritis Rheum*, **41**(4), 670–677.

76. Black, C.M., Halkier-Sorensen, L., Belch, J.J., Ullman, S., Madhok, R., Smit, A.J., *et al.* (1998). Oral iloprost in Raynaud's phenomenon secondary to systemic sclerosis: A multicentre, placebo-controlled, dose-comparison study. *Brit J rheumatol*, **37**(9), 952–960.

77. Vayssairat, M. (1999). Preventive effect of an oral prostacyclin analog, beraprost sodium, on digital necrosis in systemic sclerosis. French Microcirculation Society Multicenter Group for the Study of Vascular Acrosyndromes. *J Rheumatol*, **26**(10), 2173–2178.

78. Coleiro, B., Marshall, S.E., Denton, C.P., Howell, K., Blann, A., Welsh, K.I., *et al.* (2001). Treatment of Raynaud's phenomenon with the selective serotonin reuptake inhibitor fluoxetine. *Rheumatology (Oxford)*, **40**(9), 1038–1043.

79. Dziadzio, M., Denton, C.P., Smith, R., Howell, K., Blann, A., Bowers, E., *et al.* (1999). Losartan therapy for Raynaud's phenomenon and scleroderma: Clinical and biochemical findings in a fifteen-week, randomized, parallel-group, controlled trial. *Arthritis Rheum*, **42**(12), 2646–2655.

80. Roustit, M., Blaise, S., Allanore, Y., Carpentier, P., Caglayan, E., Cracowski, J. (2013). Phosphodiesterase-5 inhibitors for the treatment of secondary Raynaud's phenomenon: Systematic review and meta-analysis of randomised trials. *Ann Rheum Dis*, **72**(10), 1696–1699.

81. Abou-Raya, A., Abou-Raya, S., Helmii, M. (2008). Statins: Potentially useful in therapy of systemic sclerosis-related Raynaud's phenomenon and digital ulcers. *J Rheumatol*, **35**(9), 1801–1808.

82. Hummers, L., Dugowson, C., Dechow, F., Wise, R., Gregory, J., Michalek, J., *et al.* (2013). A multi-centre, blinded, randomised, placebo-controlled, laboratory-based study of MQX-503, a novel topical gel formulation of nitroglycerine, in patients with Raynaud phenomenon. *Ann Rheum Dis*, **72**(12), 1962–1967.

83. Hachulla, E., Launay, D., Yaici, A., Berezne, A., de Groote, P., Sitbon, O., *et al.* (2010). Pulmonary arterial hypertension associated with systemic sclerosis in patients with functional class II dyspnoe: Mild symptoms but severe outcome. *Rheumatology (Oxford)*, **49**(5), 940–944.

84. Condliffe, R., Kiely, D., Peacock, A., Corris, P., Gibbs, J., Vrapi, F., *et al.* (2009). Connective tissue disease-associated pulmonary arterial hypertension in the modern treatment era. *Am J Respir Crit Care Med*, **179**(2), 151–157.

85. Coghlan, J., Denton, C., Grünig, E., Bonderman, D., Distler, O., Khanna, D., *et al.* (2014). Evidence-based detection of pulmonary arterial hypertension in systemic sclerosis: The DETECT study. *Ann Rheum Dis*, **73**(7), 1340–1349.

86. Hachulla, E., Gressin, V., Guillevin, L., de Groote, P., Cabane, J., Carpentier, P., *et al.* (2004). Pulmonary arterial hypertension in systemic sclerosis: Definition of a screening algorithm for early detection (the ItinérAIR-Scléerodermie Study). *Rev Med Interne*, **25**(5), 340–347.

87. Galiè, N., Corris, P., Frost, A., Girgis, R., Granton, J., Jing, Z., *et al.* (2013). Updated treatment algorithm of pulmonary arterial hypertension. *J Am Coll Cardiol*, **62**(25 Suppl D), 60–72.

88. Channick, R.N., Simonneau, G., Sitbon, O., Robbins, I.M., Frost, A., Tapson, V.F., *et al.* (2001). Effects of the dual endothelin-receptor antagonist bosentan in patients with pulmonary hypertension: A randomised placebo-controlled study. *Lancet*, **358**(9288), 1119–1123.

89. Rubin, L.J., Badesch, D.B., Barst, R.J., Galie, N., Black, C.M., Keogh, A., *et al.* (2002). Bosentan therapy for pulmonary arterial hypertension. *New Eng J Med*, **346**(12), 896–903.

90. Humbert, M., Barst, R.J., Robbins, I.M., Channick, R.N., Galie, N., Boonstra, A., *et al.* (2004). Combination of bosentan with epoprostenol in pulmonary arterial hypertension: BREATHE-2. *Eur Respir J*, **24**(3), 353–359.

91. Barst, R.J., Langleben, D., Frost, A., Horn, E.M., Oudiz, R., Shapiro, S., *et al.* (2004). Sitaxsentan therapy for pulmonary arterial hypertension. *Am J Respir Crit Care Med*, **169**(4), 441–447.

92. Wilkins, M.R., Paul, G.A., Strange, J.W., Tunariu, N., Gin-Sing, W., Banya, W.A., *et al.* (2005). Sildenafil versus Endothelin Receptor Antagonist for Pulmonary Hypertension (SERAPH) study. *Am J Respir Crit Care Med*, **171**(11), 1292–1297.

93. Liu, C., Chen, J. (2006). Endothelin receptor antagonists for pulmonary arterial hypertension. *Cochrane Database Sys Rev*, **3**: CD004434.

94. McLaughlin, V.V. (2006). Survival in patients with pulmonary arterial hypertension treated with first-line bosentan. *Eur J Clin Invest*, **36 Suppl 3**, S10–S15.

95. Galie, N., Ghofrani, H.A., Torbicki, A., Barst, R.J., Rubin, L.J., Badesch, D., *et al.* (2005). Sildenafil citrate therapy for pulmonary arterial hypertension. *New Eng J Med*, **353**(20), 2148–2157.

96. Benza, R.L., Mehta, S., Keogh, A., Lawrence, E.C., Oudiz, R.J., Barst, R.J. (2007). Sitaxsentan treatment for patients with pulmonary arterial hypertension discontinuing bosentan. *J Heart Lung Transplant*, **26**(1), 63–69.

97. Ghofrani, H., Galiè, N., Grimminger, F., Grünig, E., Humbert, M., Jing, Z., *et al.* (2013). Riociguat for the treatment of pulmonary arterial hypertension. *New Eng J Med*, **369**(4), 330–340.

98. Oudiz, R., Schilz, R., Barst, R., Galiè, N., Rich, S., Rubin, L., *et al.* (2004). Treprostinil, a prostacyclin analogue, in pulmonary arterial hypertension associated with connective tissue disease. *Chest*, **126**(2), 420–427.

99. Olschewski, H., Simonneau, G., Galiè, N., Higenbottam, T., Naeije, R., Rubin, L., *et al.* (2002). Inhaled iloprost for severe pulmonary hypertension. *New Eng J Med*, **347**(5), 322–329.

100. Kowal-Bielecka, O., Landewé, R., Avouac, J., Chwiesko, S., Miniati, I., Czirjak, L., *et al.* (2009). EULAR recommendations for the treatment of systemic sclerosis: A report from the EULAR Scleroderma Trials and Research group (EUSTAR). *Ann Rheum Dis*, **68**(5), 620–628.

101. Badesch, D., McGoon, M., Barst, R., Tapson, V., Rubin, L., Wigley, F., *et al.* (2009). Longterm survival among patients with scleroderma-associated pulmonary arterial hypertension treated with intravenous epoprostenol. *J Rheumatol*, **36**(10), 2244–2249.

102. Badesch, D., Tapson, V., McGoon, M., Brundage, B., Rubin, L., Wigley, F., *et al.* (2000). Continuous intravenous epoprostenol for pulmonary arterial hypertension due to the scleroderma spectrum of disease. A randomized, controlled trial. *Ann Intern Med*, **132**(6), 425–434.

103. Galiè, N., Hoeper, M., Humbert, M., Torbicki, A., Vachiery, J., Barbera, J., *et al.* (2009). Guidelines for the diagnosis and treatment of pulmonary hypertension: The task force for the diagnosis and treatment of pulmonary hypertension of the European Society of Cardiology (ESC) and the European Respiratory Society (ERS), endorsed by the International Society of Heart and Lung Transplantation (ISHLT). *Eur Heart J*, **30**(20), 2493–2537.
104. Bai, Y., Sun, L., Hu, S., Wei, Y. (2011). Combination therapy in pulmonary arterial hypertension: A meta-analysis. *Cardiology*, **120**(3), 157–165.
105. Burt, R., Shah, S., Dill, K., Grant, T., Gheorghiade, M., Schroeder, J., *et al.* (2011). Autologous non-myeloablative haemopoietic stem-cell transplantation compared with pulse cyclophosphamide once per month for systemic sclerosis (ASSIST): An open-label, randomised phase 2 trial. *Lancet*, **378**(9790), 498–506.
106. van den Hoogen, F.H., Boerbooms, A.M., Swaak, A.J., Rasker, J.J., van Lier, H.J., van de Putte, L.B. (1996). Comparison of methotrexate with placebo in the treatment of systemic sclerosis: A 24 week randomized double-blind trial, followed by a 24 week observational trial. *Brit J Rheumatol*, **35**(4), 364–372.
107. Pope, J.E., Bellamy, N., Seibold, J.R., Baron, M., Ellman, M., Carette, S., *et al.* (2001). A randomized, controlled trial of methotrexate versus placebo in early diffuse scleroderma. *Arthritis Rheum*, **44**(6), 1351–1358.
108. Johnson, S.R., Feldman, B.M., Pope, J.E., Tomlinson, G.A. (2009). Shifting our thinking about uncommon disease trials: The case of methotrexate in scleroderma. *J Rheumatol*, **36**(2), 323–329.
109. Sharada, B., Kumar, A., Kakker, R., Adya, C.M., Pande, I., Uppal, S.S., *et al.* (1994). Intravenous dexamethasone pulse therapy in diffuse systemic sclerosis. A randomized placebo-controlled study. *Rheumatol Int*, **14**(3), 91–94.
110. Helfrich, D.J., Banner, B., Steen, V.D., Medsger, T.A., Jr. (1989). Normotensive renal failure in systemic sclerosis. *Arthritis Rheum*, **32**(9), 1128–1134.
111. Steen, V.D., Medsger, T.A., Jr. (1998). Case-control study of corticosteroids and other drugs that either precipitate or protect from the development of scleroderma renal crisis. *Arthritis Rheum*, **41**(9), 1613–1619.
112. DeMarco, P.J., Weisman, M.H., Seibold, J.R., Furst, D.E., Wong, W.K., Hurwitz, E.L., *et al.* (2002). Predictors and outcomes of scleroderma renal crisis: The high-dose versus low-dose D-penicillamine in early diffuse systemic sclerosis trial. *Arthritis Rheum*, **46**(11), 2983–2989.
113. Teixeira, L., Mouthon, L., Mahr, A., Agard, C., Cabane, J., Guillevin, L., *et al.* (2006). Scleroderma renal crisis: Presentation, outcome and risk factors

based on a retrospective multicenter study of 50 patients. *Arthritis Rheum*, **54 (suppl)**, s743.

114. Tashkin, D.P., Elashoff, R., Clements, P.J., Goldin, J., Roth, M.D., Furst, D.E., *et al.* (2006). Cyclophosphamide versus placebo in scleroderma lung disease. *New Eng J Medm*, **354**(25), 2655–2666.

115. Tashkin, D.P., Elashoff, R., Clements, P.J., Roth, M.D., Furst, D.E., Silver, R.M., *et al.* (2007). Effects of 1-year treatment with cyclophosphamide on outcomes at 2 years in scleroderma lung disease. *Am J Respir Crit Care Med*, **176**(10), 1026–1034.

116. Steen, V.D., Costantino, J.P., Shapiro, A.P., Medsger, T.A., Jr. (1990). Outcome of renal crisis in systemic sclerosis: Relation to availability of angiotensin converting enzyme (ACE) inhibitors. *Ann Intern Med*, **113**(5), 352–357.

117. Steen, V.D., Medsger, T.A., Jr. (2000). Long-term outcomes of scleroderma renal crisis. *Ann Intern Med*, **133**(8), 600–603.

118. Hudson, M., Baron, M., Tatibouet, S., Furst, D., Khanna, D., Investigators, ISRCS. (2014). Exposure to ACE inhibitors prior to the onset of scleroderma renal crisis-results from the International Scleroderma Renal Crisis Survey. *Semin Arthritis Rheumatism*, **43**(5), 666–672.

119. Pakozdi, A., Wilson, H., Black, C., Denton, C. (2009). Does long term therapy with lansoprazole slow progression of oesophageal involvement in systemic sclerosis? *Clin Exp Rheumatol*, **27**(3 Suppl 54), S5–S8.

120. Johnson, D., Drane, W., Curran, J., Benjamin, S., Chobanian, S., Karvelis, K., *et al.* (1987). Metoclopramide response in patients with progressive systemic sclerosis. Effect on esophageal and gastric motility abnormalities. *Arch Intern Med*, **147**(9), 1597–1601.

121. Soudah, H., Hasler, W., Owyang, C. (1991). Effect of octreotide on intestinal motility and bacterial overgrowth in sclerodema. *New Eng J Med*, **325**(21), 1461–1467.

122. Dull, J., Raufman, J., Zakai, M., Strashun, A., Straus, E. (1990). Succesful treatment of gastroparesis with erythromycin in a patient with progressive systemic sclerosis. *Am J Med*, **89**(4), 528–530.

123. Ariyasu, H., Iwakura, H., Yukawa, N., Murayama, T., Yokode, M., Tada, H., *et al.* (2014). Clinical effects of ghrelin on gastrointestinal involvement in patients with systemic sclerosis. *Endocrine J*, **61**(7), 735–742.

124. Gasbarrini, A., Lauritano, E.C., Gabrielli, M., Scarpellini, E., Lupascu, A., Ojetti, V., *et al.* (2007). Small intestinal bacterial overgrowth: Diagnosis and treatment. *Dig Dis*, **25**(3), 237–240.

125. Nagaraja, V., Denton, C., Khanna, D. (2014). Old medications and new targeted therapies in systemic sclerosis. *Rheumatol (Oxford)*, [Epub ahead of print].

126. Wells, A.U., Latsi, P., McCune, W.J. (2007). Daily cyclophosphamide for scleroderma: Are patients with the most to gain underrepresented in this trial? *Am J Respir Crit Care Med*, **176**(10), 952–953.

127. Quillinan, N.P., Denton, C.P. (2009). Disease-modifying treatment in systemic sclerosis: current status. *Curr Opin Rheumatol*, **21**(6), 636–641.

128. Smith, V.P., Van Praet, J.T., Vandooren, B.R., Vander Cruyssen, B., Naeyaert, J.M., Decuman, S., *et al.* (2008). Rituximab in diffuse cutaneous systemic sclerosis: An open-label clinical and histopathological study. *Ann Rheum Dis*, **67**(1), 193–197.

129. Panopulos, S., Bournia, V., Trakada, G., Giavri, I., Kostopoulos, C., Sfikakis, P. (2013). Mycophenolate versus cyclophosphamide for progressive interstitial lung disease associated with systemic sclerosis: A 2-year case control study. *Lung*, **191**(5), 483–489.

130. Quillinan, N., McIntosh, D., Vernes, J., Haq, S., Denton, C. (2014). Treatment of diffuse systemic sclerosis with hyperimmune caprine serum (AIMSPRO): A phase II double-blind placebo-controlled trial. *Ann Rheum Dis*, **73**(1), 56–61.

131. Steen, V.D., Medsger, T.A. (2007). Changes in causes of death in systemic sclerosis, 1972–2002. *Ann Rheum Dis*, **66**(7), 940–944.

132. Matucci-Cerenic, M., Allanore, Y., Czirják, L., Tyndall, A., Müller-Ladner, U., Denton, C., *et al.* (2009). The challenge of early systemic sclerosis for the EULAR Scleroderma Trial and Research group (EUSTAR) community. It is time to cut the Gordian knot and develop a prevention or rescue strategy. *Ann Rheum Dis*, **68**(9), 1377–1380.

133. Cutolo, M., Smith, V. (2013). State of art on nailfold capillaroscopy: A reliable diagnostic tool and putative biomarker in rheumatology? *Rheumatology (Oxford)*, **52**: 1933–1940.

134. Smith, V., De Keyser, F., Pizzorni, C., Van Praet, J.T., Decuman, S., Sulli, A., *et al.* (2011). Nailfold capillaroscopy for day-to-day clinical use: Construction of a simple scoring modality as a clinical prognostic index for digital trophic lesions. *Ann Rheum Dis*, **70**(1), 180–183.

135. Cutolo, M., Smith, V. Nailfold capillaroscopy and other methods to assess the microvasculopathy in systemic sclerosis. In: Hachulla E, Czirjak L, editors. *EULAR Textbook on Systemic Sclerosis*. London: BMJ; (2013). p. 29–38.

136. Koenig, M., Joyal, F., Fritzler, M.J., Roussin, A., Abrahamowicz, M., Boire, G., *et al.* (2008). Autoantibodies and microvascular damage are independent predictive factors for the progression of Raynaud's phenomenon to systemic sclerosis: A twenty-year prospective study of 586 patients, with validation of proposed criteria for early systemic sclerosis. *Arthritis Rheum*, **58**(12), 3902–3912.

137. Avouac, J., Fransen, J., Walker, U.A., Riccieri, V., Smith, V., Muller, C., *et al.* (2011). Preliminary criteria for the very early diagnosis of systemic sclerosis: Results of a Delphi Consensus Study from EULAR Scleroderma Trials and Research Group. *Ann Rheum Dis*, **70**(3), 476–481.

CHAPTER 9

ADVANCES IN THERAPEUTIC STRATEGIES FOR INFLAMMATORY BOWEL DISEASE

Åsa Krantz and Sven Almer

Introduction

Inflammatory bowel disease (IBD) is a group of diseases characterized by a chronic, relapsing and progressive course of intestinal inflammation. It is classified into ulcerative colitis (UC), Crohn's disease (CD) and microscopic colitis (MC). The pathogenesis is not fully understood, but is multifactorial and thought to be a combination of dysregulated immune responses to gut bacterial antigens in the context of gut dysbiosis, genetic susceptibility and environmental triggers.[1–3] If disease-control is not reached, infectious, inflammatory and structural complications may occur. These complications add to the risk for surgery, hospitalization and impairment of health-related quality of life (HRQoL). Treatment aims to diminish these risks by reducing the inflammatory burden, change the disease course and avoid long-term complications.[2–4]

For almost two decades, the medical therapy repertoire for IBD remained unchanged, consisting of glucocorticosteroids (GCS), 5-aminosalicylic acid (5-ASA, mesalazine), antibiotics and immunomodulators such as thiopurines, methotrexate and cyclosporine. When these medications failed, treatment had to rely on more or less extensive bowel resections. In the early 21st century, biologic therapy with anti-TNF antibodies (aTNF) became available and revolutionized the treatment of IBD.[1,2,4] The first aTNF drug for IBD was infliximab, followed by adalimumab, certolizumab pegol and most recently, golimumab.[3,4] Even if aTNF is able to control disease activity in a large number of IBD patients, approximately 20–40% are primary non-responders, and of those who initially respond, 10–30% per year exhibit a loss of response (LOR).[1–3,5]

The last couple of years have been marked by landmark discoveries and advances in the understanding of the pathogenesis and components in the innate and acquired immune system response in IBD. As a consequence, new drugs with alternative and more specific modes of action have been developed or are under development.[6] Some of these have become available in the clinic in 2014, and others are in the pipeline. In addition, analyses for *therapeutic drug monitoring* (TDM) have become available. Furthermore, an improved understanding of pharmacogenetics has made it possible to optimize drug therapy and to individualize treatment better than previously.[1–4]

Here we discuss the shift in current treatment strategies and goals, the expansion of available drugs as well as optimization of already well-established therapies, and, finally, add some information on what is in the frontline for the future of IBD treatment. Table 1 provides an overview of the topics that will be dealt with in this chapter.

Treatment Goals, Concepts and Strategies

Treatment of IBD aims to treat the active inflammation and to prevent flares or reactivation of inflammation, so-called maintenance treatment. One needs to take into account the severity and extension of inflammation, the behavior of disease and any prevalent complications. The overall goal is to achieve long-term disease-control and to reduce disease-related outcomes such as hospitalization and the need for surgery by reducing the number of disease flares and emergence of complications; in other words, to change the natural course of IBD and maintain HRQoL. For all incident cases of

Table 1.   Treatment strategies in inflammatory bowel disease.

1. Early identification of patients at risk
2. Avoid tissue damage
3. From symptoms to treatment targets — 'treat-to-target'
4. Biomarkers
5. Window of opportunity
6. Rapid step-up
7. Mono or combo treatment
8. Optimization
9. Pharmacogenomics
10. If and when to stop treatment
11. New drugs

IBD, we aim to identify an effective treatment within six months, either with a relevant dose of 5-ASA, and/or an immunomodulator and/or aTNF-therapy depending on the severity of disease, so called *rapid-step-up strategy*.

The current treatment strategy for an acute flare does not differ much between UC and CD; however, in CD one also has to take into consideration the risk of abscess formation and stenosis and treat accurately. The first-line treatment for a severe attack of UC is GCS with evaluation of therapy response during the following two weeks. Depending on the clinical course, and if no adequate response is achieved, a decision about rescue-treatment with aTNF or cyclosporine is needed, aiming at *clinical* and *steroid-free remission*. In clinical practice, one should try not to prolong GCS treatment for more than three months. Thiopurines (azathioprine, 6-mercaptopurine) are, since two decades, used as steroid sparing agents both in UC and CD, *i.e.* mainly in steroid dependent chronic active disease.

The current approach for maintenance treatment of UC is a 5-ASA-based medication which is also effective in mild-to-moderate disease. In the case of repeated flares, despite optimal dosage of 5-ASA, or after a severe flare in GCS-dependent disease, an immunomodulator is indicated. If therapy fails despite optimal treatment with an immunomodulator, maintenance aTNF therapy should be considered.[7]

Since the clinical presentation in CD is more complex and diverse, the approach differs in some aspects. There is no convincing evidence that 5-ASA or cyclosporine has any effect in CD. Contrary to the situation in UC, methotrexate is a second-line immunomodulator in CD patients who fail or do not tolerate thiopurines.[8]

Recent data support that early and combined clinical and endoscopic remission is important for further disease evolution. It has been shown that symptomatic clinical remission is poorly correlated to the presence of ongoing inflammatory activity. Therefore new treat-to-target goals have been proposed. Goals that correlate better with short- and long-term outcomes are *mucosal healing* (MH) and *"deep remission"* (a combination of clinical, endoscopic and biochemical markers). Available data suggest that mucosal healing is associated with better long-term disease-control by reducing the future need for GCS, hospitalization and surgery. MH is also a predictor for maintenance of disease-free remission when aTNF therapy is stopped, as well as for reduced disability and bowel damage. These definitions are still evolving and further evidence is needed, particularly in CD where extra-luminal structures can be affected causing tissue damage and chronic disability.[1,3,4]

The *timing* of treatment with biologics is an important factor in disease control. The *step-up* approach has been the traditional strategy, meaning stepwise introduction of therapies beginning with the least systemically active medication and gradually intensifying the therapy when needed. This approach is valid for patients with mild-to-moderate disease. We have seen a shift towards so called *top-down* or *rapid-step-up* management in patients with expected severe disease outcome, especially in CD (Fig. 1). Early intervention with biologics has in many observational studies and RCT's shown to be more effective in inducing clinical remission and response.[3,5,9] There is a shift from stepwise treatment escalation to a more individualized approach trying to identify patients with increased risk for a complicated and aggressive disease course who might benefit from early biological treatment. In Crohn's disease, this approach is advocated when two or more risk factors for a disabling disease course are present (Table 2). Similar data for UC are not available, but factors to consider here are young age at diagnosis and extensive disease distribution.[3]

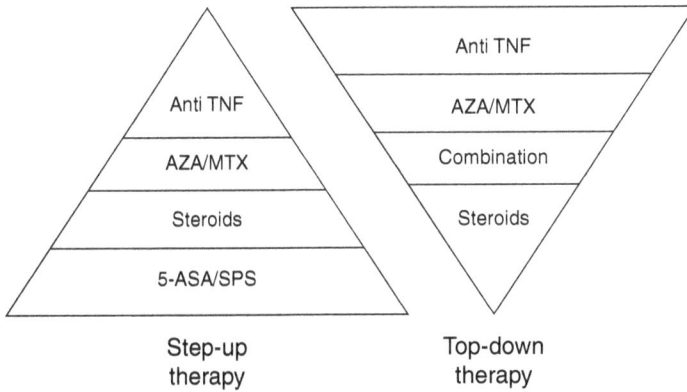

Figure 1. Schematic figure of proposed shift from Step-up therapy strategy to a top-down strategy with early aggressive treatment in a subgroup of patient with an expected aggressive disease course. AZA, azathioprine, MTX, methotrexate, 5-ASA, 5-aminosalicylic acid, SPS, sulphasalazine.

Table 2. Risk factors for disabling Crohn's disease within five years after diagnosis.[19]

Perianal disease
Ileocolonic location
Location in the upper GI-tract
Deep ulcers at endoscopy
Local complications (strictures, fistulas, or abscess)
Young age at diagnosis
Treatment of the first flare with glucocorticosteroids

To summarize, current data are pointing toward a case-by-case approach identifying those patients who would benefit from early aggressive treatment in order to reach the treat-to-target goal, mainly mucosal healing and/or stable clinical remission with normal biochemical markers, such as high-sensitive CRP and fecal calprotectin. The concept is to treat the patient before structural, irreversible damage with fibrosis development or perforation has emerged, mainly through early introduction of biologic agents which can change the natural course of the IBD. Hence, it is important to identify which patient would benefit from early intense treatment.

Personalized Medicine and Therapeutic Drug Monitoring

The immunomodulating drugs are far from being used in the most optimal way. The dosage is often standardized based on body weight; individual differences in pharmacodynamics and kinetics are not taken into consideration. One reason for this is the lack of easily accessible methods of drug monitoring in clinical practice, which includes both pharmacogenetic testing and measurement of drug levels and/or presence of antibodies towards biological drugs. At present, there is an unmet need of available *therapeutic drug monitoring* (TDM) methods which can help to individualize drug treatment in a more systematic way. Furthermore, a deepened understanding of pharmacodynamics and kinetics will make it possible to rationalize and tailor treatment to the individual patient.[1–4]

Thiopurines

Pharmacogenetic testing in clinical use for IBD is at the moment limited to thiopurine methyl transferase (TPMT) genotyping, often in combination with enzyme activity assays before initiating thiopurine treatment.[10] Approximately 10% of subjects have a heterozygous phenotype and they are at an increased risk for adverse events when introducing thiopurines in normal dose.[11] Less than 1% display a defective homozygous TPMT genotype translating into almost no TPMT activity. These patients are at a very high risk for fatal myelosuppression if treated.

Monitoring of thiopurine metabolites (6-TGN, 6-MMP) is available at many centres. The application of these assays has to some extent been hampered by a reported overlap between patients with active disease and those in remission with respect to the 6-TGNs that relate to anti-inflammatory effect and the 6-MMP that relates to the emergence of adverse events, such as myelosuppression and liver toxicity.[12] However, this discrepancy is mainly due to the use of different assays; when using well-validated assays, 6-TGN levels correlate with clinical remission.[13] Approximately one in seven patients have a 'skewed' or 'aberrant' metabolism,[14] meaning formation of excess of the methylated metabolites (meTIMP, MMP) to the detriment of phosphorylated metabolites (6-TGNs). These patients are at increased risk of lack of response and emergence of adverse events but can be "saved" back to effective treatment by combining low-dose thiopurine (25–30% of conventional doses) with the xanthine oxidase inhibitor, allopurinol.[15,16] By tradition, the combination of thiopurines with allopurinol has been given as absolutely contraindicated in pharmaceutical references due to the possible emergence of severe toxicity. However, when using TPMT and metabolite measurements, almost all of this risk is circumvented and long-term follow-up of these patients shows very low toxicity.

Overall, monitoring of thiopurine metabolism is indicated (1) when suspecting non-compliance; (2) in lack of efficacy, including skewed metabolism; (3) when contemplating use of higher than normal dosing; and (4) in the differential diagnosis of thiopurine related adverse events.[17]

Anti-TNF-antibodies

Even if therapy with aTNF has dramatically changed the treatment of moderate to severe IBD, approximately 20–40% of patients are primary non-responders and the occurrence of LOR in maintenance treatment ranges from 10% to 30% per year.[1–3,5]

aTNF serum drug levels correlate with the efficacy of treatment, both in rates of clinical remission and mucosal healing.[1,2,4,5,18] We have obtained a better understanding of factors that affect the clearance, drug concentration and primary response to aTNFs. Presence of severe bowel inflammation increases drug clearance. High CRP and low albumin levels correlate with lower serum drug concentrations. Several factors account for this; aTNF drug can be lost in faeces, an increased catabolism of aTNF in the reticuloendothelial system (RES) and antibody-associated neutralization of the drug. The disease phenotype has also been shown to influence aTNF clearance, where UC patients compared to CD patients more often exhibit undetectable trough levels. High weight and BMI are associated with low serum levels and early LOR. Age has been negatively associated with adalimumab clearance. In clinical practice, these factors are not systematically taken into consideration when deciding which dose of drug should be given[1,2] but observational studies suggest the use of increased infliximab dosing when treating an acute severe attack of UC, either with shortened dosing intervals or with an increase in dose to 10 mg or occasionally 20 mg per kg body weight.

A dilemma in the treatment with aTNF and other biologics is the development of *anti-drug antibodies* (ADA), which are associated with lower drug concentrations and hence loss of response. Besides increasing the risk of allergic reactions and anaphylaxis, ADA increase the drug clearance via formation of immune complexes eliminated in the RES and directly neutralize the biological activity of the drug.[1–3,5,18] ADA are associated with worse clinical symptoms and higher CRP levels independent of serum aTNF concentration, suggesting that immunogenicity disrupts efficacy beyond direct effects on drug concentrations. However, ADA do not consistently predict LOR, and ADA-formation may be associated with poorer clinical outcome in a titer and time dependent manner. For example, persistent ADA are associated with significantly higher ADA titers than transient ADA, and this conferred a much higher risk of LOR.[1–3]

Before aTNF drug assays became available, in LOR the strategy relied on intensification of treatment either by shortening of administration intervals or dose escalation (sometimes both) which recaptures response for a while but often LOR occurs again. Another option is to switch drugs either within the same class (another aTNF) or switch between drug classes.[1,2] Based on the access to TDM, new strategies and algorithms are emerging to support more rational decision-making when optimizing the use of anti-TNF therapy, mainly when LOR occurs. For example in patients with signs of ongoing inflammatory activity or LOR, one might have the following considerations: in case of high-titer ADA, one should switch drugs within class; in case of low-titer ADA and sub-therapeutic drug levels, one should consider dose escalation, switch within class or addition of an immunomodulator; if ADA testing is negative and drug levels are sub-therapeutic, one could consider dose escalation and addition of an immunomodulator; and lastly, if ADA testing is negative and drug levels are therapeutic, the most logical step would be to change drug class (Fig. 2). This type of risk-stratification-guided treatment has shown to be cost-effective,[1,2,4] but further data are required to clarify optimal treatment strategies.

Combination therapy with infliximab and the immunomodulator azathioprine has shown to be superior to monotherapy in inducing GCS-free and sustained remission, in CD as well as in UC.[3,9,18,19] The combined use of aTNF with methotrexate has not been shown to be superior to monotherapy. When combining two immunosuppressors, continuing attention

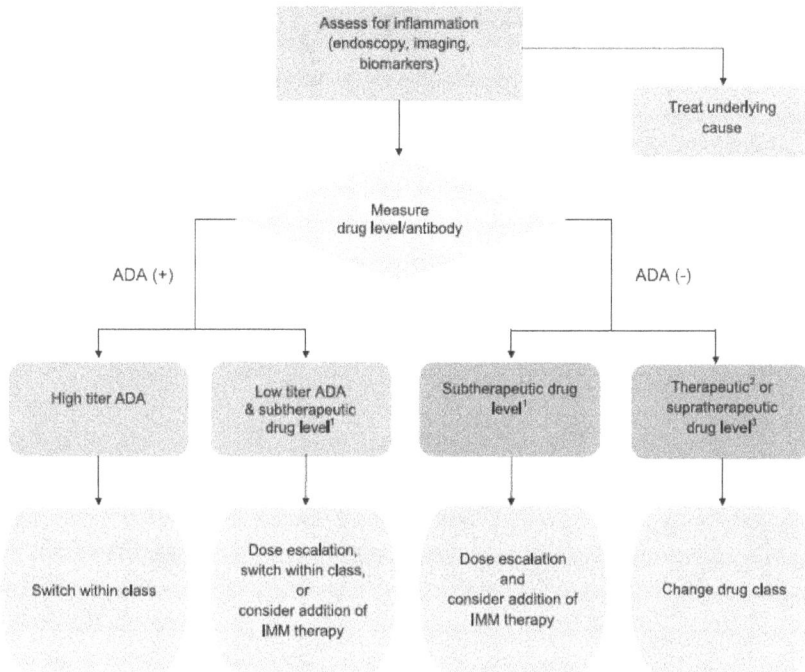

Figure 2.   Therapeutic drug monitoring to manage loss of response to anti–TNF therapy. ADA = anti-drug antibodies.[2]

needs to be taken to the risk of adverse events, such as severe infections or malignancy.[20]

Several mechanisms for the superior effect of combination therapy have been suggested, in addition to reduced immunogenicity and ADA formation. In contrast to adalimumab, infliximab has been shown to increase the levels of active thiopurine metabolites (6-TGN), hence optimizing thiopurine therapy.[21] Conversely, thiopurines may have a similar effect on infliximab turnover, increasing its trough levels.[22] Lastly, when using two immuno-suppressive agents with different modes of action, the anti-inflammatory spectrum becomes wider with an increased propensity to control inflammation. At present, the recommendation is shifting toward more frequent use of combination therapy in a selected subgroup of patients, decided on an individual basis weighing risks against benefits. A suggested approach to the use of combination therapy in clinical practice is shown in Fig. 3.[20] Further investigations are necessary to clarify the optimal duration of com-

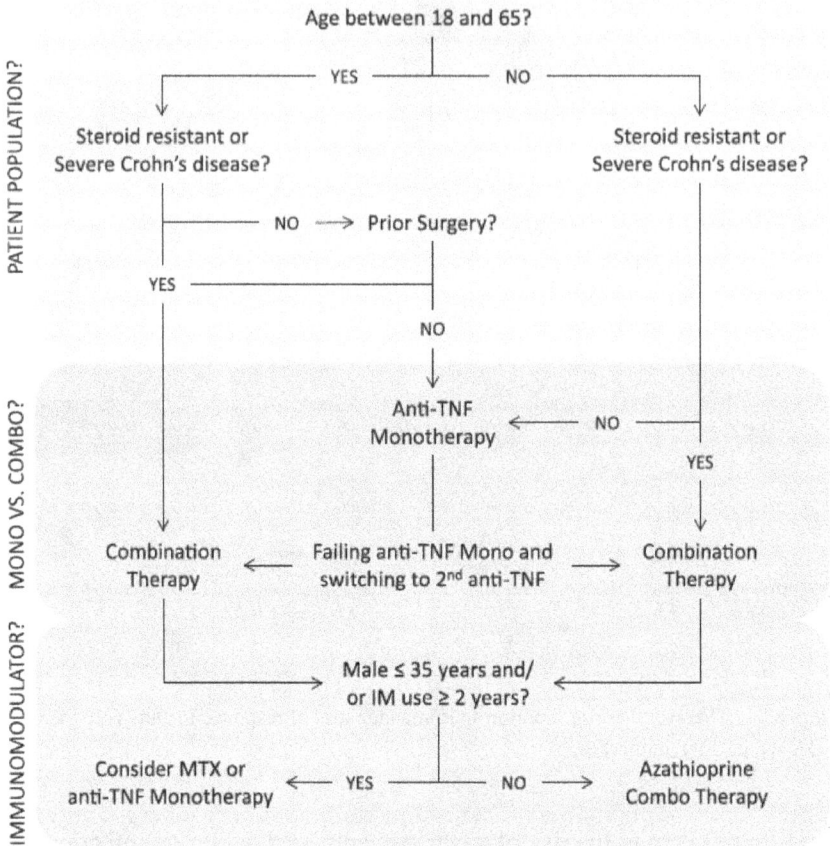

Figure 3.　Suggested approach to the use of combination therapy with an aTNF agent and thiopurines in clinical practice. Ultimately, the decision should be made on an individual basis after carefully weighing risks and benefits of each strategy. aTNF therapies are Infliximab, Adalimumab, Certolizumab pegol and Golimumab. IM, immunomodulator. MONO, monotherapy, COMBO, combination therapy.[20]

bination therapy with regards to efficacy versus risks associated with long-term double immunosuppressive therapy.[3,9,18,19]

In Table 3, we summarize some unresolved questions when individualizing treatment options. An important issue under debate is when to stop aTNF therapy. Long-term treatment with aTNF is expensive and exposes the patient to an increased risk of infections and some malignancies, but many

Table 3.   Unanswered questions in the treatment of inflammatory bowel disease.

Are there convincing advantages to phenotype-style strategies (PTSS), dissecting genetic correlates to individual phenotypes, when choosing treatment?

Is early drug introduction beneficial? If so, for whom, which drug and when?

Should dosing strategies be based on previous bowel resection or not?

Can we predict efficacy and/or adverse events with molecular signatures (biomarkers, mRNA-expression, etc)?

Where should appropriate biomarkers be measured — in the blood? In biopsies?

Is there potential clinical use for measuring "pharmacogenes", for example those related to drug transporters, or "immunogenes" related to the immune response?

Can combining half-dose drug A + half-dose drug B provide a full effect and fewer adverse events?

Head-to-head-comparisons within drug-classes and between drug-classes are lacking.

In patients with ongoing combined maintenance treatment ('combo-treatment') who are in durable remission: which drug to stop and when?

patients who stop aTNF treatment have a relapse of disease. In one study, approximately 52% relapsed within two years, while another study showed that patients who were in remission and discontinued aTNF treatment maintained remission for a median time of 13 months in patients with CD and 16 months in patients with UC.[36] Several factors could predict the risk of relapse, such as absence of mucosal healing at therapy cessation, elevated inflammatory indices, smoking and high infliximab trough levels. The STORI study sought to identify such risk factors, and in a selected subgroup of patients with low relapse risk, 90% were able to maintain stable remission for 24 months. This indicates that in patients with stable remission for at least six months and especially in those without biochemical or endoscopic evidence of active inflammation, withdrawal of aTNF therapy might be a viable option while continuing monotherapy with a thiopurine.[19,37]

New Therapeutic Targets — New Drugs on the Horizon

Due to advances in our understanding of the immune response in IBD, new therapeutic targets have been identified and translated into drugs with

Table 4. New treatment possibilities in inflammatory bowel disease.

Golimumab (Simponi) — in ulcerative colitis
Vedolizumab (Entyvio) — antibody to α4β7-integrin — in ulcerative colitis and Crohn's disease
aTNF-biosimilars (Inflectra, Remsima)
Etrolizumab — antibody to β7-integrin — in ulcerative colitis (and Crohn's disease?)
(Natalizumab (Tysabri) — antibody to α4-integrin — in Crohn's disease)
Ustekinumab (Stelara) — antibody to p40 IL12/IL23 — in refractory Crohn's disease
Tofacitinib — oral JAK-1/3-blocker — in ulcerative colitis

new modes of action. Some of these have been introduced into clinical practice during 2014 and others are underway. These new drugs and their modes of action are shown in Table 4; they include the integrin/CAM-inhibitors vedolizumab and etrolizumab; the p40-IL-12/23 blocker usteki-numab; and the small molecule JAK-1/3 inhibitors tofacitinib.[23, 24]

Integrin/CAM-inhibitors

Natalizumab, vedolizumab and etrolizumab are integrin inhibitors that block the interaction between T-cells (expressing integrin α4β7) and the adhesion molecule MAdCAM-1, disabling recruitment of T-cells to the gut and thereby decreasing the inflammation. The first effective integrin inhibitor was natalizumab, an α4-integrin-inhibitor. It was effective in inducing remission in CD, but its use has been limited because of the risk of progressive multifocal leukoencephalopathy (PML) based on its non-selectivity, also targeting lymphocyte trafficking to the central nervous system. The second-generation anti-trafficking agent, vedolizumab, is a gut-selective α4β7 integrin inhibitor that restricts leukocyte influx to the intestine. It became available for clinical use in 2014. Vedolizumab has in phase III trials shown promising results for the induction and maintenance of clinical response and remission with mucosal healing, both in CD and UC. Patients naive to aTNF as well as those who had failed aTNF treatment responded, but results were better in aTNF-naive patients. Its safety profile is reassuring with so far no increased risk of PML and, since it is gut-selective, a reduced risk of systemic infections.[24–26] A third-generation β7-integrin inhibitor, etrolizumab, has been tested in phase III trials of UC-patients.

Ustekinumab (IL-12/23 blocker)

Ustekinumab is a human monoclonal immunoglobin targeting the pro-inflammatory cytokines IL-12 and IL-23 by blocking the p40 subunit present in both IL-12 and IL-23.[27] IL-12 and IL-23 are involved primarily in the immunological pathogenesis of CD. In phase II trials, ustekinumab has shown high response rates in patients with moderate to severe CD who previously failed aTNF treatment, while remission rates were not statistically different from those on placebo.[24,28–30] Patients who had a clinical response in the induction phase maintained clinical response at week 22 and the rates of clinical remission became higher.[28,29] Safety data do not show an increased risk of serious adverse events. Ustekinumab has been used for the treatment of psoriasis for a longer time, and safety data in trials up to five years indicates no higher risk of malignancy or cardiovascular events, which initially was a concern.[28] The results of phase III trials in IBD are not yet available.

JAK-1/3 inhibitors: tofacitinib

Tofacitinib is an oral JAK-1/3 inhibitor. It acts by blocking the intracellular Janus kinases (JAK) 1/3 responsible for transducing signals from pro-inflammatory cytokines that play a crucial role in cell growth, survival, development and differentiation of immune cells. In phase II trials, a dose-dependent improvement in both clinical response and remission rates were found in moderate to severe UC. However, in CD tofacitinib showed no clinically significant response compared to placebo, although it was well tolerated. In the United States and many other countries, it has been approved for the treatment of rheumatoid arthritis.[6,23,24,27] The safety profile seems most similar to IL-6 blocking biologic therapies. Tofacitinib has been associated with a potential risk of opportunistic infections, lipid abnormalities, bone marrow suppression and lymphoma.[6,23,24,27] Other JAK inhibitors with different specificities and side-effect profiles are being studied in IBD.[6,24,27]

Biosimilars

Infliximab was the first aTNF approved for treatment of IBD. As the patent expires, *biosimilars* will enter the market. An infliximab biosimilar

(Inflectra, Remsima) is already available in most European countries. The advantage of a biosimilar is that it will be less expensive than the originator drug. Biosimilars are "versions" of the originator drug with enough similarities to be used in the same clinical indications, expecting similar efficacy and safety. However, biologics are very complex molecules in comparison to traditional generic drugs which are usually simple molecules with a highly reproducible way of manufacturing. Because of the complexity of biologics, one can expect differences between two different batches of the same drug. This raises questions about "identity" and "similarity" to the originator drug. Many regulatory authorities (*e.g.*, WHO, EMA, FDA) and scientific societies have agreed upon stringent criteria to assure quality data on efficacy and risks for humans in at least one of the diseases for which the originator previously has been approved. Another issue at hand is the relevance of giving full market authorization to a biosimilar for all indications approved for the originator in the absence of comparative clinical trials. Despite these issues, biosimilars are likely to become an important part in treating IBD patients in the future.[31]

On the Horizon

Cell-based therapy aims to restore the dysregulation or imbalance in the immune response in IBD. The different cell-based therapies that have been tested in IBD are *hematopoietic stem cell transplantation (HSCT)* in CD, *mesenchymal stem cell transplantation (MSC)* in refractory fistulizing and luminal CD, and injection of regulatory T cells *(Tregs)*.[23,32] HSCT has been effective in severe, highly refractory CD patients, although the long-term duration of drug-free remission is unknown. On the other hand safety concerns remain, since serious adverse events are common with mortality rates as high as 2–10%. Therefore more data are needed to investigate early and late effects of this treatment, which the ASTIC multicenter trial has addressed.[32,39] The infusion of MSCs is a well-tolerated therapy, but results on efficacy are inconsistent. The mode of action of MSCs is by immune modulatory properties to increase Tregs (anti-inflammatory) and decrease activated effector T cells (pro-inflammatory) in combination with tissue repair capacity. More clinical trials to evaluate these therapies are needed.

Therapy with injection of Tregs has been evaluated in early phase I/IIa trials and has shown promising results in patients refractory to conventional therapy. It was well tolerated and demonstrated dose-related efficacy.[32,33]

The application of antisense oligonucleotides (ASON) for the modulation of the inflammatory cascade is another, new treatment possibility. Systemic administration of alicaforsen, an ASON to ICAM-1, has not been successful in CD.[40] However, topical application may be useful in UC and pouchitis patients.[41] Recently, mongersen, an oral SMAD7 ASON that increases TGF-1β signaling, showed impressive efficacy in a short-term trial of CD without severe adverse events.[42] Further trials are underway and ASON might represent an important addition to the therapeutic armamentarium of IBD.

The involvement of the *microbiota* in the pathogenesis of IBD has received considerable attention during the last five years. In IBD, there is an imbalance in the composition of the microbiota in the gut with less diversity compared to healthy subjects, so called dysbiosis. Despite large efforts in identifying therapeutic targets and trying to restore the microbiota, at present there are no clinical therapies available.[34] Hopefully, new therapeutic avenues within this area will come in the future.

In CD, development of *intestinal fibrosis* with stricture formation and stenosis is a relatively frequent consequence of chronic inflammation. At the moment, these complications can be treated with endoscopic dilatation or surgery. Up to 80% of CD patients undergo surgery at least once during the course of their disease, and in up to 50% fibrotic strictures are the indication. Since extensive surgery increases the risk for short-bowel syndrome with diarrhea and malabsorption, it would be attractive to treat fibrosis medically to "save bowel". Indirectly, fibrosis development can be treated with effective anti-inflammatory therapies, but that is mainly before the fibrosis manifests. At present, there is no approved or effective medical therapy for treating fibrosis in IBD. There is ongoing research on anti-fibrotic therapy in scleroderma, lung, kidney and liver fibrosis with strategies based on interference with TGFβ expression, the use of tyrosine kinase blockers, and inhibition of specific molecules by microRNA.[35]

References

1. Altwegg, R., Vincent, T. (2014). TNF blocking therapies and immunomonitoring in patients with inflammatory bowel disease. *Mediators Inflamm,* **2014**, 7.
2. Lin, K., Mahadevan, U. (2014). Pharmacokinetics of biologics and the role of therapeutic monitoring. *Gastroenterol Clin North Am,* **43**(3), 565–579.
3. Singh, S., Pardi, D.S. (2014). Update on anti-tumor necrosis factor agents in crohn disease. *Gastroenterol Clin North Am,* **43**(3), 457–478.
4. Samaan, M.A., Bagi, P., Casteele, N.V., D'Haens, G.R., Levesque, B.G. (2014). An update on anti-TNF agents in ulcerative colitis. *Gastroenterol Clin North Am,* **43**(3), 479–494.
5. Cornillie, F., Hanauer, S.B., Diamond, R.H., Wang, J., Tang, K.L., Xu, Z., *et al.* (2014). Postinduction serum infliximab trough level and decrease of C-reactive protein level are associated with durable sustained response to infliximab: a retrospective analysis of the ACCENT I trial. *Gut,* **63**(11), 1721–1727.
6. Boland, B.S., Sandborn, W.J., Chang, J.T. (2014). Update on janus kinase antagonists in inflammatory bowel disease. *Gastroenterol Clin North Am,* **43**(3), 603–617.
7. Dignass, A., Lindsay, J.O., Sturm, A., Windsor, A., Colombel J-F, Allez, M., *et al.* (2012). Second European evidence-based consensus on the diagnosis and management of ulcerative colitis part 2: current management. *J Crohn's Colitis,* **6**(10), 991–1030.
8. Van Assche, G., Dignass, A., Panes, J., Beaugerie, L., Karagiannis, J., Allez, M., *et al.* (2010). The second European evidence-based Consensus on the diagnosis and management of Crohn's disease: Definitions and diagnosis. *J Crohn's Colitis,* **4**(1), 7–27.
9. Panccione, R., Ghosh, S., Middleton, S., Marquez, J.R., Khalif, I., Flint, L., *et al.* (2011). Infliximab, azathioprine, or infliximab+ azathioprine for treatment of moderate to severe ulcerative colitis: the UC SUCCESS trial. *Gastroenterology,* **140**(5), S–134.
10. Hindorf, U., Appell, M.L. (2012). Genotyping should be considered the primary choice for pre-treatment evaluation of thiopurine methyltransferase function. *J Crohn's Colitis,* **6**(6), 655–659.
11. Hindorf, U., Lindqvist, M., Peterson, C., Söderkvist, P., Ström, M., Hjortswang, H., *et al.* (2006). Pharmacogenetics during standardised initiation of thiopurine treatment in inflammatory bowel disease. *Gut,* **55**(10): 1423–1431.
12. Osterman, M.T., Kundu, R., Lichtenstein, G.R., Lewis, J.D. (2006). Association of 6-thioguanine nucleotide levels and inflammatory bowel disease activity: a meta-analysis. *Gastroenterology,* **130**(4), 1047–1053.

13. Moreau, A.C., Paul, S., Del Tedesco, E., Rinaudo-Gaujous, M., Boukhadra, N., Genin, C., *et al.* (2014). Association between 6-thioguanine nucleotides levels and clinical remission in inflammatory disease: a meta-analysis. *Inflamm Bowel Dis,* **20**(3), 464–471.

14. Appell, M.L., Wagner, A., Hindorf, U. (2013). A skewed thiopurine metabolism is a common clinical phenomenon that can be successfully managed with a combination of low-dose azathioprine and allopurinol. *J Crohn's Colitis,* **7**(6), 510–513.

15. Almer, S., Wagner, A., Måhl, M., Hindorf, U. (2014). P573 A combination of low-dose thiopurine and allopurinol (ThioComp) is long-term efficacious and well-tolerated in IBD patients. *J Crohn's Colitis,* 8, S307.

16. Sparrow, M.P., Hande, S.A., Friedman, S., Cao, D., Hanauer, S.B. (2007) Effect of allopurinol on clinical outcomes in inflammatory bowel disease nonresponders to azathioprine or 6-mercaptopurine. *Clin Gastroenterol Hepatol,* **5**(2), 209–214.

17. Chouchana, L., Narjoz, C., Beaune, P., Loriot, M.A., Roblin, X. (2012). Review article: the benefits of pharmacogenetics for improving thiopurine therapy in inflammatory bowel disease. *Alim Pharmacol Ther,* **35**(1), 15–36.

18. Colombel, J.F., Sandborn, W.J., Reinisch, W., Mantzaris, G.J., Kornbluth, A., Rachmilewitz, D., *et al.* (2010). Infliximab, azathioprine, or combination therapy for Crohn's disease. *N Eng J Med,* **362**(15), 1383–1395.

19. Louis, E., Mary, J.Y., Vernier–Massouille, G., Grimaud, J.C., Bouhnik, Y., Laharie, D., *et al.* (2012). Maintenance of remission among patients with Crohn's disease on antimetabolite therapy after infliximab therapy is stopped. *Gastroenterology,* **142**(1), 63–70. e5.

20. Parambir, S., Dulai, C.A.S., Laurent Peyrin-Biroulet. (2014). Anti–tumor necrosis factor-a monotherapy versus combination therapy with an Immunomodulator in IBD. *Gastroenterol Clin North Am,* 43(3), 441–456.

21. Roblin, X., Serre-Debeauvais, F., Phelip, J.M., Bessard, G., Bonaz, B. (2003). Drug interaction between infliximab and azathioprine in patients with Crohn's disease. *Alim Pharmacol Ther,* **18**(9), 917–925.

22. Reinisch, W., Colombel J.-F., Sandborn, W.J., Mantzaris, G.J., Kornbluth, A., Adedokun, O.J., *et al.* (2014). Factors associated with short- and long-term outcomes of therapy for crohn's disease. *Clin Gastroenterol Hepatol.*

23. Danese, S. (2012). New therapies for inflammatory bowel disease: from the bench to the bedside. *Gut,* **61**(6), 918–932.

24. Torres, J., Danese, S., Colombel, J.-F. (2013). New therapeutic avenues in ulcerative colitis: thinking out of the box. *Gut,* **62**(11), 1642–1652.

25. Feagan, B.G., Rutgeerts, P., Sands, B.E., Hanauer, S., Colombel, J.-F., Sandborn, W.J., *et al.* (2013). Vedolizumab as induction and maintenance therapy for ulcerative colitis. *N Eng J Med,* **369**(8), 699–710.

26. Sandborn, W.J., Feagan, B.G., Rutgeerts, P., Hanauer, S., Colombel, J.-F., Sands, B.E., *et al.* (2013). Vedolizumab as induction and maintenance therapy for Crohn's disease. *N Eng J Med,* **369**(8), 711–721.

27. Sandborn, W.J., Ghosh, S., Panes, J., Vranic, I., Su, C., Rousell, S., *et al.* (2012). Tofacitinib, an oral Janus kinase inhibitor, in active ulcerative colitis. *N Eng J Med,* **367**(7), 616–624.

28. Leung, Y., Panaccione, R. (2014). Update on ustekinumab for the treatment of crohn's disease. *Gastroenterol Clin North Am,* **43**(3), 619–630.

29. Sandborn, W.J., Gasink, C., Gao, L.-L., Blank, M.A., Johanns, J., Guzzo, C., *et al.* (2012). Ustekinumab induction and maintenance therapy in refractory Crohn's disease. *N Eng J Med,* **367**(16), 1519–1528.

30. Toedter, G.P., Blank, M., Lang, Y., Chen, D., Sandborn, W.J., de Villiers, W.J. (2009). Relationship of C-reactive protein with clinical response after therapy with ustekinumab in Crohn's disease. *Am J Gastroenterol,* **104**(11), 2768–2773.

31. Rinaudo-Gaujous, M., Paul, S., Tedesco, E., Genin, C., Roblin, X., Peyrin-Biroulet, L. (2013). Review article: biosimilars are the next generation of drugs for liver and gastrointestinal diseases. *Alim Pharmacol Ther,* **38**(8), 914–924.

32. Lanzoni, G., Roda, G., Belluzzi, A., Roda, E., Bagnara, G.P. (2008). Inflammatory bowel disease: moving toward a stem cell-based therapy. *World J Gastroenterol,* **14**(29): 4616–4626.

33. Voswinkel, J., Francois, S., Simon, J.-M., Benderitter, M., Gorin, N.-C., Mohty, M., *et al.* (2013). Use of mesenchymal stem cells (MSC) in chronic inflammatory fistulizing and fibrotic diseases: a comprehensive review. *Clin Rev Allergy Immunol,* **45**(2), 180–192.

34. Satokari, R. (2015). Contentious host-microbiota relationship in inflammatory bowel disease — can foes become friends again? *Scand J Gastroenterol,* **50**(1), 34–42.

35. Rosenbloom, J., Mendoza, F.A., Jimenez, S.A. (2013). Strategies for anti-fibrotic therapies. *Biochimica et Biophysica Acta (BBA)-Mol Basis Dis,* **1832**(7), 1088–1103.

36. Armuzzi, A., Marzo, M., Felice, C., De Vincentis, F., Andrisani, G., Mocci *et al.* (2010). Long-term scheduled therapy with infliximab in inflammatory bowel disease: a single-centre observational study. *Gastroenterology,* **138**(5):691–692.

37. Ben-Horin, S., Kopylov, U., Chowers, Y. (2014). Optimizing anti-TNF treatments in inflammatory bowel disease. *Autoimmun Rev,* **13**(1):24–30.

38. Molander, P., Färkkilä, M., Salminen, K., Kemppainen, H., Blomster, T., Koskela, R. *et al.* (2014). Outcome after discontinuation of TNF-blocking therapy in patients with inflammatory bowel disease in deep remission. *Inflamm Bowel Dis*, **20**(6):1021–1028.

39. Hawkey, C. , Allez, M., Clark, M., Labopin, M., Lindsay, J., Ricart, E. *et al.* (2015). Prolonged deep remission of ileocolonic crohn's disease following autologous haemopoetic stem cell transplantation, presented on behalf of all the ASTIC trialists. *J Crohns Colitis*,**9**(Suppl 1):S11–12.

40. Yacyshyn, B., Chey, W.Y., Wedel, M.K., Yu, R.Z., Paul, D., Chuang, E. (2007). A randomized, double-masked, placebo-controlled study of alicaforsen, an antisense inhibitor of intercellular adhesion molecule 1, for the treatment of subjects with active Crohn's disease. *Clin Gastroenterol Hepatol*, **5**(2):215–220.

41. Vegter, S., Tolley, K., Wilson Waterworth, T., Jones, H., Jones, S., Jewell, D. (2013). Meta-analysis using individual patient data: efficacy and durability of topical alicaforsen for the treatment of active ulcerative colitis. *Aliment Pharmacol Ther*, **38**(3):284–293.

42. Monteleone, G., Neurath, M.F., Ardizzone, S., Di Sabatino, A., Fantini, M.C., Castiglione, F., Scribano, M.L., Armuzzi, A., Caprioli, F., Sturniolo, G.C., Rogai, F., Vecchi, M., Atreya, R., Bossa, F., Onali, S., Fichera, M., Corazza, G.R., Biancone, L., Savarino, V., Pica, R., Orlando, A., Pallone, F. (2015). Mongersen, an oral SMAD7 antisense oligonucleotide, and Crohn's disease. *N Engl J Med*, **372**(12):1104–1113.

CHAPTER 10

SKIN, A DISPLAY ORGAN FOR THE IMMUNE SYSTEM — AN UPDATE ON PUTATIVE THERAPY TARGETS

Liv Eidsmo and Mona Ståhle

The skin provides a canvas for clinicians and researchers where induction and resolution of diseases, and thus the effect of novel treatments, can be followed by the naked eye. Topical or systemic corticosteroid treatment is still the dominating therapy in inflammatory diseases of the skin and induces unspecific and broad dampening of the skin immune system. Over the last few decades, basic research has enhanced our understanding of the immunopathology underlying common and rare dermatoses. In this chapter, we highlight a few skin diseases that arise due to chronic and exaggerated immune reactions in the skin and where increased knowledge of basic immunopathology has identified new therapeutic targets.

An Introduction to the Skin as an Immunological Organ

The skin forms a large physical barrier to the external environment and is covered by microbiota that adds an additional protective layer preventing colonization with pathogenic microbes. Recent studies have shown that microbiota constantly compromise the skin barrier. During normal homeostatic conditions, an effective immune system is able to control the microbial burden within the skin[1] whereas a hyperreactive immune system may cause inflammatory disorders in response to the normal microbiome in the absence of infective pathogens.[2] The skin epithelium, epidermis, is inhabited by traditional immune cells such as Langerhans cells and tissue resident T cells. Keratinocytes, in addition to serving as the structural backbone of the epithelium, are also capable of mounting immune responses upon activation, in particular by TLR driven inflammasome activation and IL-1β and IL-36 production. The underlying dermis harbours a multitude of cells: different populations of dendritic cells, T cells, innate lymphoid cells, mast cells and macrophages. The highly vascularised dermis permits rapid recruitment of neutrophils, eosinophils and monocytes upon inflammatory signals.[3] It seems that inflammatory skin disorders may arise from disruption of homeostasis of the skin immune system due to a mixture of environmental and genetic factors.

Autoinflammatory Skin Diseases are Caused by Mutations Enhancing Inflammasome Activity or IL-1β Signaling

Autoinflammatory diseases share the common skin phenotype of urticaria-like or pustular skin lesions with pronounced neutrophilic infiltration and these diseases also cause inflammation of bone, joints, gut or eyes in combination with systemic symptoms such as arthralgia and episodic fevers. Genetic and functional analyses have recently pin-pointed the exact alterations affecting the inflammasome and IL-1β system in a number of different autoinflammatory syndromes. The inflammasome is formed through intracellular assembly of proteins such as NLRP1, NLRP3, NLRC4 with caspase-1 and functions as first-line response to danger signals in peripheral tissues and facilitates the cleavage of pro-IL-1β to its active form. In homeostasis, IL-1β signaling through IL-1R, which is ubiquitously expressed, is controlled by IL-1R antagonists. IL-1β induces epithelial expression of another member of the IL-1 family, IL-36, which in turn is controlled by the IL-36R antagonist in homeostasis. Inflammasomes were initially

Autoinflammatory skin diseases

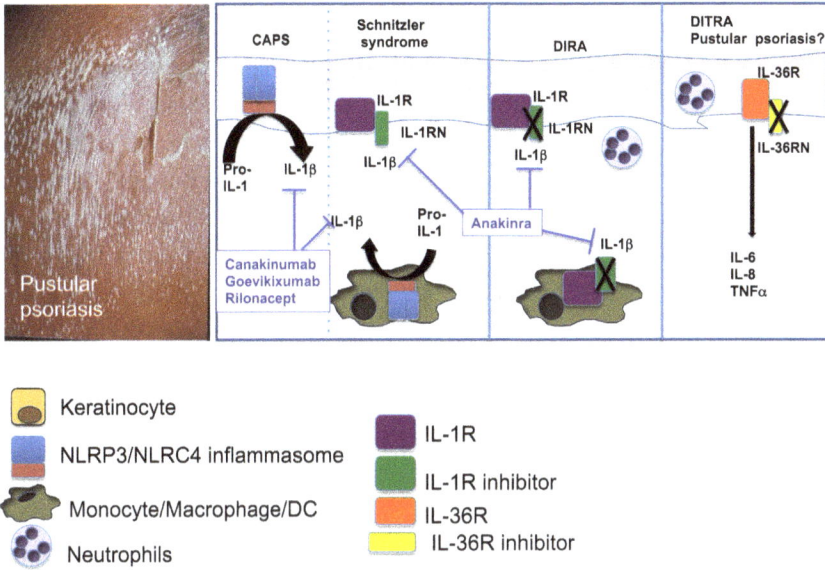

Figure 1. Autoinflammatory skin diseases are caused by mutations enhancing inflamma-some activity or IL-1β signaling.

Clinical picture of infiltration of neutrophils into the epidermis in pustular psoriasis (far left). In CAPS (cryopyrin-associated periodic syndromes) and Schnitzler syndrome, muta-tions of NLRP3/NLRC4 lead to increased production of IL-1β. As the name implies, a functional IL-1R antagonist deficiency causes DIRA (Deficiency of the Interleukin 1 Receptor Antagonist) whereas deficiencies in the IL-36 receptor antagonist have been shown in DITRA (Deficiency of the IL-36R antagonist) and a few cases of pustular psoria-sis. Monoclonal antibody therapies blocking IL-1β (canakinumab and geovikizumab), the recombinant IL-1R antagonist anakinra and the soluble IL-1β receptor rilonacept are avail-able therapies for CAPS, Schnitzler syndrome and DIRA.

identified in hematopoetic cells such as macrophages and dendritic cells, but keratinocytes also express NLRP1, NLRP3 and AIM2 and are effective in inflammasome activation and IL-1β signaling.[4] In autoinflammatory diseases, normal stimuli such as the constant and homeostatic interaction with the microbiota or other danger signals will lead to an exaggerated activation of the inflammasome and IL-1β and IL-36 signaling and thus cause skin pathology.

Missense mutations of the NLRP3 inflammasome protein leads to inflammasome over-activation in the cryopyrin-associated periodic syndromes (CAPS) with intermittent fevers and cold-induced urticaria.[5] CAPS was recently linked to mutations in another inflammasome protein, NLRC4, in a Japanese study.[6] The Schnitzler syndrome is associated with chronic urticaria, IgM gammopathy, bone pain, arthralgia and systemic inflammation with IL-1β over-expression in peripheral blood mononuclear cells. Exome sequencing revealed myeloid lineage-restricted somatic mosaicism of NLRP3 mutations whereas keratinocytes were not affected in three Schnitzler patients.[7] These results have initiated a discussion within the field of dermatology of whether the Schnitzler syndrome is a variant of CAPS. Through a candidate gene approach and sequencing of IL-1RN, the rare autosomal recessive disease Deficiency of the Interleukin 1 Receptor Antagonist (DIRA) was characterised in a number of families from the Netherlands, Libanon, Puerto Rico and Newfoundland.[8] The functional IL-1R antagonist deficiency presents with severe pustular skin eruptions, nail dystrophy and skeletal malformations and DIRA is often lethal already in childhood. A valuable outcome of these recent insights in the pathogenesis of autoinflammatory diseases caused by mutations both in the inflammasome or IL-1R is that these diseases often respond to monoclonal antibody therapies targeting IL-1β. The recombinant IL-1R antagonist anakinra, which blocks IL-1R1, the monoclonals canakinumab and geovikizumab which block IL-1β, and the soluble IL-1β receptor rilonacept are currently available.[5]

Another group of patients affected by severe pustular skin disease with familial segregation is linked to mutations in the IL-36 R antagonist and was first described in Tunisian families.[9] In parallel, the same mutation was found in sporadic cases of generalised pustular psoriasis linked to over-expression of IL-1 and other inflammatory cytokines such as IL-6, IL-8 and TNF.[10] This condition has been named DITRA (Deficiency of the IL-36R antagonist) and in line with the strict expression of IL-36R in the skin, DITRA-patients do not display bone involvement. Experiments in mice suggested that blocking IL-1 would not dampen DITRA and this would be consistent with reports that only a fraction of DITRA patients respond to anti-IL-1 treatment. It is conceivable that IL-36 may induce pathology downstream of IL-1 but further research is needed to fully clarify this. Hopefully, direct inhibition of the IL-36 signaling system will be available shortly and ideally would offer a novel and effective treatment in the case of DITRA.

DIRA and DITRA are rare diseases but may pave the way to understanding more common manifestations of highly inflammatory and pustular lesions in psoriasis. The severe and hard-to-treat condition known as Acrodermatitis continua Hallopeau affecting fingers and toes may represent a local variant of DITRA.[11] Thus, these insights may open our eyes for new disease-driving mechanisms in diseases that currently pose a clinical problem due to the lack of effective treatments.

Blistering Skin Diseases are Associated with Autoantibodies and Cytotoxic T Cells

In blistering skin diseases, physical separation of cells within the epidermis or separation of the epidermis from the dermis leads to loss of temperature and fluidic control as well as a loss of the immunological barrier function of the skin. Blistering skin diseases often cause acute, severe symptoms and may be lethal when the disease affects large areas of the skin. Pemphigus vulgaris or foliaceus are painful blistering disorders where antibodies to the adhesive proteins desmoglein 1 and 3 are bound to keratinocytes in the basal layers of epidermis at the site of keratinocyte acanthosis and the epidermal split. Bullous pemphigoid (BP) presents with severe itching, sometimes for several years prior to the onset of blisters, and typically affects older, frail patients. Antibodies specific to the hemidesmosomal antigens BP180 or BP230 can be detected in serum and induce degradation of the basal membrane and separation of the epidermis and dermis.

Traditionally, both pemphigus and pemphigoid were treated long term with potent topical and oral corticosteroids associated with side effects in the form of secondary diabetes, osteoporosis and skin atrophy. In bullous pemphigoid, other immunosuppressive treatments like dapsone and cyclosporine can be successful and in particular low dose metotrexate treatment has shown excellent clinical results with limited side effects[12] and is routinely used as a first-line therapy in our hospital. The treatment of pemphigus is more challenging but in an attempt to deplete pathogenic antibodies, dermatologists have turned to off-label usage of rituximab, an anti-CD-20 antibody. The evaluation of off-label usage of novel treatments is complicated

Blistering skin diseases

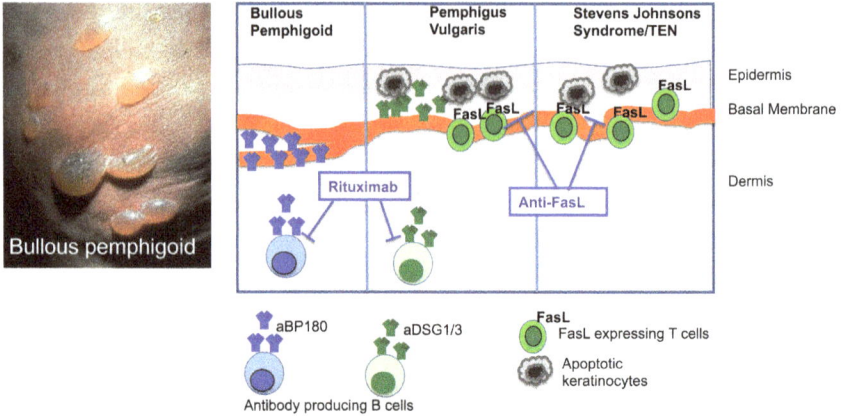

Figure 2. Blistering skin diseases are associated with autoantibodies and cytotoxic T cells. Clinical picture of the separation of epidermis and dermis at the level of the basal cell membrane in bullous pemphigoid (left). Autoreactive antibodies produced by B cells expressing CD20 are directed against the basal membrane antigen BP180 in bullous pemphigoid and against the intraepithelial antigens DSG-1 and -3 in pemphigus. The anti-CD20 antibody therapy rituximab leads to depletion of the pathogenic B cells. FasL expressing cytotoxic T cells are present in the skin in both pemphigus vulgaris and in Stevens-Johnson syndrome and TEN (toxic epidermal necrolysis) and here, anti-FasL blocking antibodies could be a potential future treatment strategy.

but in a six-year follow-up of 22 rituximab-treated pemphigus patients, two-thirds of the patients reported long-lasting effect of the treatment and nine patients obtained long-term remission with no need for further pemphigus treatment.[13] Importantly, although the circulating B cell compartment was skewed towards immature B cells as long as six years after treatment in the responders, IgG levels of anti-tetanus toxin or pneumococcal antigens, as a marker of immunity induced prior to the B cell depleting treatment, was not affected. Although one treated patient died due to sepsis 18 months after the initial treatment, increased incidence of severe infections was not detected in the responders.[13] In another study, eight out of 15 patients treated with low-dose rituximab showed long-term remission.[14] With all the limitations associated with these off-label, observational studies, depletion of B cells emerges as an important therapeutic alternative in pemphigus and potentially also in recalcitrant bullous pemphigoid.

The exact mechanism of the antibody driven epidermal acantholysis (cell death) in pemphigus is not clarified but cytotoxic T cells infiltrate the affected skin[15] and FasL mediated apoptosis has been suggested.[16] In toxic epidermal necrolysis and Stevens-Johnson syndrome, both of which are severe and acute systemic drug reactions, blistering of large areas of the skin leads to mortality ranging between 25–35%. In these diseases, drug-specific T cells are found in the skin and FasL mediated apoptosis has been shown to play a role in the pathophysiology.[17,18] Treatment with intravenous immunoglobulins (IVIG) has shown contradictory results and this has been linked to different amounts of FasL-neutralizing antibodies in the different batches of IVIG.[19] Thus, the monoclonal anti-FasL antibody PC11 planned for a phase I trial in pemphigus is a potential therapeutic agent also in drug induced blistering diseases such as TEN and Stevens-Johnson syndrome.

Atopic Dermatitis — Inhibition of IL-4 and IL-13 Signaling is Emerging as The Master Switch of Atopic Dermatitis

Atopic dermatitis (AD) affects 10–15% of children of the industrialized world and involves pro-allergic Th2 type responses within the skin coupled to high serum IgE levels. AD is often linked to allergic asthma and pollen allergy and the inflammation in the airways and skin display similar pathophysiologies. Both genetic and environmental factors precipitate the disease[20] and in particular the epidermal barrier function is often severely impaired by mutations of the protein filaggrin, which leads to an increased microbial burden and activation of keratinocytes.[21] As a result of constant immune activation, several keratinocyte-, eosinophil- or basophil-derived cytokines such as IL-25,[22] IL-33,[23,24] and thymic stromal lymphopoietin (TSLP)[25] are elevated in the skin and participate in development and/or maintenance of skin pathology. Several studies have been performed with the aim to change the composition of the gut microbiota through ingestion of oral probiota in an attempt to decrease skin inflammation in AD. To date, such efforts have shown contradictory results and there is currently no solid rational for utilizing probiotics in AD (summarized in Ref. [26]). Interestingly, one study propose that topical alteration of the skin microbiota

Atopic dermatitis

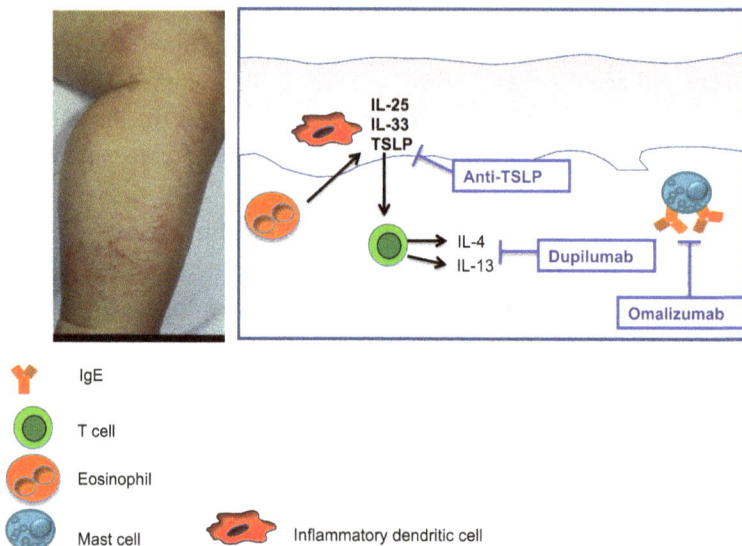

Figure 3. Atopic dermatitis — inhibition of IL-4 and IL-13 signaling is emerging as the master switch of atopic dermatitis.

Clinical picture of atopic dermatitis. The keratinocyte-, eosinophil- or basophil-derived cytokines TSLP, IL-25 and IL-33 are emerging as master-regulators of atopic inflammation and a clinical trial blocking TSLP is underway. Taking the high levels of serum IgE in atopic dermatitis, omalizumab, a humanised monoclonal anti-IgE antibody has been evaluated in small proof-of-concept studies and may become an effective treatment alternative for subgroups of patients lacking filaggrin mutations. Presently, the most promising biologic therapy is targeting the alpha chain of the IL-4 receptor and thus blocking both IL-13 and IL-4 signaling with the fully human monoclonal antibody dupilumab.

may skew the local inflammatory milieu[27] in a way that reduces atopic dermatitis.[28] Circulating T cells show strict specificity for different organs.[29] Elegant studies in germ-free mouse models of infections have shown that the effect of microbiota on the tissue resident immune system is organ specific and local microbiota composition at the site of infection elicits appropriate responses to infections. Thus, microbiota in the gut did not affect local immune responses in the skin.[30] These findings would explain the lack of convincing success with attempts to dampen skin inflammation by changing the gut microbiota.

In the early phase of eczema formation, Th2 responses dominate whereas a mixture of Th1 and Th2 immune cells and cytokines are seen in chronic AD.[31] In comparison to psoriasis, the development of targeted therapies is lagging behind in AD. However, after many frustrating years of negative results in clinical AD trials targeting IL-5, IL-6, CD20, TNF, and IL-23, there are several novel treatments in the pipe-line that show great promise. Given the high levels of serum IgE in atopic dermatitis, omalizumab, a humanised monoclonal anti-IgE antibody has been tested in atopic dermatitis. Although serum IgE, TSLP, OX40L and IL-9 levels were strikingly decreased in children with severe refractory atopic dermatitis, no significant impact on clinical scores or itching was found in a pilot study with eight patients in total.[32] Another study tested omalizumab treatment followed by rituximab in the case of refractory AD but again the study group would have to be increased for any conclusive data on the clinical effects of such strategy.[33] In another small and open-label study with omalizumab in adult AD, patients carrying a filaggrin mutation did not respond to IgE neutralization whereas patients lacking filaggrin mutations all showed a clinical response to the therapy.[34] The latter study is very promising and encourages larger and placebo controlled trials based upon the genetic background of the patients. In the future, stringent classification of patients based on clinical phenotypes and genotypes is likely to enhance efficacy of tailored treatments in clinically heterogenous diseases including AD.

TSLP, IL-25 and IL-33 are emerging as master-regulators of atopic inflammation. Although no clinical trials targeting IL-33 and IL-25 have been reported to our knowledge, phase I trials of blocking TSLP-signaling are underway. In addition to a compromised skin barrier and chronic inflammation, patients with atopic dermatitis suffer from pronounced itching and recently a direct link between TSLP and activation of peripheral neurons to induce itch was shown in a murine model of dermatitis.[32] Although clinical data from trials in AD are lacking, TSLP-inhibition has shown promising results in allergic asthma[35] and it will be interesting to follow the results on itch in the on-going phase I trials in AD.

Currently the most promising approach in AD is to simultaneously block IL-4 and IL-13 signaling. A recent double-blind and placebo controlled clinical trial with dupilumab showed remarkable effects utilizing a fully human monoclonal antibody targeting the alpha chain of the IL-4 receptor and thus blocking both IL-13 and IL-4 signaling.[36] Transcriptomic comparison of lesional skin biopsies before and after dupilumab showed consistent normalization of the molecular signature in the skin in parallel with the clinical improvement.[37] Thus it seems that after many years of failed trials, there will be effective and targeted systemic treatment available for severe atopic dermatitis.

Psoriasis — A Success-Story When it Comes to Implementing Novel Biological Treatments in Dermatology

Psoriasis is a chronic and relapsing inflammatory skin disease affecting 2–3% of the world-wide population with significantly lower prevalence in both Asia and within indigenous populations in Australia, South America and the Arctic area. The majority of patients have limited disease but at least 10–15% display severe disease with a need for systemic therapy. Treatment of severe psoriasis was revolutionized by an observant gastro-enterologist who noticed that systemic blocking of TNF was effective in treating psoriasis as well as inflammatory bowel disease. Today, first-line biologic treatments for severe psoriasis are different variants of TNF neutralization; soluble TNF receptor (etanercept) or anti-TNF antibodies (infliximab or adalimumab). In psoriasis, T cell infiltration of the skin maintains chronic inflammation and systemic ablation of T cells induces remission of disease.[38] The lesional infiltrate is dominated by IFNγ producing T cells, but a small and significant population of IL-17 producing T cells is present in the inflamed skin[39] and both neutrophils and mast cells produce IL-17 in lesional skin.[40] The clinical effect of ustekinumab, a monoclonal antibody blocking signaling through the common IL-23 and IL-12 receptor, is excellent in severe psoriasis of the skin with limited effects on psoriatic arthritis.[41] The efficacy of ustekinumab indicated that the downstream cytokine IL-17 might drive the disease and the pathogenic importance of IL-17 in psoriasis was recently formally proven by excellent efficacy in three clinical trials using antibodies targeting IL-17A and -17F,[42] IL-17-A alone[43] or the IL-17 receptor.[44] In addition to IL-17,

Psoriasis

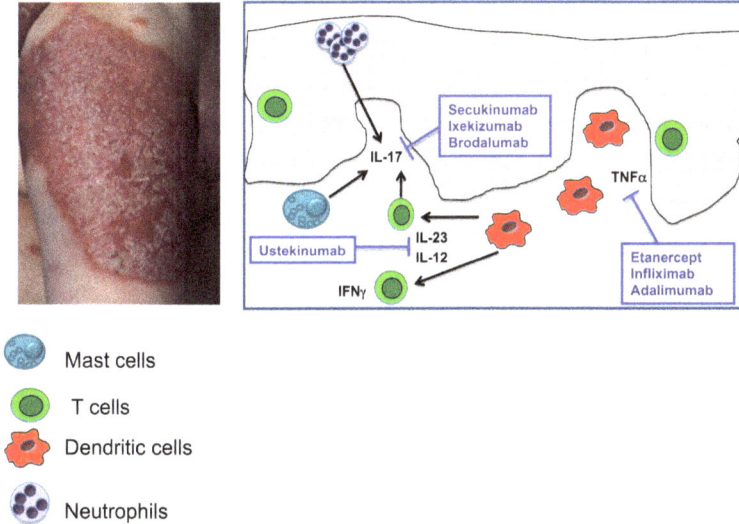

Mast cells

T cells

Dendritic cells

Neutrophils

Figure 4. Psoriasis — a success-story when it comes to implementing novel biological treatments in dermatology.

Clinical picture of well-demarcated psoriasis plaque. Different variants of TNF neutralization; soluble TNF receptor (etanercept) or anti-TNF antibodies (infliximab or adalimumab) have revolutionized the treatment of severe psoriasis. IL-17 is produced by infiltrating neutrophils, mast cells and T cells in epidermis and dermis and ustekinumab inhibit both IL-12 and IL-23 signaling through the common receptor p40. Direct IL-17 inhibition is a novel therapeutic strategy where the different strategies of inhibiting IL-17A alone (secukinumab), both IL-17A and IL-17F (ixekizumab) or blocking the IL-17R (brodalumab) will have to be compared in the clinical setting once the clinical trials are finished.

IL-22 overexpression was shown in psoriasis and we have linked mutations in the IL-22 promotor to overexpression of IL-22 in circulating T cells and an increased risk of onset of psoriasis in early childhood.[45] Thus IL-22 could serve as another potential drug target in psoriasis, but a phase I trial testing IL-22 blockade in psoriasis was recently withdrawn, potentially due to the protective role of IL-22 in the gut. Unfortunately, biologic therapies are long-term, come at a high cost and are associated with potential severe side-effects in terms of infections and malignancies. The failure to induce long-term remission could be explained by the presence of tissue resident T cells prone to produce IL-17 and IL-22 upon activation in sites of previous inflammation in psoriasis.[46] It would be desirable to eradicate such disease memory in recurrent inflammatory diseases of the skin. Thus, there is still a need for novel therapies in psoriasis despite the success of systemic inhibition of several different cytokines.

Another major drawback with antibody-based therapies is the lack of possibilities for topical application whereas small molecules, such as *e.g.*, Janus kinase JAK inhibitors, affecting intracellular signaling, readily penetrate the skin barrier. Oral treatment with tofacitinib that inhibits JAK1 and JAK3 signaling has shown promising results in phase II trials.[47] Topical ointments containing either tofacitinib or ruxolitinib inhibiting JAK1 and JAK2 offer potentially viable alternatives to the dominating corticosteroid and vitamin D treatment in limited disease.[48]

Recently, the selective inhibitor of phosphodiesterase 4 apremilast (Otezla) was approved for the treatment of psoriasis (and psoriatic arthritis). In several large randomized controlled trials apremilast achieved significant clinical efficacy compared to placebo, and it appears to have a good safety and tolerability profile with gastro-intestinal adverse events being the most common.[49–51] It is given as an oral dose with a slow up-titration to 30 mg twice daily in order to minimize side-effects. How it compares to other systemic therapies for psoriasis has not yet been studied. Given the molecular structure, there may be a potential for developing a topical formulation which would be welcome for treatment of more limited skin lesions.

Conclusions

The toolbox of treatments in dermatology is growing as the pathogenesis of rare and severe dermatological disorders is clarified in parallel to the development of novel therapies targeting different parts of the immune system. In autoinflammatory diseases, IL-1β is emerging as a key driver of inflammation and we hope that future therapies targeting IL-36 will become available and show consistent effect in DITRA. In pemphigus, long-term remission can be obtained by depletion of pathogenic B cells and it is possible that targeting other mechanisms of pathology such as FasL or cytotoxicity could have a future role in the treatment of drug induced skin diseases. In T cell driven diseases such as atopic eczema and psoriasis, clinical trials have shown that the most efficient treatment strategy is to address overexpressing cytokines, potentially as these cytokines are expressed by more than one cell type.

Wanted for the Future: Topical Treatments Beyond Corticosteroids and Short-Term Systemic Treatments

Current highly effective systemic therapies and the promising pipeline for a number of severe dermatoses have changed the life for many patients in dermatology. Still, the majority of patients with more limited yet highly disturbing symptoms represent a clinical dilemma. Biologic therapies may not be justified and the toolbox of topical therapies is quite restricted. The development of small molecules targeting the disease pathways are underway, of which the most advanced are JAK/STAT inhibitors that block signaling through various cytokine receptors. Given the probable triggering potential of local microbiota in several inflammatory disorders of the skin, one attractive future strategy would be to tailor and transplant therapeutic microbiota in limited disease.

References

1. Nakatsuji, T., Chiang, H.I., Jiang, S.B., Nagarajan, H., Zengler, K., and Gallo, R.L. (2013). The microbiome extends to subepidermal compartments of normal skin. *Nat Comm*, **4**, 1431.
2. Belkaid, Y., and Segre, J.A. (2014). Dialogue between skin microbiota and immunity. *Science*, **346**, 954–959.
3. Pasparakis, M., Haase, I., and Nestle, F.O. (2014). Mechanisms regulating skin immunity and inflammation. *Nat Rev Immunol*, **14**, 289–301.
4. Lamkanfi, M., and Dixit, V.M. (2014). Mechanisms and functions of inflammasomes. *Cell* 157: 1013–1022.
5. Beer, H.D., Contassot, E., and French, L.E. (2014). The inflammasomes in autoinflammatory diseases with skin involvement. *J Invest Dermatol*, **134**, 1805–1810.
6. Kitamura, A., Sasaki, Y., Abe, T., Kano, H., and Yasutomo, K. (2014). An inherited mutation in NLRC4 causes autoinflammation in human and mice. *J Exp Med.*

7. de Koning, H.D., van Gijn, M.E., Stoffels, M., Jongekrijg, J., Zeeuwen, P.L., Elferink, M.G., Nijman, I.J., Jansen, P.A., Neveling, K., van der Meer, J.W., Schalkwijk, J., and Simon, A. (2014). Myeloid lineage-restricted somatic mosaicism of NLRP3 mutations in patients with variant Schnitzler syndrome. *J Allergy Clin Immunol.*

8. Aksentijevich, I., Masters, S.L., Ferguson, P.J., Dancey, P., Frenkel, J., van Royen-Kerkhoff, A., Laxer, R., Tedgard, U., Cowen, E.W., Pham, T.H., Booty, M., Estes, J.D., Sandler, N.G., Plass, N., Stone, D.L., Turner, M.L., Hill, S., Butman, J.A., Schneider, R., Babyn, P., El-Shanti, H.I., Pope, E., Barron, K., Bing, X., Laurence, A., Lee, C.C., Chapelle, D., Clarke, G.I., Ohson, K., Nicholson, M., Gadina, M., Yang, B., Korman, B.D., Gregersen, P.K., van Hagen, P.M., Hak, A.E., Huizing, M., Rahman, P., Douek, D.C., Remmers, E.F., Kastner, D.L., and Goldbach-Mansky, R. (2009). An autoinflammatory disease with deficiency of the interleukin-1-receptor antagonist. *New Eng J Med*, **360**, 2426–2437.

9. Marrakchi, S., Guigue, P., Renshaw, B.R., Puel, A., Pei, X.Y., Fraitag, S., Zribi, J., Bal, E., Cluzeau, C., Chrabieh, M., Towne, J.E., Douangpanya, J., Pons, C., Mansour, S., Serre, V., Makni, H., Mahfoudh, N., Fakhfakh, F., Bodemer, C., Feingold, J., Hadj-Rabia, S., Favre, M., Genin, E., Sahbatou, M., Munnich, A., Casanova, J.L., Sims, J.E., Turki, H., Bachelez, H., and Smahi, A. (2011). Interleukin-36-receptor antagonist deficiency and generalized pustular psoriasis. *New Eng J Med*, **365**, 620–628.

10. Onoufriadis, A., Simpson, M.A., Pink, A.E., Di Meglio, P., Smith, C.H., Pullabhatla, V., Knight, J., Spain, S.L., Nestle, F.O., Burden, A.D., Capon, F., Trembath, R.C., and Barker, J.N. (2011). Mutations in IL36RN/IL1F5 are associated with the severe episodic inflammatory skin disease known as generalized pustular psoriasis. *Am J Hum Genet*, **89**, 432–437.

11. Abbas, O., Itani, S., Ghosn, S., Kibbi, A.G., Fidawi, G., Farooq, M., Shimomura, Y., and Kurban, M. (2013). Acrodermatitis continua of Hallopeau is a clinical phenotype of DITRA: evidence that it is a variant of pustular psoriasis. *Dermatology*, **226**, 28–31.

12. Kjellman, P., Eriksson, H., and Berg, P., (2008). A retrospective analysis of patients with bullous pemphigoid treated with methotrexate. *Arch Dermatol*, **144**, 612–616.

13. Colliou, N., Picard, D., Caillot, F., Calbo, S., Le Corre, S., Lim, A., Lemercier, B., Le Mauff, B., Maho-Vaillant, M., Jacquot, S., Bedane, C., Bernard, P., Caux, F., Prost, C., Delaporte, E., Doutre, M.S., Dreno, B., Franck, N., Ingen-Housz-Oro, S., Chosidow, O., Pauwels, C., Picard, C., Roujeau, J.C., Sigal, M., Tancrede-Bohin, E., Templier, I., Eming, R., Hertl, M.,

D'Incan, M., Joly, P., and Musette, P. (2013). Long-term remissions of severe pemphigus after rituximab therapy are associated with prolonged failure of desmoglein B cell response. *Sci Transl Med*, **5**, 175ra130.

14. Horvath, B., Huizinga, J., Pas, H.H., Mulder, A.B., and Jonkman, M.F., 2012. Low-dose rituximab is effective in pemphigus. *Brit J Dermatol*, **166**, 405–412.

15. Grando, S.A., Glukhenky, B.T., Drannik, G.N., Kostromin, A.P., Boiko, Y., and Senyuk, O.F. (1989). Autoreactive cytotoxic T lymphocytes in pemphigus and pemphigoid. *Autoimmunity*, **3**, 247–260.

16. Lotti, R., Marconi, A., and Pincelli, C. (2012). Apoptotic pathways in the pathogenesis of pemphigus: targets for new therapies. *Curr Pharm Biotech*, **13**, 1877–1881.

17. Viard, I., Wehrli, P., Bullani, R., Schneider, P., Holler, N., Salomon, D., Hunziker, T., Saurat, J.H., Tschopp, J., and French, L.E. (1998). Inhibition of toxic epidermal necrolysis by blockade of CD95 with human intravenous immunoglobulin. *Science*, **282**, 490–493.

18. Fu, M., Gao, Y., Pan, Y., Li, W., Liao, W., Wang, G., Li, C., Li, C., Gao, T., and Liu, Y. (2012). Recovered patients with Stevens-Johson syndrome and toxic epidermal necrolysis maintain long-lived IFN-gamma and sFasL memory response. *PloS One*, **7**, e45516.

19. French, L.E., Trent, J.T., and Kerdel, F.A. (2006). Use of intravenous immunoglobulin in toxic epidermal necrolysis and Stevens-Johnson syndrome: our current understanding. *Int Immunopharmacol*, **6**, 543–549.

20. Eyerich, K., and Novak, N. (2013). Immunology of atopic eczema: overcoming the Th1/Th2 paradigm. *Allergy*, **68**, 974–982.

21. Guttman-Yassky, E., Nograles, K.E., and Krueger, J.G. (2011). Contrasting pathogenesis of atopic dermatitis and psoriasis--part II: immune cell subsets and therapeutic concepts. *J Allergy Clin Immunol*, **127**, 1420–1432.

22. Wang, Y.H., Angkasekwinai, P., Lu, N., Voo, K.S., Arima, K., Hanabuchi, S., Hippe, A., Corrigan, C.J., Dong, C., Homey, B., Yao, Z., Ying, S., Huston, D.P., and Liu, Y.J. (2007). IL-25 augments type 2 immune responses by enhancing the expansion and functions of TSLP-DC-activated Th2 memory cells. *J Exp Med*, **204**, 1837–1847.

23. Shimizu, M., Matsuda, A., Yanagisawa, K., Hirota, T., Akahoshi, M., Inomata, N., Ebe, K., Tanaka, K., Sugiura, H., Nakashima, K., Tamari, M., Takahashi, N., Obara, K., Enomoto, T., Okayama, Y., Gao, P.S., Huang, S.K., Tominaga, S., Ikezawa, Z., and Shirakawa, T. (2005). Functional SNPs in the distal promoter of the ST2 gene are associated with atopic dermatitis. *Hum Mol Genet*, **14**, 2919–2927.

24. Savinko, T., Matikainen, S., Saarialho-Kere, U., Lehto, M., Wang, G., Lehtimaki, S., Karisola, P., Reunala, T., Wolff, H., Lauerma, A., and Alenius, H.

(2012). IL-33 and ST2 in atopic dermatitis: expression profiles and modulation by triggering factors. *J Invest Dermatol*, **132**, 1392–1400.

25. Soumelis, V., Reche, P.A., Kanzler, H., Yuan, W., Edward, G., Homey, B., Gilliet, M., Ho, S., Antonenko, S., Lauerma, A., Smith, K., Gorman, D., Zurawski, J., Abrams, S., Menon, S., McClanahan, T., de Waal-Malefyt Rd, R., Bazan, F., Kastelein, R.A., and Liu, Y.J. (2002). Human epithelial cells trigger dendritic cell mediated allergic inflammation by producing TSLP. *Nat Immunol*, **3**, 673–680.

26. Kim, S.O., Ah, Y.M., Yu, Y.M., Choi, K.H., Shin, W.G., and Lee, J.Y. (2014). Effects of probiotics for the treatment of atopic dermatitis: a meta-analysis of randomized controlled trials. *Ann Allergy Asthma Immunol*, **113**, 217–226.

27. Volz, T., Skabytska, Y., Guenova, E., Chen, K.M., Frick, J.S., Kirschning, C.J., Kaesler, S., Rocken, M., and Biedermann, T. (2014). Nonpathogenic bacteria alleviating atopic dermatitis inflammation induce IL-10-producing dendritic cells and regulatory Tr1 cells. *J Invest Dermatol*, **134**, 96–104.

28. Gueniche, A., Knaudt, B., Schuck, E., Volz, T., Bastien, P., Martin, R., Rocken, M., Breton, L., and Biedermann, T. (2008). Effects of nonpathogenic gram-negative bacterium Vitreoscilla filiformis lysate on atopic dermatitis: a prospective, randomized, double-blind, placebo-controlled clinical study. *Brit J Dermatol*, **159**, 1357–1363.

29. Comerford, I., Kara, E.E., McKenzie, D.R., and McColl, S.R., (2014). Advances in understanding the pathogenesis of autoimmune disorders: focus on chemokines and lymphocyte trafficking. *Brit J Haematol*, **164**, 329–341.

30. Naik, S., Bouladoux, N., Wilhelm, C., Molloy, M.J., Salcedo, R., Kastenmuller, W., Deming, C., Quinones, M., Koo, L., Conlan, S., Spencer, S., Hall, J.A., Dzutsev, A., Kong, H., Campbell, D.J., Trinchieri, G., Segre, J.A., and Belkaid, Y. (2012). Compartmentalized control of skin immunity by resident commensals. *Science*, **337**, 1115–1119.

31. Gittler, J.K., Shemer, A., Suarez-Farinas, M., Fuentes-Duculan, J., Gulewicz, K.J., Wang, C.Q., Mitsui, H., Cardinale, I., de Guzman Strong, C., Krueger, J.G., and Guttman-Yassky, E. (2012). Progressive activation of T(H)2/T(H)22 cytokines and selective epidermal proteins characterizes acute and chronic atopic dermatitis. *J Allergy Clin Immunol*, **130**, 1344–1354.

32. Wilson, S.R., The, L., Batia, L.M., Beattie, K., Katibah, G.E., McClain, S.P., Pellegrino, M., Estandian, D.M., and Bautista, D.M. (2013). The epithelial cell-derived atopic dermatitis cytokine TSLP activates neurons to induce itch. *Cell*, **155**, 285–295.

33. Sanchez-Ramon, S., Eguiluz-Gracia, I., Rodriguez-Mazariego, M.E., Paravisini, A., Zubeldia-Ortuno, J.M., Gil-Herrera, J., Fernandez-Cruz, E.,

and Suarez-Fernandez, R. (2013). Sequential combined therapy with omalizumab and rituximab: a new approach to severe atopic dermatitis. *J Invest Allergol Clin Immunol*, **23**, 190–196.

34. Hotze, M., Baurecht, H., Rodriguez, E., Chapman-Rothe, N., Ollert, M., Folster-Holst, R., Adamski, J., Illig, T., Ring, J., and Weidinger, S. (2014). Increased efficacy of omalizumab in atopic dermatitis patients with wild-type filaggrin status and higher serum levels of phosphatidylcholines. *Allergy*, **69**, 132–135.
35. Gauvreau, G.M., P.M., O'Byrne, Boulet, L.P., Wang, Y., Cockcroft, D., Bigler, J., FitzGerald, J.M., Boedigheimer, M., Davis, B.E., Dias, C., Gorski, K.S., Smith, L., Bautista, E., Comeau, M.R., Leigh, R., and Parnes, J.R. (2014). Effects of an anti-TSLP antibody on allergen-induced asthmatic responses. *N Eng J Med*, **370**, 2102–2110.
36. Beck, L.A., Thaci, D., Hamilton, J.D., Graham, N.M., Bieber, T., Rocklin, R., Ming, J.E., Ren, H., Kao, R., Simpson, E., Ardeleanu, M., Weinstein, S.P., Pirozzi, G., Guttman-Yassky, E., Suarez-Farinas, M., Hager, M.D., Stahl, N., Yancopoulos, G.D., and Radin, A.R. (2014). Dupilumab treatment in adults with moderate-to-severe atopic dermatitis. *N Eng J Med*, **371**, 130–139.
37. Hamilton, J.D., Suarez-Farinas, M., Dhingra, N., Cardinale, I., Li, X., Kostic, A., Ming, J.E., Radin, A.R., Krueger, J.G., Graham, N., Yancopoulos, G.D., Pirozzi, G., and Guttman-Yassky, E. (2014). Dupilumab improves the molecular signature in skin of patients with moderate-to-severe atopic dermatitis. *J Allergy Clin Immunol*, **134**, 1293–1300.
38. Prinz, J., Braun-Falco, O., Meurer, M., Daddona, P., Reiter, C., Rieber, P., and Riethmuller, G. (1991). Chimaeric CD4 monoclonal antibody in treatment of generalised pustular psoriasis. *Lancet*, **338**, 320–321.
39. Lowes, M.A., Kikuchi, T., Kikuchi, T., Fuentes-Duculan, J., Fuentes-Duculan, J., Cardinale, I., Cardinale, I., Zaba, L.C., Zaba, L.C., Haider, A.S., Haider, A.S., Bowman, E.P., Bowman, E.P., Krueger, J.G., and Krueger, J.G. (2008). Psoriasis vulgaris lesions contain discrete populations of Th1 and Th17 T cells. *J Invest Dermatol*, **128**, 1207–1211.
40. Res, P.C.M., Piskin, G., de Boer, O.J., van der Loos, C.M., Teeling, P., Bos, J.D., and Teunissen, M.B.M. (2010). Overrepresentation of IL-17A and IL-22 producing CD8 T cells in lesional skin suggests their involvement in the pathogenesis of psoriasis. *PloS One*, **5**, e14108.
41. Leonardi, C.L., Kimball, A.B., Papp, K.A., Yeilding, N., Guzzo, C., Wang, Y., Li, S., Dooley, L.T., and Gordon, K.B. (2008). Efficacy and safety of ustekinumab, a human interleukin-12/23 monoclonal antibody, in patients with psoriasis: 76-week results from a randomised, double-blind, placebo-controlled trial (PHOENIX 1). *Lancet*, **371**, 1665–1674.

42. Leonardi, C., Matheson, R., Zachariae, C., Cameron, G., Li, L., Edson-Heredia, E., Braun, D., and Banerjee, S. (2012). Anti-interleukin-17 monoclonal antibody ixekizumab in chronic plaque psoriasis. *New Eng J Med*, **366**, 1190–1199.
43. Hueber, W., Patel, D.D., Dryja, T., Wright, A.M., Koroleva, I., Bruin, G., Antoni, C., Draelos, Z., Gold, M.H., Durez, P., Tak, P.P., Gomez-Reino, J.J., Foster, C.S., Kim, R.Y., Samson, C.M., Falk, N.S., Chu, D.S., Callanan, D., Nguyen, Q.D., Rose, K., Haider, A., and Di Padova, F. (2010). Effects of AIN457, a fully human antibody to interleukin-17A, on psoriasis, rheumatoid arthritis, and uveitis. *Sci Trans Med*, **2**, 52ra72.
44. Papp, K.A., Leonardi, C., Menter, A., Ortonne, J.P., Krueger, J.G., Kricorian, G., Aras, G., Li, J., Russell, C.B., Thompson, E.H., and Baumgartner, S. (2012). Brodalumab, an anti-interleukin-17-receptor antibody for psoriasis. *N Eng J Med*, **366**, 1181–1189.
45. Nikamo, P., Cheuk, S., Lysell, J., Enerback, C., Bergh, K., Xu Landen, N., Eidsmo, L., and Stahle, M. (2013). Genetic variants of the IL22 promoter associate to onset of psoriasis before puberty and increased IL-22 production in T Cells. *J Invest Dermatol*, **134**(6), 1535–1541.
46. Cheuk, S., Wiken, M., Blomqvist, L., Nylen, S., Talme, T., Stahle, M., and Eidsmo, L. (2014). Epidermal th22 and tc17 cells form a localized disease memory in clinically healed psoriasis. *J Immunol*, **192**, 3111–3120.
47. Papp, K.A., Menter, A., Strober, B., Langley, R.G., Buonanno, M., Wolk, R., Gupta, P., Krishnaswami, S., Tan, H., and Harness, J.A. (2012). Efficacy and safety of tofacitinib, an oral Janus kinase inhibitor, in the treatment of psoriasis: a Phase 2b randomized placebo-controlled dose-ranging study. *Brit J Dermatol*, **167**, 668–677.
48. Hsu, L., and Armstrong, A.W. (2014). JAK inhibitors: treatment efficacy and safety profile in patients with psoriasis. *J Immunol Res*, **2014**, 283617.
49. Papp, K., Cather, J.C., Rosoph, L., *et al.* (2012). Efficacy of apremilast in the treatment of moderate to severe psoriasis: a randomised controlled trial. *Lancet*, **380**, 738–746.
50. Gottlieb, A.B., Matheson, R.T., Menter, A., *et al.* (2013). Efficacy, tolerability, and pharmacodynamics of apremilast in recalcitrant plaque psoriasis: a phase II open-label study. *J Drugs Dermatol*, **12**, 888-97.
51. Gottlieb, A.B., Strober, B., Krueger, J.G., *et al.* (2008). An open-label, single-arm pilot study in patients with severe plaque-type psoriasis treated with an oral anti-inflammatory agent, apremilast. *Curr Med Res Opin*, **24**, 1529–1538.

CHAPTER 11

ADVANCES IN THERAPY FOR CUTANEOUS LUPUS ERYTHEMATOSUS

Annegret Kuhn and Aysche Landmann

Introduction

Lupus erythematosus (LE) is an inflammatory autoimmune disorder, which may encompass various systemic organ manifestations (systemic lupus erythematosus, SLE), but may also affect primarily the skin (cutaneous lupus erythematosus, CLE).[1] A small percentage of patients with CLE develop systemic organ involvement during the course of their disease, but cutaneous manifestations appear also in 73–85% of patients with SLE and may occur at any stage of the disease.[2] The broad variety of skin lesions in CLE has led to the practice of identifying different subtypes of the disease: acute cutaneous LE (ACLE), subacute cutaneous LE (SCLE) (Figs. 1 and 2), chronic cutaneous LE (CCLE), including discoid LE (DLE) (Fig. 3), LE panniculitis (LEP), and chilblain LE (CHLE), and intermittent cutaneous LE (ICLE), including LE tumidus (LET).[3] Due to the broad spectrum of cutaneous manifestations, it is a challenge to define therapeutic strategies for all different subtypes of the disease. To our knowledge, therapeutic guidelines for CLE developed by an interdisciplinary group are only available in the German literature.[4] Moreover, no drugs have been licensed specifically for the treatment of CLE and only a few agents are supported by evidence from randomized controlled trials.[5,6] In contrast, several agents, such as hydroxychloroquine (HCQ), chloroquine (CQ), cyclophosphamide and azathioprine are approved for the treatment of SLE, including the novel monoclonal antibody belimumab, a B lymphocyte

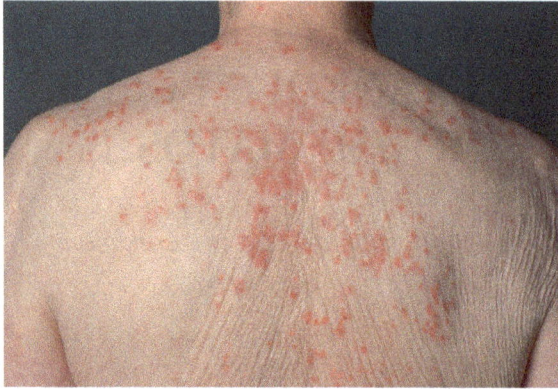

Figure 1. Erythematous papules on the upper back of subacute cutaneous lupus erythematosus (SCLE).

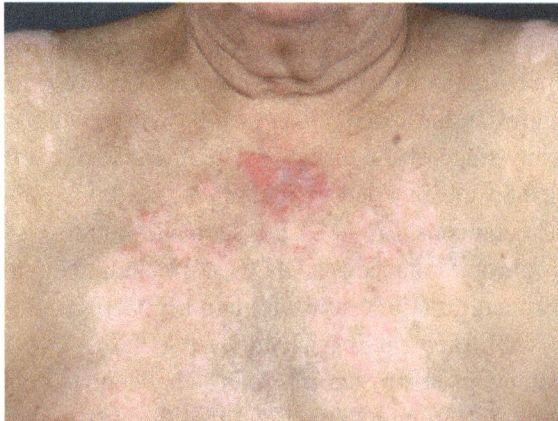

Figure 2. Vitiligo-like hypopigmentation with erythematous papules on the upper chest of subacute cutaneous lupus erythematous (SCLE).

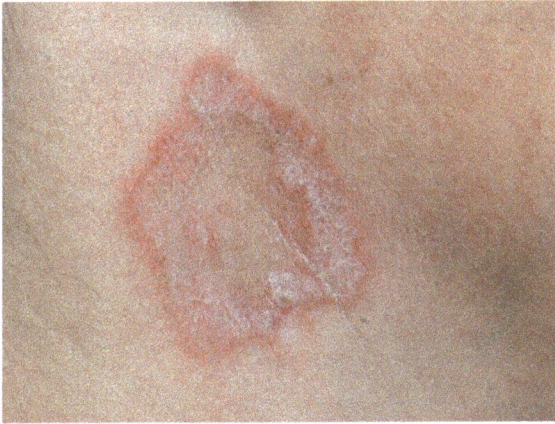

Figure 3. Discoid plaque with erythematous atrophic border and central hyperpigmentation on the neck of discoid lupus erythematosus (DLE).

stimulator specific inhibitor.[7] Therefore, topical and systemic agents are commonly used off-label for most patients with CLE.

Prevention

As early as in the 19th century, photosensitivity was described as a characteristic feature in patients with SLE. Nowadays, ultraviolet (UV) light has been accepted as an important environmental factor in the pathogenesis of the disease.[8,9] It has been shown that different CLE subtypes can be triggered and exacerbated by sun exposure and that systemic organ involvement can also be worsened by UV irradiation.[10,11] Therefore, the education of patients with regard to avoidance of sun exposure (including sunbathing and visiting tanning salons), continuous photoprotection by physical measures, such as protective clothing and daily application of broad-spectrum sunscreens with a high sun protection factor, as well as avoidance of potentially photosensitizing drugs are required (Table 1).[12] Furthermore, it has long been known that smoking does not only impact skin health in many different ways, but also has a negative influence on skin manifestations in SLE.[13,14] Recently, a multicenter analysis of 1002 patients with CLE in Europe assessed by the EUSCLE Core Set Questionnaire confirmed that smoking is a risk factor for the disease, in particular for the development

Table 1.   Preventive and therapeutic options in CLE.

First-line Systemic Treatment	Second-line Systemic Treatment	Further Systemic Treatment Options
	alternatively or additionally to first-line treatment	alternatively or additionally to first-/second-line treatment
• Antimalarials (Hydroxychloroquine, Chloroquine, Quinacrine) • Systemic Glucocorticosteroids (highly acute skin lesions)	• Methotrexate • Mycophenolate Mofetil (MMF, MPS) • Retinoids • Dapsone	• Belimumab • Further Biologicals and Experimental Therapies

Topical and Physical Treatment

• Corticosteroids (topical, occlusive, intralesional)
• Topical Calcineurin Inhibitors (Pimecrolimus, Tacrolimus)
• Further Topical Agents (R-Salbutamol)

Prevention

• UV Protection
• Other Preventive Strategies (e.g., Nicotine abstinence, Elimination of photosensitizing drugs)

of LET.[15] Moreover, several studies have suggested that smoking interferes with the efficacy of antimalarials.[15–18] Therefore, patients with CLE should be motivated to cease smoking, but even a reduction in smoking can improve disease activity.[19] As CLE may also be triggered by several drugs, such as terbinafine, hydrochlorothiazide, or TNF antagonists, the avoidance of these medications is an important preventive measure.[20] The most frequent drug-induced subtype is SCLE, while drug-induced DLE and LET have only been reported in single cases.[21]

Topical Treatment

Topical corticosteroids (CS)

Topical corticosteroids are the first-line treatment for skin lesions of all CLE subtypes.[5] According to the Cochrane Database of Systematic Review, only one randomized controlled study for DLE exists, which compares the efficacy of 0.05% fluocinonide (a high-potency CS cream) with 1% hydrocortisone (a low-potency CS cream) in 78 patients.[22,23] The results of this trial showed that high-potency topical CS are more effective than low-potency topical CS. In order to evaluate the efficacy of other treatment options, more recent studies applied topical CS as reference treatment in patients with CLE. For example, 0.05% clobetasole propionate ointment (ultrahigh-potency CS) was applied once daily for six weeks in 21 DLE patients from Thailand resulting in a greater improvement of disease activity than the twice-daily application of 0.1% tacrolimus ointment.[24] In a recent analysis by EUSCLE assessing therapeutic strategies in 1002 patients with CLE, topical CS were applied in 81.5% of the patients with an efficacy of 88.4%; the highest efficacy was observed in patients with ACLE compared to all other subtypes.[25] The choice of the corticosteroid class depends on the location and the activity of the skin lesion,[26] but due to the well-known side effects, such as atrophy, telangiectasia, and steroid-induced rosacea-like dermatitis, treatment with topical CS should be applied intermittently and not exceed an application of more than a few weeks.

In hairy areas, such as the scalp, CS solutions, lotions, or foams can be applied. The efficacy and penetration of CS may be increased by occlusive techniques (*e.g.*, plastic food wrap, hydrocolloid dressings) and salicylic acid. In skin manifestations of localized DLE, intralesional injection of CS (triamcinolone acetonide 5–10 mg/ml) can be used with high efficacy; however, the risk of subcutaneous atrophy has to be considered.[5]

Calcineurin inhibitors (CI)

In recent years, topical CI, such as tacrolimus and pimecrolimus, have been shown to be effective in patients with CLE.[26] A retrospective study applied a specially formulated preparation of 0.3% tacrolimus in 0.05% clobetasol propionate ointment in 13 therapy-resistant patients with CLE and compared its efficacy with the efficacy of 0.1% tacrolimus ointment in five patients with CLE.[27] The results of this study suggest that the combined preparation is more effective than the monotherapy with 0.1% tacrolimus ointment. In a multicenter, randomized, double-blind, vehicle-controlled trial, tacrolimus 0.1% ointment was applied in 30 patients with various CLE subtypes and resulted in a significantly higher response rate compared to the vehicle.[28] A clear and significant improvement was observed in edematous lesions of patients with ACLE, SCLE, and LET, compared with skin lesions treated with the vehicle.

In an open-label and uncontrolled study, 11 patients with different subtypes of CLE were treated with 1% pimecrolimus cream twice daily for three weeks under semiocclusive conditions (overnight occlusion with hydrocolloid dressings); the skin lesions of all patients improved.[29] A further randomized, double-blind pilot study applied 1% pimecrolimus cream and topical 0.1% betamethasone 17-valerate cream in 10 patients with moderate to severe manifestations of DLE and observed significant improvement in both groups.[30] After eight weeks of treatment, a decrease of 86% and 73% in the clinical disease severity score was observed with 1% pimecrolimus and 0.1% betamethasone 17-valerate cream, respectively. To date, tacrolimus ointment and pimecrolimus cream are only approved for the treatment of atopic dermatitis in children and adults.[31] Despite their off-label use, CI are recommended for topical application in CLE, particularly in atrophy-prone areas such as the face or in intertriginous zones.

R-salbutamol (ASF-1096)

The β2-adrenergic receptor agonist R-Salbutamol inhibits the activity of CD4+ T lymphocytes and other cells with a high density of β2 receptors such as Langerhans cells, monocytes, and macrophages.[32] A multicenter, double-blind, randomized, placebo-controlled phase II trial applied 0.5% R-Salbutamol cream for eight weeks twice daily in 37 patients with DLE.[33] Compared to the placebo-treated group, scaling/hypertrophy, pain, itching, and patient global assessment were observed to be significantly reduced in the R-Salbutamol-treated group. However, further phase III trials are warranted to evaluate the efficacy of R-Salbutamol in CLE.

Other topical treatment options

Treatment with topical retinoids, such as tazarotene, tretinoin, or tocoretinate, has only been described in single case reports of patients with therapy-refractory hypertrophic CLE and localized or disseminated DLE.[34–36] In a patient with DLE, 5% imiquimod cream was administered once daily in two cycles over three weeks and resulted in an improvement in erythema and follicular scaling of the scalp.[37] However, as imiquimod is a toll-like receptor agonist, there may be a theoretical risk of exacerbating the cutaneous disease.

Systemic Treatment

Antimalarials

Antimalarials, such as HCQ, CQ, and quinacrine (synonym: mepacrine) are used since the 1950s and are considered the first-line treatment for disfiguring and widespread skin manifestations in patients with CLE, irrespective of the subtype of the disease.[38] Moreover, antimalarials are often recommended as standard therapy in all SLE patients;[39] in particular, the application of HCQ is associated with higher rates of remission, fewer relapses, and reduced damage in the course of the disease, even in lupus nephritis.[40,41]

To date, only one multicenter, randomized, placebo-controlled study exists in CLE comparing HCQ (400 mg/day, 30 patients) with acitretin (50 mg/day, 28 patients).[42] About 50% of patients with CLE treated with HCQ and 46% of patients treated with acitretin improved, but more side effects were seen in the acitretin group. In general, HCQ has been suggested to be better tolerated than CQ but less effective, which might be due to the fact that especially in earlier case series, HCQ was used in lower doses than CQ; comparative studies have not yet been performed. Recently, Japanese groups[43–45] evaluated the efficacy of HCQ in different CLE subtypes: within four months, 82% of all patients (32/39) responded to the treatment, but only 22% (6/27) showed a complete or almost complete resolution of the cutaneous manifestations. In 2012, a French multicenter, prospective study of 300 patients with refractory CLE evaluated HCQ treatment given for at least three months; after this period, 38% of the patients were in complete remission, 29% in partial remission (clearing of > 50% of skin manifestations) and 33% of patients were refractory to HCQ.[46] In the recent analysis by EUSCLE, 799 of 1002 CLE patients used antimalarials (as monotherapy or in combination with any topical agent) with an efficacy of 84.3%.[25]

The maximal oral daily dosages are 6–6.5 mg/kg ideal bodyweight for HCQ and 3.5–4 mg/kg ideal bodyweight for CQ; treatment with higher dosages should be time-limited.[38] Oral dosages of 100 mg/day quinacrine (one tablet) should not be exceeded. After obtaining a good response (usually within 3–6 months), the dosage of quinacrine should be tapered to maintenance dosages of one to three tablets per week. In case of adverse reactions, the daily dosage of quinacrine may be reduced to 25–50 mg. The most feared side effect of HCQ and CQ treatment is irreversible retinal damage; to avoid this side effect, the dosage should comply with the ideal body weight of adults and children, and the visual status should be evaluated before and during treatment.[5] Moreover, several studies statistically confirmed that smoking interferes with the efficacy of antimalarials and some mechanisms by which smoking may alter the antimalarial metabolism have been proposed.[15,16] In contrast, other studies suggest that cigarette smoking does not have any significant influence on the response to HCQ and/or CQ.[47] Therefore, prospective investigations are necessary to evaluate whether smoking influences the efficacy of treatment with antimalarials.[48]

Systemic corticosteroids (CS)

In SLE, systemic CS are a cornerstone of treatment, in particular in lupus nephritis; as these agents show rapid and distinct clinical effects, systemic CS may be also indicated until the onset of antimalarials and/or for acute flare-ups of CLE.[49,50] In the recent analysis by EUSCLE, systemic CS were applied in 41.3% of the included 1002 CLE patients and were effective in 94.3% of cases.[25] The highest efficacy was observed in patients with ACLE.

The usual dose of systemic CS is 0.5–1mg/kg bodyweight/day for 2–4 weeks followed by tapering to the lowest possible dosages.[5] Alternatively, a successful 3-day intravenous pulse therapy (1g methylprednisolone) has been described in patients with therapy-refractory CLE.[51] However, due to their well-known side effects (*e.g.*, osteoporosis, Cushing's syndrome, arterial hypertension and type II diabetes), the application of CS should be time-limited and intermittent.[5,52]

Methotrexate (MTX)

MTX has been successfully applied as second-line treatment in therapy-refractory SCLE and DLE[6] and is broadly used as therapeutic option in SLE.[53] The efficacy of MTX for different skin lesions of recalcitrant CLE was confirmed in a study including 43 patients.[54] The skin manifestations improved in 98% of patients treated with low-dose MTX, administered either orally or intravenously (i.v.). In patients with SCLE and localized DLE, a greater improvement was observed compared to patients with disseminated DLE. In a follow-up study, the application of MTX i.v. was modified to subcutaneous (s.c.) application in 15 of the 43 patients with CLE. Due to the easier and self-administered injection, s.c. application was tolerated better than the i.v. administration, and a comparable efficacy was observed.[55] In the analysis by EUSCLE, MTX was used in 77 (7.7% of 1002) patients;[25] compared with the previous studies, the patients showed lower efficacy with a success rate of only 65.6%.

MTX should be given in a dosage of 7.5–25 mg per week preferably via s.c. injection; folic acid supplementation may additionally be administered to prevent gastrointestinal side effects.[26]

Retinoids

Retinoids (such as acitretin and isotretinoin) are listed as second-line treatment options for CLE in the Guidelines of the American Academy of Dermatology, primarily based on the good results (especially in patients with DLE and SCLE) achieved in several prospective trials conducted since 1985 and due to their relatively innocuous side-effect profile.[56] A recent case report described high efficacy of the new retinoid, alitretinoin, in three patients with different subtypes of CLE.[58] The recommended oral dosage of alitretinoin is 10–30 mg/day, the oral dosages of acitretin and isotretinoin is 0.2–1.0 mg/kg bodyweight/day. The response to retinoid therapy usually occurs within the first 2–6 weeks of treatment.[59] As retinoids are teratogenic, effective contraception is essential during and after treatment (alitretinoin, isotretinoin: 1 month; acitretin: 2 years). Due to their shorter half-life, alitretinoin and isotretinoin are preferable in female patients with childbearing potential. Further side effects of retinoids include dryness of skin and mucous membranes (*e.g.*, xerophthalmia, xerostomia), gastrointestinal disturbances, skeletal toxicity, muscle pain, and arthralgia are less common.[60] Treatment with retinoids may further result in hyperlipidemia and altered liver function tests, but severe hepatotoxic reactions have only been observed in single cases.

Dapsone

Dapsone has been described to be effective in patients with SCLE, LEP, urticarial vasculitis, oral ulcerations, and in bullous eruptions complicating SLE.[60–62] Bullous SLE was treated with dapsone in combination with CQ, and an ongoing remission of the disease was described.[63,64] Moreover, dapsone combined with HCQ and CS was reported to be effective in a patient with methimazole-induced bullous SLE and multiple oral ulcerations, but the generalized annular patches showed only partial response.[65] Several studies also demonstrated the efficacy of dapsone in DLE.[6]

Therapeutic dosages of dapsone range from 25–150 (maximum 200) mg/day; it is recommended to start with a low dose and to taper the dose gradually. To minimize possible side effects, such as agranulocytosis, hemolysis and methemoglobinemia, the lowest effective dose should be applied.

Mycophenolate mofetil (MMF) and mycophenolate sodium (EC-MPS)

MMF is an immunosuppressive drug, which has been observed to be effective in single case reports of SCLE, DLE, and CHLE, and is particularly recommended as initial treatment of lupus nephritis (class III–IV).[66] In 2002, MMF was applied in four therapy-resistant patients with SLE and various skin lesions, resulting in a complete remission of the cutaneous manifestations within three months.[67] These results could not be confirmed by Pisoni *et al.* several years later,[68] who used MMF in SLE patients with various skin manifestations. In 2011, Gammon *et al.*[69] published a retrospective analysis on the use of MMF in combination with oral CS and/or HCQ in 24 patients with CLE refractory to antimalarial therapy. The addition of MMF to the existing regimen resulted in an improvement of all patients. In an open-pilot study, the enteric-coated form of MMF (EC-MPS) was administered in 10 SCLE patients, who had been resistant to at least one standard therapy.[70] The treatment demonstrated significant improvement of the skin lesions, while no serious side effects were observed.

MMF should be given in dosages between 1 g and 3 g/day. The highest efficacy may be achieved with 2 g to 3 g/day, but due to its delayed onset it may take 1 to 2 months until clinical effects become visible. In general, MMF is well tolerated by most patients.[6]

Further immunosuppressive agents (azathioprine, cyclosporine, cyclophosphamide)

Immunosuppressive agents, such as azathioprine, cyclosporine, and cyclophosphamide, have been widely used for the management of SLE and treatment-resistant forms of CLE (generalized discoid lesions and severe DLE of palms and soles) since the early 1960s.[6] Due to the lack of consistent data on its efficacy and its side effect profile (*e.g.*, hepatotoxicity and bone marrow toxicity), azathioprine is not recommended in patients with CLE.[6] The efficacy of cyclosporine in CLE has only been evaluated in a few reports.[71–73] Malar rash improved after treatment with cyclosporine,[74] but another case report described the ineffectiveness of this drug in two patients with DLE.[75] Due to the rare and contradictory reports and its insufficient efficacy, cyclosporine is also not recommended as therapeutic option in CLE.[6] For many years, intermittent intravenous pulses of cyclophosphamide combined with intravenous prednisolone have been the standard therapy for lupus nephritis and severe SLE.[76,77] However, only some case reports exist in the literature indicating that cyclophosphamide may be effective in severe, refractory SCLE;[78] therefore, this agent is not recommended in patients with CLE.[6]

Fumaric acid esthers (FAEs)

FAEs are licensed in Germany for moderate to severe psoriasis vulgaris, if topical treatment is not sufficient.[84] In 2011, a mono-center, open-label, prospective pilot study was initiated to assess the efficacy and safety of FAEs in patients with CLE. Eleven patients with different disease subtypes were included in the study, and the efficacy was evaluated by the Revised Cutaneous Lupus Erythematosus Disease Area and Severity Index (RCLASI), the Patient Assessment of Global Improvement (PAGI), and by a Visual Analog Scale (VAS) to evaluate itch and pain (ClinicalTrials.gov Identifier: NCT01352988). Preliminary published data show that FAEs are highly effective in the treatment of CLE; the disease activity of one patient with DLE decreased from 17 points to 8 points which was a clear improvement after six months of treatment.[85] Further results of the study are currently in preparation for publication.

Belimumab

Belimumab, a monocolonal antibody that inhibits the B-lymphocyte stimulator, is the first of a new class of immunomodulators with a novel mechanism of action, which was approved for SLE in 2011 based on two phase III studies (BLISS-52 and BLISS-76).[79,80] This agent was applied in a dosage of 1 mg/kg or 10 mg/kg i.v. and the efficacy of belimumab or placebo was assessed by the SLE Responder Index (SRI) at week 52 and week 76, respectively. In 2012, a post hoc analysis was performed on these 1684 autoantibody-positive SLE patients included in the phase III trials and SLE disease activity was assessed by the Safety of Estrogens in Lupus National Assessment-Systemic Lupus Erythematosus Disease Activity Index (SELENA-SLEDAI) and the British Isles Lupus Assessment Group score (BILAG).[7] The data demonstrated that belimumab plus standard therapy showed a significantly higher efficacy than placebo plus standard therapy for mucocutaneous manifestations in SLE. However, the mucocutaneous manifestations were not further specified and a validated skin activity and damage score, *e.g.*, the RCLASI,[81] was not applied in these phase III trials. Therefore, it is difficult to evaluate and reproduce the efficacy of belimumab on mucocutaneous lesions in SLE patients and future prospective studies using a validated skin score are required. Currently, a randomized, double-blind, placebo-controlled study was initiated to evaluate the safety of belimumab in estimated 5000 SLE patients who receive concomitant standard therapy.[82] In addition, a further randomized, double-blind, controlled study will assess the efficacy and safety of belimumab in pediatric patients with SLE.[83]

Rituximab

Several open-label studies have demonstrated the efficacy of rituximab, a monoclonal antibody against CD20, in the treatment of therapy-refractory SLE patients; however, based on the trial data it has never been approved for this disease.[86] Rituximab was applied in single cases of refractory SCLE and in SLE patients with cutaneous involvement.[6] Due to insufficient clinical experience and contradictory results, this agent cannot — up to date — be recommended for the treatment of CLE.[6]

Sirukumab (anti-IL6) and tocilizumab (anti-IL6R)

Sirukumab, a human monoclonal antibody targeting interleukin 6, was used in 31 CLE patients and 15 SLE patients in a two-part, phase I, double blind, placebo-controlled trial.[87] The study was designed to evaluate the safety and pharmacokinetics of multiple intravenous infusions of sirukumab, but not the efficacy of this agent. However, the agent was well-tolerated in patients with mild, stable, and active disease. Tocilizimab, a human monoclonal antibody targeting the interleukin 6 receptor, was given to a patient with therapy-refractory CLE and urticarial vasculitis; the patient responded favorably with a remission of fever, arthritis, and skin manifestations.[88] Further studies are warranted to evaluate the efficacy of sirukumab and tocilizumab in patients with CLE.

Summary

To date, no systemic medications have been licensed specifically for the treatment of CLE; however, several agents are approved for the treatment of SLE, including the novel monoclonal antibody belimumab. Topical CS have proven to be a very effective treatment for single skin lesions in all disease subtypes, but they are of limited value due to their well-known side effects, such as atrophy and telangiectasia. In recent years, topical CI, such as tacrolimus and pimecrolimus, were applied successfully in patients with CLE and are particularly recommended in atrophy-prone areas such as the face. Antimalarials, in particular HCQ, are the first-line treatment for all patients with CLE, irrespective of the disease subtype, and are recommended in all SLE patients as baseline treatment. The application of these agents results in higher rates of remission, fewer relapses, and reduced damage in the course of the disease, even in lupus nephritis. In contrast to other immunosuppressive agents, such as azathioprine, cyclophosphamide, and cyclosporine, only methotrexate has received more attention in the treatment of CLE. Further second-line treatment options include retinoids, dapsone, and mycophenolate mofetil. In addition to belimumab, which is approved for antibody-positive SLE, other biologicals such as rituximab, sirukumab, and tocilizumab have also been suggested to be effective for the treatment of skin manifestations in the disease. Single case reports and a recent pilot have further demonstrated that FAEs could be a new alternative therapeutic option for patients with CLE. In summary, several advances have been made in improving the treatment of CLE, but only some agents are supported by evidence from randomized controlled trials.

Acknowledgements

The figures were kindly provided by the Photographic Laboratory (with thanks to J. Bueckmann and P. Wissel), Department of Dermatology, University of Muenster, Germany.

References

1. Gronhagen, C.M., Nyberg, F. (2014). Cutaneous lupus erythematosus: An update. *Indian Dermatol Online J,* **5**, 7–13.
2. Jimenez, S., Cervera, R. *et al.* (2004). The epidemiology of cutaneous lupus erythematosus. In: Kuhn, A. Lehmann, P. *et al.* (eds), *Cutaneous Lupus Erythematosus*, pp. 45–52. Springer-Verlag, Berlin.
3. Kuhn, A., Ruzicka, T. (2004). Classification of cutaneous lupus erythematosus. In: Kuhn, A., Lehmann, P. *et al.* (eds), *Cutaneous Lupus Erythematosus*, pp. 53–58. Springer-Verlag, Heidelberg.
4. Kuhn, A., Aberer, E. *et al.* (2009). Leitlinien Kutaner Lupus Erythematosus (Entwicklungsstufe 1). In: Korting, H., Callies, R. *et al.* (eds), *Dermatologische Qualitätssicherung: Leitlinien und Empfehlungen*, pp. 214–257. ABW Wissenschaftsverlag GmbH, Berlin.
5. Kuhn, A., Ruland, V. *et al.* (2011). Cutaneous lupus erythematosus: Update of therapeutic options Part I. *J Am Acad Dermatol,* **65**, e179–193.
6. Kuhn, A., Ruland, V. *et al.* (2011). Cutaneous lupus erythematosus: Update of therapeutic options part II. *J Am Acad Dermatol,* **65**, e195–213.
7. Manzi, S., Sanchez-Guerrero, J. *et al.* (2012). Effects of belimumab, a B lymphocyte stimulator-specific inhibitor, on disease activity across multiple organ domains in patients with systemic lupus erythematosus: combined results from two phase III trials. *Ann Rheum Dis,* **71**, 1833–1838.
8. Kuhn, A., Beissert, S. (2005). Photosensitivity in lupus erythematosus. *Autoimmunity,* **38**, 519–529.
9. Millard, T.P., Hawk, J.L. *et al.* (2000). Photosensitivity in lupus. *Lupus,* **9**, 3–10.
10. Schmidt, E., Tony, H.P. *et al.* (2007). Sun-induced life-threatening lupus nephritis. *Ann N Y Acad Sci,* **1108**, 35–40.

11. Vila, L.M., Mayor, A.M. *et al.* (1999). Association of sunlight exposure and photoprotection measures with clinical outcome in systemic lupus erythematosus. *P R Health Sci J*, **18**, 89–94.

12. Patsinakidis, N., Wenzel, J. *et al.* (2012). Suppression of UV-induced damage by a liposomal sunscreen: a prospective, open-label study in patients with cutaneous lupus erythematosus and healthy controls. *Exp Dermatol*, **21**, 958–961.

13. Bourre-Tessier, J., Peschken, C.A. *et al.* (2013). Association of smoking with cutaneous manifestations in systemic lupus erythematosus. *Arthritis Care Res (Hoboken)*, **65**, 1275–1280.

14. Metelitsa, A.I., Lauzon, G.J. (2010). Tobacco and the skin. *Clin Dermatol*, **28**, 384–390.

15. Kuhn, A., Sigges, J. *et al.* (2014). Influence of smoking on disease severity and antimalarial therapy in cutaneous lupus erythematosus: analysis of 1002 patients from the EUSCLE database. *Br J Dermatol*, **171**, 571–579.

16. Kreuter, A., Gaifullina, R. *et al.* (2009). Lupus erythematosus tumidus: response to antimalarial treatment in 36 patients with emphasis on smoking. *Arch Dermatol*, **145**, 244–248.

17. Jewell, M.L., McCauliffe, D.P. (2000). Patients with cutaneous lupus erythematosus who smoke are less responsive to antimalarial treatment. *J Am Acad Dermatol*, **42**, 983–987.

18. Rahman, P., Gladman, D.D. *et al.* (1998). Smoking interferes with efficacy of antimalarial therapy in cutaneous lupus. *J Rheumatol*, **25**, 1716–1719.

19. Hugel, R., Schwarz, T. *et al.* (2007). Resistance to hydroxychloroquine due to smoking in a patient with lupus erythematosus tumidus. *Br J Dermatol*, **157**, 1081–1083.

20. Marzano, A.V., Tavecchio, S. *et al.* (2014). Drug-induced lupus erythematosus. *G Ital Dermatol Venereol*, **149**, 301–309.

21. Sifuentes Giraldo,W.A., Ahijon Lana, M. *et al.* (2012). Chilblain lupus induced by TNF-alpha antagonists: a case report and literature review. *Clin Rheumatol*, **31**, 563–568.

22. Jessop, S., Whitelaw, D.A. *et al.* (2009). Drugs for discoid lupus erythematosus. *Cochrane Database Syst Rev*: CD002954.

23. Roenigk, H.H., Jr., Martin, J.S. *et al.* (1980). Discoid lupus erythematosus. Diagnostic features and evaluation of topical corticosteroid therapy. *Cutis*, **25**, 281–285.

24. Pothinamthong, P., Janjumratsang, P. (2012). A comparative study in efficacy and safety of 0.1% tacrolimus and 0.05% clobetasol propionate ointment in discoid lupus erythematosus by modified cutaneous lupus erythematosus disease area and severity index. *J Med Assoc Thai*, **95**, 933–940.

25. Sigges, J., Biazar, C. *et al.* (2013). Therapeutic strategies evaluated by the European Society of Cutaneous Lupus Erythematosus (EUSCLE) Core Set Questionnaire in more than 1000 patients with cutaneous lupus erythematosus. *Autoimmun Rev,* **12**, 694–702.

26. Kuhn, A., Ochsendorf, F. *et al.* (2010). Treatment of cutaneous lupus erythematosus. *Lupus,* **19**, 1125–1136.

27. Madan, V., August, P.J. *et al.* (2010). Efficacy of topical tacrolimus 0.3% in clobetasol propionate 0.05% ointment in therapy-resistant cutaneous lupus erythematosus: a cohort study. *Clin Exp Dermatol,* **35**, 27–30.

28. Kuhn, A., Gensch, K. *et al.* (2011). Efficacy of tacrolimus 0.1% ointment in cutaneous lupus erythematosus: a multicenter, randomized, double-blind, vehicle-controlled trial. *J Am Acad Dermatol,* **65**, 54–64.

29. Kreuter, A., Gambichler, T. *et al.* (2004). Pimecrolimus 1% cream for cutaneous lupus erythematosus. *J Am Acad Dermatol.,* **51**, 407–410.

30. Barikbin, B., Givrad, S. *et al.* (2009). Pimecrolimus 1% cream versus betamethasone 17-valerate 0.1% cream in the treatment of facial discoid lupus erythematosus: a double-blind, randomized pilot study. *Clin Exp Dermatol,* **34**, 776–780.

31. Nghiem, P., Pearson, G. *et al.* (2002). Tacrolimus and pimecrolimus: from clever prokaryotes to inhibiting calcineurin and treating atopic dermatitis. *J Am Acad Dermatol,* **46**, 228–241.

32. Prenner, B.M. (2008). Role of long-acting beta2-adrenergic agonists in asthma management based on updated asthma guidelines. *Curr Opin Pulm Med,* **14**, 57–63.

33. Jemec, G.B., Ullman, S. *et al.* (2009). A randomized controlled trial of R-salbutamol for topical treatment of discoid lupus erythematosus. *Br J Dermatol,* **161**, 1365–1370.

34. Edwards, K.R., Burke, W.A. (1999). Treatment of localized discoid lupus erythematosus with tazarotene. *J Am Acad Dermatol,* **41**, 1049–1050.

35. Seiger, E., Roland, S. *et al.* (1991). Cutaneous lupus treated with topical tretinoin: a case report. *Cutis,* **47**, 351–355.

36. Terao, M., Matsui, S. *et al.* (2011). Two cases of refractory discoid lupus erythematosus successfully treated with topical tocoretinate. *Dermatol Online J,* **17**, 15.

37. Gerdsen, R., Wenzel, J. *et al.* (2002). Successful treatment of chronic discoid lupus erythematosus of the scalp with imiquimod. *Dermatology,* **205**, 416–418.

38. Ochsendorf, F.R. (2010). Use of antimalarials in dermatology. *J Dtsch Dermatol Ges,* **8**, 829–844.

39. Bertsias, G., Ioannidis, J.P. *et al.* (2008). EULAR recommendations for the management of systemic lupus erythematosus. Report of a Task Force of the

EULAR Standing Committee for International Clinical Studies Including Therapeutics. *Ann Rheum Dis,* **67**, 195–205.

40. Costedoat-Chalumeau, N., Leroux, G. *et al.* (2010). Why all systemic lupus erythematosus patients should be given hydroxychloroquine treatment? *Joint Bone Spine,* **77**, 4–5.

41. Fessler, B.J., Alarcon, G.S. *et al.* (2005). Systemic lupus erythematosus in three ethnic groups: XVI. Association of hydroxychloroquine use with reduced risk of damage accrual. *Arthritis Rheum,* **52**, 1473–1480.

42. Ruzicka, T., Sommerburg, C. *et al.* (1992). Treatment of cutaneous lupus erythematosus with acitretin and hydroxychloroquine. *Br J Dermatol,* **127**, 513–518.

43. Ikeda, T. Kanazawa, N. *et al.* (2012). Hydroxychloroquine administration for Japanese lupus erythematosus in Wakayama: a pilot study. *J Dermatol,* **39**, 531–535.

44. Momose, Y., Arai, S. *et al.* (2013). Experience with the use of hydroxychloroquine for the treatment of lupus erythematosus. *J Dermatol,* **40**, 94–97.

45. Yokogawa, N., Tanikawa, A. *et al.* (2013). Response to hydroxychloroquine in Japanese patients with lupus-related skin disease using the cutaneous lupus erythematosus disease area and severity index (CLASI). *Mod Rheumatol,* **23**, 318–322.

46. Frances, C., Cosnes, A. *et al.* (2012). Low blood concentration of hydroxy-chloroquine in patients with refractory cutaneous lupus erythematosus: a French multicenter prospective study. *Arch Dermatol,* **148**, 479–484.

47. Wahie, S., Daly, A.K. *et al.* (2011). Clinical and pharmacogenetic influences on response to hydroxychloroquine in discoid lupus erythematosus: a retrospective cohort study. *J Invest Dermatol,* **131**, 1981–1986.

48. Dutz, J., Werth, V.P. (2011). Cigarette smoking and response to antimalarials in cutaneous lupus erythematosus patients: evolution of a dogma. *J Invest Dermatol,* **131**, 1968–1970.

49. Ziemer, M., Milkova, L. *et al.* (2014). Lupus erythematosus. Part II: Clinical picture, diagnosis and treatment. *J Dtsch Dermatol Ges,* **12**, 285–301.

50. Chang, A.Y., Werth, V.P. (2011). Treatment of cutaneous lupus. *Curr Rheumatol Rep,* **13**, 300–307.

51. Goldberg, J.W., Lidsky, M.D. (1984). Pulse methylprednisolone therapy for persistent subacute cutaneous lupus. *Arthritis Rheum,* **27**, 837–838.

52. Winkelmann, R.R., Kim, G.K. *et al.* (2013). Treatment of cutaneous lupus erythematosus: review and assessment of treatment benefits based on oxford centre for evidence-based medicine criteria. *J Clin Aesthet Dermatol,* **6**, 27–38.

53. Miyawaki, S., Nishiyama, S. *et al.* (2013). The effect of methotrexate on improving serological abnormalities of patients with systemic lupus erythematosus. *Mod Rheumatol,* **23**, 659–666.

54. Wenzel, J., Brahler, S. *et al.* (2005). Efficacy and safety of methotrexate in recalcitrant cutaneous lupus erythematosus: results of a retrospective study in 43 patients. *Br J Dermatol,* **153**, 157–162.

55. Huber, A., Tuting, T. *et al.* (2006). Methotrexate treatment in cutaneous lupus erythematosus: subcutaneous application is as effective as intravenous administration. *Br J Dermatol,* **155**, 861–862.

56. Drake, L.A., Dinehart, S.M. *et al.* (1996). Guidelines of care for cutaneous lupus erythematosus. American Academy of Dermatology. *J Am Acad Dermatol,* **34**, 830–836.

57. Ruzicka, T., Lynde, C.W. *et al.* (2008). Efficacy and safety of oral alitretinoin (9-cis retinoic acid) in patients with severe chronic hand eczema refractory to topical corticosteroids: results of a randomized, double-blind, placebo-controlled, multicentre trial. *Br J Dermatol,* **158**, 808–817.

58. Kuhn, A., Patsinakidis, N. *et al.* (2012). Alitretinoin for cutaneous lupus erythematosus. *J Am Acad Dermatol,* **67**, e123–126.

59. Ruzicka, T., Meurer, M. *et al.* (1988). Efficiency of acitretin in the treatment of cutaneous lupus erythematosus. *Arch Dermatol,* **124**, 897–902.

60. Bacman, D., Kuhn, A. *et al.* (2004). Dapsone and retinoids. In: Kuhn, A. Lehmann, P., *et al.* (eds), *Cutaneous Lupus Erythematosus,* pp. 373–390. Springer-Verlag, Berlin.

61. Ludgate, M.W., Greig, D.E. (2008). Bullous systemic lupus erythematosus responding to dapsone. *Australas J Dermatol,* **49**, 91–93.

62. Ujiie, H., Shimizu, T. *et al.* (2006). Lupus erythematosus profundus successfully treated with dapsone: review of the literature. *Arch Dermatol.,* **142**, 399–401.

63. Grover, C., Khurana, A. *et al.* (2013). Bullous systemic lupus erythematosus. *Indian J Dermatol,* **58**, 492.

64. Nasongkhla, P. Pratchyapruit, W. *et al.* (2012). Bullous systemic lupus erythematosus induced by UVB: report a case. *J Med Assoc Thai,* **95**, 969–973.

65. Seo, J.Y., Byun, H.J. *et al.* (2012). Methimazole-induced bullous systemic lupus erythematosus: a case report. *J Korean Med Sci,* **27**, 818–821.

66. Bertsias, G.K., Tektonidou, M. *et al.* (2012). Joint European League Against Rheumatism and European Renal Association-European Dialysis and Transplant Association (EULAR/ERA-EDTA) recommendations for the management of adult and paediatric lupus nephritis. *Ann Rheum Dis,* **71**, 1771–1782.

67. Hanjani, N.M., Nousari, C.H. (2002). Mycophenolate mofetil for the treatment of cutaneous lupus erythematosus with smoldering systemic involvement. *Arch Dermatol,* **138**, 1616–1618.
68. Pisoni, C.N., Obermoser, G. *et al.* (2005). Skin manifestations of systemic lupus erythematosus refractory to multiple treatment modalities: poor results with mycophenolate mofetil. *Clin Exp Rheumatol,* **23**, 393–396.
69. Gammon, B., Hansen, C. *et al.* (2011). Efficacy of mycophenolate mofetil in antimalarial-resistant cutaneous lupus erythematosus. *J Am Acad Dermatol,* **65**, 717–721.
70. Kreuter, A., Tomi, N.S. *et al.* (2007). Mycophenolate sodium for subacute cutaneous lupus erythematosus resistant to standard therapy. *Br J Dermatol,* **156**, 1321–1327.
71. Dammacco, F., Della Casa Alberighi, O. *et al.* (2000). Cyclosporine-A plus steroids versus steroids alone in the 12-month treatment of systemic lupus erythematosus. *Int J Clin Lab Res,* **30**, 67–73.
72. Klein, A., Vogt, T. *et al.* (2011). Cyclosporin combined with methotrexate in two patients with recalcitrant subacute cutaneous lupus erythematosus. *Australas J Dermatol,* **52**, 43–47.
73. Saeki, Y., Ohshima, S. *et al.* (2000). Maintaining remission of lupus erythematosus profundus (LEP) with cyclosporin A. *Lupus,* **9**, 390–392.
74. Caccavo, D., Lagana, B. *et al.* (1997). Long-term treatment of systemic lupus erythematosus with cyclosporin A. *Arthritis Rheum,* **40**, 27–35.
75. Yell, J.A., Burge, S.M. (1994). Cyclosporin and discoid lupus erythematosus. *Br J Dermatol,* **131**, 132–133.
76. Baskin, E., Ozen, S. *et al.* (2010). The use of low-dose cyclophosphamide followed by AZA/MMF treatment in childhood lupus nephritis. *Pediatr Nephrol,* **25**, 111–117.
77. Takada, K., Illei, G.G. *et al.* (2001). Cyclophosphamide for the treatment of systemic lupus erythematosus. *Lupus,* **10**, 154–161.
78. Raptopoulou, A., Linardakis, C. *et al.* (2010). Pulse cyclophosphamide treatment for severe refractory cutaneous lupus erythematosus. *Lupus,* **19**, 744–747.
79. Furie, R., Petri, M. *et al.* (2011). A phase III, randomized, placebo-controlled study of belimumab, a monoclonal antibody that inhibits B lymphocyte stimulator, in patients with systemic lupus erythematosus. *Arthritis Rheum,* **63**, 3918–3930.
80. Navarra, S.V., Guzman, R.M. *et al.* (2011). Efficacy and safety of belimumab in patients with active systemic lupus erythematosus: a randomised, placebo-controlled, phase 3 trial. *Lancet,* **377**, 721–731.

81. Kuhn, A., Meuth, A.M. *et al.* (2010). Revised Cutaneous Lupus Erythematosus Disease Area and Severity Index (RCLASI): a modified outcome instrument for cutaneous lupus erythematosus. *Br J Dermatol*, **163**, 898–899.

82. HGS Inc. (2014). Belimumab Assessment of Safety in SLE (BASE). ClinicalTrials.gov [Internet]. Bethesda (MD): National Library of Medicine (US). (NCT01705977). Retrieved 11/06/2014 https://clinicaltrials.gov/ct2/show/NCT01705977?term=lupus+erythematosus&recr=Recruiting&no_unk=Y&rank=27

83. GlaxoSmithKline. (2014). Pediatric Lupus Trial of Belimumab Plus Background Standard Therapy (PLUTO). (NCT01649765). Retrieved 11/06/2014 https://clinicaltrials.gov/ct2/show/NCT01649765?term=belimumab+lupus&rank=11

84. Nast, A., Boehncke, W.H. *et al.* (2012). S3 — Guidelines on the treatment of psoriasis vulgaris (English version). Update. *J Dtsch Dermatol Ges,* **10 Suppl 2**, S1–95.

85. Tsianakas, A., Herzog, S. *et al.* (2014). Successful treatment of discoid lupus erythematosus with fumaric acid esters. *J Am Acad Dermatol*, **71**, e15–17.

86. Garcia-Carrasco, M., Jimenez-Hernandez, M. *et al.* (2009). Use of rituximab in patients with systemic lupus erythematosus: an update. *Autoimmun Rev,* **8**, 343–348.

87. Szepietowski, J.C., Nilganuwong, S. *et al.* (2013). Phase I, randomized, double-blind, placebo-controlled, multiple intravenous, dose-ascending study of sirukumab in cutaneous or systemic lupus erythematosus. *Arthritis Rheum,* **65**, 2661–2671.

88. Makol, A., Gibson, L.E. *et al.* (2012). Successful use of interleukin 6 antagonist tocilizumab in a patient with refractory cutaneous lupus and urticarial vasculitis. *J Clin Rheumatol,* **18**, 92–95.

CHAPTER 12

ADVANCES IN THERAPIES FOR INTERSTITIAL LUNG DISEASES

Giovanni Ferrara and Magnus Sköld

Introduction

Diffuse parenchymal lung diseases (DPLD, also called interstitial lung diseases, ILD) are a group of respiratory diseases affecting the interstitial space in the lung. These diseases often lead to a restrictive ventilatory deficiency and can progress to respiratory failure as a result of diffuse remodelling of the lung parenchyma. The most aggressive forms lead to death within a short period of time. The definition includes a number of different diseases, with different pathogeneses and mechanisms, and are often idiopathic. Most of them are considered rare and classified as orphan diseases of the lung, due to the very low incidence (around 4–8 patients/100 000 for idiopathic pulmonary fibrosis, IPF). A new classification of ILD has recently been published and is illustrated in Fig. 1.[1]

Knowledge and interest about ILD increased in the 80's, mostly due to to the technical innovation brought by the flexible bronchoscopy and the bronchoalveolar lavage (BAL) technique. The possibility of obtaining samples from the peripheral parts of the lung with a relatively non-invasive method boosted a number of studies on the cellularity and cellular activation

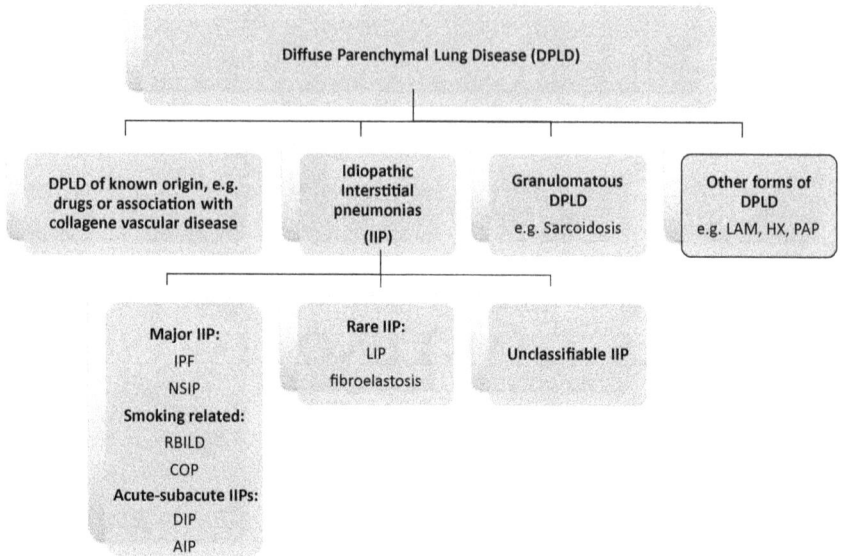

Figure 1. Classification of Diffuse Parenchymal Lung Disease (American Thoracic Society 2002–2013).
LAM: Lymphangioleyomiomatosis; HX: Histiocytosis X; PAP: Pulmonary Alveolar Proteinois; IPF: Idiopathic Pulmonary Fibrosis; NSIP: Nonspecific Interstitial Pneumonia; RBILD: Respiratory Bronchiolitis Interstitial Lung Disease; COP: Cryptogenic Organising Pneumonia; DIP: Desquamative Interstitial Pneumonia; AIP: Acute Interstitial Pneumonia; LIP: Lymphocytic Interstitial Pneumonia.

in a variety of ILD. In particular, a number of papers dealing with the pathogenesis of inflammatory granulomatous diseases such as sarcoidosis and berylliosis were published.[2–5] In both of these diseases, the expansion of specific subpopulations of cells recovered in BAL (*i.e.* CD4 T cells) and their specific activation with a Th1 profile seemed to offer the basis for a common understanding of all ILD. The hypothesis was introduced that an unknown cause could trigger a specific uncontrolled inflammation in the alveolar space and in the lung interstitium. This was thought to result in remodelling of the parenchyma with fibrotic changes replacing the normal architecture leading to pathophysiological changes responsible for the clinical manifestations of the diseases.[6] In the same model (*i.e.* berylliosis), a specific genetic susceptibility could be identified and the mechanisms of the disease elucidated.[7] This has given the illusion that all ILD referred to an inflammatory pathogenesis, and has resulted in the concept that most of these conditions can be treated with immunosuppressive drugs despite the very different clinical and radiological presentations.

Only during the 90's did the development of mini-invasive techniques to obtain lung tissues (such as Video-Assisted-Thoracoscopy, VATS) allow us to study the detailed pathology of the lung in the course of interstitial lung diseases *ex vivo*. In parallel, significant improvements in imaging techniques such as high resolution computerized tomography (HRCT) led to a better understanding of the differences and similarities of the ILD and could, in many disease entities, replace the need for open or thoracoscopic lung biopsy. At the end of the 90's, a revision of all the clinical, radiological and pathological features of the ILD led to a systematic classification that highlighted the differences among the inflammatory ILD and other forms of idiopathic diseases.[8] It then became clear that most of the ILD were closer to proliferative diseases than to inflammatory ones and it took almost 15 years to develop and register the first drugs with an anti-fibrotic effect for the foremost fibrotic lung disease, idiopathic pulmonary fibrosis (IPF).[9]

In this chapter, we will discuss the current pharmacological approaches for the most common ILD, with a special focus on recent randomized clinical trials. We will also discuss the current approaches to some other rare lung diseases, and the importance of the orphan drug designation for new compounds.

The New Paradigm of Idiopathic Pulmonary Fibrosis (IPF)

Idiopathic pulmonary fibrosis (IPF) is the most common form of the idiopathic interstitial pneumonias with an estimated prevalence of 14–16/ 100 000. The increasing knowledge about the pathophysiology and clinical course of IPF has completely changed the approach to its management and treatment. In the 1980's, IPF was considered to be the result of uncontrolled inflammation in the lung. The finding of increased numbers of inflammatory cells (especially neutrophils) in BAL of patients with IPF supported this hypothesis and resulted in a small number of clinical trials including immunosuppressive treatments, which did not show any real effect. Small studies suggested in the 1990's a potential effect on IPF of a combination therapy including three anti-inflammatory drugs, including low dose prednisolone, azathioprine and N-acetylcysteine (NAC).[10] However a multicenter randomised controlled trial demonstrated that this "triple therapy" was even associated with a higher morbility and mortality compared with placebo.[11] In addition, it was recently shown[79] that treatment with high-dose NAC as single therapy was not favourable compared to placebo.

The lack of a shared definition and diagnostic criteria for the disease made it difficult for researchers and investigators to compare data until the end of the 1990's, when a revised classification of ILD was presented. Based on consistent pathological findings, it was made clear that inflammation was not the main feature of IPF.[12] An abnormal proliferation of fibroblasts resulting in extended fibrosis of the lung became the hallmark of the disease. New theories based on the activation of cell growth factors resulted in clinical trials with alternative approaches. One of the first was interferon-γ, the main cytokine of the Th1-mediated response. Since this cytokine has the ability to revert the activation of Transforming Growth Factor (TGF)-beta, it was hypothesized that interferon-γ would slow disease progression. However, a large study, in fact the only study performed so far with mortality as a primary endpoint, was not able to show any advantages as compared to placebo.[13]

Idiopathic pulmonary fibrosis is certainly the interstitial lung disease that has attracted most research in the last 10 years. The increasing interest in the disease led to a shared evidence-based definition and to guidelines endorsed by the American Thoracic Society, European Respiratory Society, Japanese Respiratory Society and other major respiratory scientific societies.[14] IPF is today defined as a chronic and progressive fibrotic process of unknown origin, limited to the lung, occurring primarily in older adults, and associated with the histopathological and/or radiologic pattern of usual interstitial pneumonia (UIP) (Fig. 2). Strict diagnostic criteria and parameters for follow-up are still being discussed, but it is now clear that IPF is a proliferative disorder of the lung, with fibroblasts as the main cells involved, rather than the result of an enduring inflammation.[8,12,14]

New insights in the pathogenesis and disease course of IPF resulted in a number of clinical trials (Table 1), the first being published in 2004.[15]

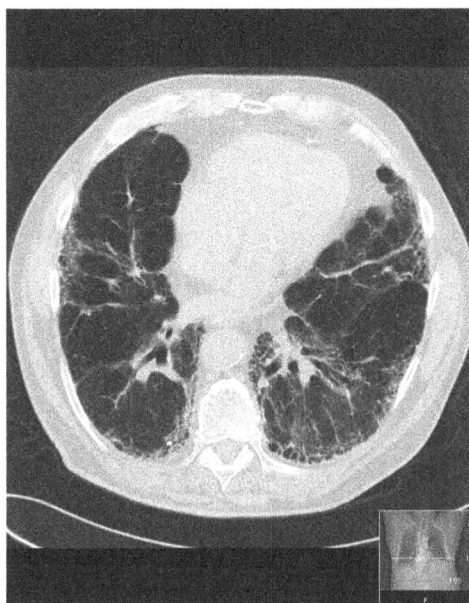

Figure 2. High Resolution Computerized Tomography (HRCT) of a patient with idiopathic pulmonary fibrosis (IPF). Peripheral fibrosis, mostly symmetrical in the lower lobes, traction bronchiectasis and honey combing are easily recognised in the scan.

Unfortunately, most of these trials were negative, with some exceptions. Thus, the first drug being registered was pirfenidone which became available in Japan in 2007 and in the EU in 2011.

In 2014, two drugs, pirfenidone and nintedanib, received the Breakthrough Therapy Designation from the Food and Drug Administration (FDA) in the United States. Both compounds have an anti-fibrotic and inhibitory effects on cell proliferation, even though they have completely different modes of action.

Pirfenidone

Pirfenidone, a pyridine [5-methyl-1-phenyl-2-(1H)-pyridone], is a small molecule that was developed initially as an anthelminthic and antipyretic drug. Due to its small structure and chemical properties, it is very easily absorbed from the gastrointestinal tract and it is able to move through cell membranes without requiring a receptor. It has a very short half-life, which

Table 1. Randomized clinical trials published for idiopathic pulmonary fibrosis (IPF).

Study	Lenght (weeks)	N of patients	Intervention	Primary outcome	Result
Raghu *et al.* *NEJM* 2004[15]	58	330	IFN-γ	FVC, PaO$_2$	NEG
Azuma *et al.* *AJRCCM* 2005[69]	63	107	Pirfenidone	SpO$_2$ 6MWT	NEG
IFIGENIA *NEJM* 2005[70]	52	182	NAC per os	FVC, DlCO	POS
Raghu *et al.* *AJRCCM* 2008[71]	48	88	Etanercept	FVC	NEG
BUILD-1 *AJRCCM* 2008[72]	52	158	Bosentan	6MWT	NEG
INSPIRE *Lancet* 2009[13]	64	826	IFN- γ	Mortality	NEG
STEP-IPF *NEJM* 2010[73]	12	180	Sildenafil	6MWT	NEG
Daniels *et al.* *AJRCCM* 2010[74]	96	119	imatinib	FVC	NEG
Taniguchi *et al.* *ERJ* 2010[18]	52	275	Pirfenidone	VC	POS
BUILD-3 *AJRCCM* 2011[75]	52	616	Bosentan	FVC, DlCO	NEG
CAPACITY I and II *Lancet* 2011[9]	72	779	Pirfenidone	FVC	POS
TOMORROW *NEJM* 2011[23]	52	432	Nintedanib	FVC	NEG
Homma *et al.* *Respirology* 2012[76]	48	76	NAC, inhaled	FVC	NEG
ACE-IPF *AJRCCM* 2012[77]	48	145	Warfarin	Death, hospitalisation, FVC	NEG
ARTEMIS-IPF *Ann Intern Med* 2013[78]	34	492	Ambrisentan	Death, hospitalisation, progession	NEG

(Continued)

Table 1. (*Continued*)

Study	Lenght (weeks)	N of patients	Intervention	Primary outcome	Result
PANTHER-IPF *NEJM* 2014[11,79]	60	155	Prednisolone, AZA, NAC/ NAC alone	FVC	NEG
MUSIC *ERJ* 2013[80]	52	178	Macitentan	FVC	NEG
ASCEND *NEJM* 2014[81]	52	555	Pirfenidone	FVC, death	POS
INPULSIS *NEJM* 2014[24]	52	1066	Nintedanib	FVC	POS

means that multiple administrations over the day are necessary to keep a therapeutic concentration in the blood. Pirfenidone is metabolized in the liver, with two metabolites (hydroxypirfenidone and carboxypirfenidone), eliminated mainly through urine. This contributes to potential interactions with other drugs inducing or inhibiting hepatic cytochromes and limits the use of the drug in patients with reduced kidney function (creatinine clearance <30 ml/min). Its rapid absorption and diffusion through all cell membranes is also responsible for the most common sides effects, such as headache, nausea and dizziness.[16] A summary of the main side effects is reported in Table 2.

Pirfenidone is believed to work on fibrogenesis via three main effects: reducing oxidative stress, reducing TGF-beta activation and expression and by directly reducing the deposition of collagen in the tissues. The drug was able to reduce the development of fibrosis in animal models of pulmonary fibrosis with experiments showing reduction of different pro-inflammatory cytokines and growth factors. However, it is still unknown exactly how pirfenidone is able to exert its anti-fibrotic effects in IPF.[16,17]

Small open label studies and a small randomised controlled trial (RCT) suggested that pirfenidone could slow down the progression of the disease with a significant reduction in the loss of Vital Capacity (VC) over time.[18] Three multicentre multinational double blind RCTs have shown that pirfenidone was effective in reducing the decline of lung function

Table 2. Comparison of adverse events reported for pirfenidone and nintedanib.[19,24]

	Pirfenidone	Nintedanib
Nausea	36%	24.4%
Headache	25.9%	NR
URTI	21.9%	9.1%
Fatigue	20.9%	NR
Rash	28.1%	NR
Cough	25.2%	13.4%
Diarrhea	22.3%	62.3%
Dizziness	17.6%	NR
Dyspepsia	17.6%	NR
Anorexia	15.8%	10.6%
Dyspnoea	14.7%	7.6%
Vomiting	12.9%	11.6%
Nasopharyngitis	11.9%	13.6%
Gastroesofagal reflux	11.9%	NR
Back Pain	10.8%	NR
Decrease in weight	12.6%	9.6%
Constipation	11.5%	NR
Bronchitis	14%	10.5%
Worsening of IPF	9.4%	10%
Insomnia	11.2%	NR

URTI: upper respiratory tract infection.

compared to placebo, measured as change in percent of predicted FVC from baseline to 56 weeks. Also, a significant effect on slowing down disease progression was shown, defined as time to $\geq 10\%$ decline in percent predicted FVC, $>15\%$ decline in percent predicted diffusion capacity for carbon monoxide (DLCO), or death.[9,19] Data on safety and efficacy in long-survivors have shown a good tolerability profile and the possibility to treat patients for over seven years, still having an effect on the course of the disease.[20] Since 2011 the drug is already registered and available in Europe, and was recently approved by the Food and Drug Administration for marketing in the United States.

Nintedanib

The second drug that has recently been approved for use both in Europe and United States is nintedanib. This is a triple tyrosine kinase inhibitor originally developed to treat prostatic cancer as a result of its anti-angio-genic properties (angiokinase inhibitor class). It is effective in inhibiting the downstream pathways of three receptors: the vascular endothelial growth factor receptor (VEGFR), the platelet derived growth factor receptor (PDGFR) and the fibroblast growth factor receptor (FGFR).[21,22] It is tested in combined regimens with taxanes (docetaxel or placitexel) for the treatment of various cancers including lung, breast and colon cancer. Especially in non-small cell lung cancer, a multinational phase III RCT showed very promising results in patients experiencing disease-progression after first-line chemotherapy: an overall survival benefit of 2.5 months in a subgroup of patients with adenocarcinoma was observed compared with conventional second-line treatment.[23]

Nintedanib is easily absorbed and can be administered orally, with maximum plasma concentration occurring mainly 1–4 h after administration and a terminal half-life of 19 h. Furthermore, data from *in vitro* experiments showed that the inhibitory effect at a cellular level can be sustained up to 32 h after exposure to nintedanib for 1 hour. The drug is converted to its active form by methyl ester cleavage and is mainly excreted via the liver.[21,22]

The peculiar effect on FGFR and fibroblasts provided a rationale to test nintedanib in the treatment of patients with IPF: one phase II study and two identical phase III studies were completed and published between 2011 and 2014, showing that the drug is effective in slowing down the loss of FVC with a sustained effect over time.[24,25]

Main side effects of nintedanib are nausea, diarrhea, vomiting and elevation of liver enzymes. In particular, diarrhea was experienced by 60% of the patients in the phase III trials (Table 2).

An update of the American Thoracic/European Respiratory Society Guidelines on IPF is pending and it is expected to include evidence-based recommendations on the use of pirfenidone and nintedanib.

Other Potential Drugs in Development for IPF

It is likely that the different characteristics and targets of pirfenidone and nintedanib will increase the possibilities to tailor treatments to patients with IPF. Studies looking at the possibility to combine the two drugs are also warranted. At least 16 new compounds and drugs approved for use in other medical conditions (Table 3) are currently being tested in clinical trials for the treatment of IPF.[26] Molecular markers and genetic testing will hopefully be validated in the near future. This will probably allow us to enter an era of personalized precision medicine in the field of interstitial lung diseases, and it may shift the paradigm of IPF from a deadly disorder to a chronic lung disease.

Lung Transplantation

To date, the only intervention that has a proven effect on survival is lung transplantation. All patients fulfilling inclusion criteria for a transplantation should be considered for short-listing on a waiting list at an early stage, in some cases at the time of diagnosis. Inclusion criteria and short-listing criteria vary by country as do the upper age limit for transplantation and period on waiting list, which in Sweden is 3–6 months. Extracorporeal membrane oxygenation (ECMO) has been described as a bridge to lung transplantation for patients who are rapidly deteriorating.[27]

Lymphangioleyomiomatosis (*LAM*) and Pulmonary Alveolar Proteinosis (PAP): When Proliferation of Blasts and Cell Maturation Matter

Lymphangioleiomyomatosis (*LAM*) is a rare progressive disease of the lung, affecting almost exclusively women in their fertile period, and is characterised by a progressive cystic destruction of the lung (Fig. 3) and by the association with mutations in the tuberous sclerosis complex (TSC) genes.[29]

Often the clinical course of the disease is complicated by recurrent pneumothorax, chylous pleural effusions and abdominal tumours, such as

Table 3. New compounds being tested for idiopathic pulmonary fibrosis.

Compound	Mechanism	Administration route	Company	Phase
Bardoxolone methyl	Nrf2 agonist, PDJ2 mimetic	Oral	Abbott/Reatta	III
Thalidomide	Unknown, reduces collagen production	Oral	Celgene	II
CC-930	JNK inhibitor	Oral	Celgene	II
GS-6624	Anti-LOXL2 monoclonal antibody	i.v.	Gilead/Arresto	I
IFN-α	Anti-inflammatory	Oral	Amarillo Biosciences	II
Zileuton (Zyflo)	Leukotriene synthesis inhibitor, 5-LO inhibitor	Oral	Cornerstone Therapeutics/ Skyepharma	II
Tetrathiomolybdate (Coprexa)	Copper chelator	Oral	Adeona/Pipex Therapeutics	II
CNTO-888	Anti-CCL2 monoclonal antibody	i.v.	Centocor	II
QAX576	IL-13 inhibitor	i.v.	Novartis	II
PXS25	Leukocyte extravasation inhibitor	i.v.	Pharmaxis	II
Vasoactive intestinal peptide (VIP)	Anti-inflammatory	Inhaled	Mondobiotech	II
GC-1008 (fresolimumab)	Anti-TGF-β monoclonal antibody	i.v.	Genzyme	II
FG-3019	Anti-CTGF human monoclonal antibody	i.v.	FibroGen	II
STX-100	Anti–αvβ6 integrin monoclonal antibody	i.v.	Stromedix	II
PRM-151	Recombinant human SAP, monocyte inhibitor	i.v.	Promedior	Ib
Unknown	Anti-IL-4/IL-13 receptor monoclonal antibody	i.v.	Bristol-Myers Squibb	I

CTGF, connective tissue growth factor; FGFR, fibroblast growth factor receptor; IFN, interferon; IL, interleukin; IV, intravenous; SAP, serum amyloid protein; subcut., subcutaneous; TGF, transforming growth factor; TNF, tumor necrosis factor.

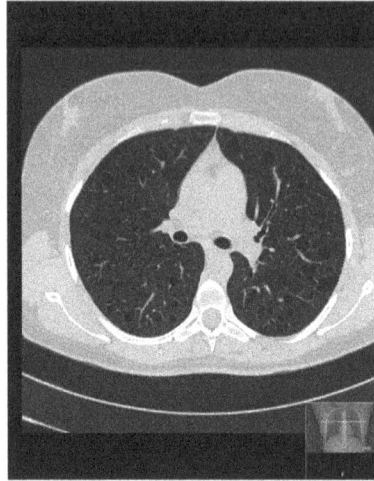

Figure 3. High Resolution Computerized Tomography (HRCT) of a female patient with lymphangioleiomyomatosis (LAM). The scan is characterised by multiple cystic lesions spread all over the parenchyma of the lung.

angiomyolipomas and lymphangiomyomas. Sporadic forms are the most common but familiar forms associated with tuberous sclerosis exist. Most of the mutations target a highly evolutionarily preserved GTPase-activating protein: tuberin (encoded by TSC2 genes). Another protein, which heterodimerizes with tuberin and hamartin (TSC1 genes), contributes to regulate the activity of the mammalian target of the rapamycin complex (mTORC) 1 and 2. The downstream pathway of mTORC1 and 2 is involved in the signalling and regulation of a number of processes such as autophagy, apoptosis, angiogenesis and lymphangiogenesis. The mutation of the TSC results in the acquisition of anti-apoptotic properties and the capacity of LAM-cells to invade and spread via lymphatic vessels, despite a benign microscopic phenotype. This causes the typical clinical course of the disease that often leads to death within 10–20 years from the first diagnosis.[29,30]

Sirolimus (also known as rapamycin) is a macrolide discovered in 1999 on the Easter Island Rapa Nui. Sirolimus is produced by the bacteria *Streptomyces hygroscopicus* and it was originally developed as an antifungal agent. Due to its potent immunosuppressive and anti-proliferative properties, sirolimus is today used as immunosuppressant in kidney-transplantation and as coronary stent coating.[31]

Sirolimus binds a cytosolic protein, the FK-binding protein 12 (FKBP12). The resulting complex binds to and inhibits mTORC1 and 2. The discovery of the association of mTORC in LAM supported the hypothesis of using sirolimus in clinical trials in LAM.[32] The first trial was designed to study the effect of sirolimus on angiomyolipomas in LAM and the tuberous sclerosis complex (TSC). The volume of angiomyolipomas decreased by about 50% in the study population during the treatment period. It was also observed that sirolimus slowed the decline rate of lung function.[33] The results prompted the design of a new trial, the Multicenter International LAM Efficacy of Sirolimus (MILES) study, which was designed to test if sirolimus could slow down progression of decline in lung function and reduce its complications. The trial met its primary endpoint and was also associated with a reduction of symptoms and improvement in quality of life. Furthermore, a marker of disease-activity, Vascular Endothelial Growth Factor-D (VGEF-D) was reduced in the blood in the treated patients. Adverse events, mostly dermatological and gastrointestinal, were more common in the treatment arm, but the occurrence of severe side effects was not different between the treatment group and placebo.[34]

Preliminary data also showed that sirolimus may reduce the rate of recurrence of LAM in patients receiving lung transplantation.[35] Taken together, the data suggested that sirolimus and everolimus will be therapeutic options in the treatment of complicated LAM associated with TSC-1 and -2 genes, although no evidence-based guidelines are available. A number of other drugs like Rheb inhibitors (*e.g.*, farnesyltransferase inhibitors and statins), selective estrogen antagonists (*e.g.*, fispemifene), tyrosine kinase inhibitors (*e.g.*, imatinib mesylate), metalloproteinase inhibitors (*e.g.*, doxycycline), angiogenesis inhibitors (*e.g.*, bevacizumab), and lymphangiogenesis inhibitors (*e.g.*, anti-VEGF-D antibody) are already approved for other diseases and it is likely that they will be tested for LAM/TSC in the near future.[29,30,32]

Pulmonary alveolar proteinosis (PAP) is a rare disease of the lung characterised by the accumulation of surfactant components in the alveoli and terminal airways. The disease is caused by the inhibition of maturation and consequent reduced scavenger activity of alveolar macrophages. Its incidence is around 3–6 cases/1 000 000 inhabitants and the autoimmune/idiopathic form represents approximately 90% of the patients with PAP. Secondary and congenital forms of the disease make up the rest of the cases.[36,37]

The autoimmune form is characterised by circulating antibodies against the granulocyte and monocyte colony stimulating factor (GM-CSF), a cytokine playing a key role in the differentiation and maturation of circulating monocytes into alveolar macrophages.[36]

The clinical presentation is characterised by a history of dyspnea that has occurred for several weeks. In advanced disease, severe respiratory failure with shunt effects will develop. Patients often seek doctors when respiratory failure is already established, due to the slowly progressive dyspnea over several weeks and lack of other symptoms. Radiologically, a typical appearance of "crazy-paving" on computerized tomography of the lung can be observed.[38]

Exclusion of other causes and presence of antibodies against GM-CSF is necessary for the diagnosis of autoimmune PAP. In addition, a typical bronchoalveolar lavage cell finding or compatible finding on surgical lung biopsy and a typical clinical and radiological picture are required.[36,38] Whole lung lavage is still the main treatment for PAP, even with extracorporeal membrane oxygenation support,[39,40] but other strategies aiming to reduce the inhibitory effect of autoimmune antibodies against GM-CSF are currently tested. The administration of GM-CSF subcutaneously[41,42] or via aerosol[43] has proved to be effective in some patients with PAP, but recurrence after discontinuation of the treatment is frequent. Other investigators have tried to "clean" the autoimmune antibodies by selective depletion of B-lymphocytes with rituximab[44] or by plasmapheresis.[45] These strategies have been tested alone or in combination with whole lung lavage with an efficacy of 40–80%.[36] The data mostly originate from single centres and with relatively limited cohorts of patients, due to the rarity of the disease. No evidence-based guidelines are available at the moment, and it is generally believed that patients with autoimmune PAP have a lower survival compared to the general population (about 68% at 10 years), but reliable representative data are not available.[36,37]

"Cross-Over" Diseases and New Therapy Approaches: Systemic Sclerosis and Dermatomyositis/Polymyositis

The lung is often the target of inflammatory processes in the course of connective tissue disease (CTD), resulting in fibrosis and remodelling of the whole lung architecture, which are typical for a group of ILD called CTD-ILD.[1,12] These processes eventually lead to significant morbidity and complications, and often to death by respiratory failure. A number of mechanisms take part in these events. Alveolar epithelial damage can be triggered by innate, non-specific mechanisms and by acquired immunity with effector cells and antibodies targeting antigens in the lung. Both these mechanisms can result in the activation or overexpression of growth-factors, such as transforming growth factor (TGF)-β and connective tissue growth factor (CTGF), leading to fibroblast proliferation and connective tissue deposition.[46,47]

Systemic sclerosis

Involvement of the lung is particularly frequent in systemic sclerosis (SSc). Although this disease is more often limited to the skin, the diffuse form can also involve visceral organs and may have a very aggressive course, with an overall 10-year survival of 50%. The mechanisms leading to lung fibrosis in SSc are still unknown, but it is likely that the SSc-antibodies and other subtypes of anti-nuclear antibodies (anti-RNA polymerase III, anti-topoisomerase, anti-U11/U12, anti-Th/To ribonucleoprotein-antibodies) might have a role in triggering the initial inflammatory response in the lung, leading to proliferation of fibroblasts and collagen deposition. The most frequent histologic pattern in ILD associated with SSc is nonspecific interstitial pneumonia (NSIP), highlighting the relation between inflammation and fibrosis in this particular disease.[48]

In 2006, a multicentre RCT showed that oral cyclophosphamide was able to stabilise the course of the disease by reducing the loss of lung function compared to placebo.[49] Further studies have demonstrated that cyclophosphamide is better tolerated when administrated intravenously as pulse therapy and that its effect is limited to the period of administration.[50] Other immunosuppressive drugs have been tested, including the combination azathioprine-prednisolone and methotrexate,[48] but the current treatment strategy is based on an induction phase with i.v. cyclophosphamide and maintenance with mycophenolate mofetil, which is well tolerated and can be used for long periods without severe side effects.[51]

Polymyositis-dermatomyositis is the second most common CTD affecting the lung. The disease can have more variable pathological patterns with organizing pneumonia, NSIP and even UIP. The use of high-dose corticos-teroids is justified only in the presentation with a pattern of organizing pneumonia, due to the fact that high-dose steroids are associated with a high risk for renal crisis in SSc. For all other presentations (NSIP and UIP), cyclophosphamide is recommended in the induction phase, followed by another more tolerable immunosuppressive drug combined with steroids. The use of these drugs is still justified even in forms with a UIP-pattern, due to the inflammatory pathogenesis of the diseases. Nevertheless, the real efficacy of these treatments in rheumatoid arthritis and in other CTD-ILD presenting with UIP-pattern is not proven. Other approaches have been suggested, including pirfenidone for SSc and rituximab for patients with polymyositis-dermatomyositis with severe forms of lung involvement. Autologous hematopoietic stem cell transplantation has recently been inves-tigated for the treatment of advanced SSc, but conclusive results on efficacy and safety are not available.[52,53]

Idiopathic Interstitial Pneumonias

Idiopathic Interstitial Pneumonias (IIP) is a group of diseases of the lung of unknown pathogenesis, which enter the differential diagnostic flow-chart of IPF and of the other ILD[1,11] (Fig. 1). *Idiopathic non specific interstitial pneumonia (NSIP)* is characterised by fibrosis and concomitant inflamma-tion involving different areas of the lung, resulting in fibrosis and ground glass opacities on HRCT scans and a relative absence of honey combing. The histopathology can be divided into a cellular or a fibrotic form, depending on the presence of inflammatory cells; the latter carries a worse prognosis. Treatment of NSIP is entirely based on expert opinion and case reports as no RCT has been performed. The current treatment strategy include a com-bination of steroids and an immunosuppressive, usually azathioprine. The results of a recent study showing a higher mortality with "triple therapy" in IPF[11] has prompted an international discussion on the appropriateness of this therapy in NSIP.

Respiratory bronchiolitis-ILD (RB-ILD) and *desquamative interstitial pneumonia (DIP)* are two entities characterised by proliferation of alveolar macrophages in alveolar and peri-bronchiolar spaces, induced by smoking. The clinical presentation is usually mild with combined restrictive and obstructive lung function impairment. Smoking cessation is usually enough to treat these conditions and to ensure a complete recovery.

Acute interstitial pneumonia (AIP) is an idiopathic condition characterized by rapidly worsening respiratory failure, diffuse ground-glass infiltrates on HRCT and infiltration of interstitial spaces with inflammatory cells. The condition mimics adult respiratory distress syndrome (ARDS) and corresponds histopathologically to diffuse alveolar damage, DAD. The condition has a mortality of more than 50% in small reported series, and immunosuppressive therapy is ineffective.

Cryptogenic organizing pneumonia (COP) is probably more common than previously thought. Patients with COP present with a history of 2–4 months of variable degrees of cough and dyspnea, with typical patchy and often migratory subpleural and peribronchial consolidation, commonly associated with ground-glass opacity on HRCT. Histology shows a patchy process with organizing pneumonia involving alveolar ducts and alveoli with and without intraluminal polyps. No RCT are available and the treatment is based on expert opinion. Most patients recover with steroids, but relapses are common. Methotrexate and anti-TNF drugs have been used in anecdotal cases, but no real proof exists of their efficacy.[54]

Lung transplantation can be discussed in patients with IIP who might fill all the selection criteria; the efficacy, long-term survival and risk of relapse are still unknown due to the relatively small case-series reported.

Notes on New Approaches for Sarcoidosis

Sarcoidosis is a multisystem disease characterized by a granulomatous inflammation of unknown origin, which is able to affect any organ of the human body. The clinical presentation of sarcoidosis can vary from completely asymptomatic to organ-specific symtoms and signs, to severely invalidating and life-threatening conditions. The main feature of sarcoidosis is the presence of well-formed, non-necrotizing granulomas in the absence of any known cause or diagnosis. The lung is the organ that is most commonly affected by sarcoidosis, with typical radiological presentations (Fig. 4).

The natural history of the disease is variable, from acute self-limiting forms (Löfgren's syndrome) to chronic forms causing progressive damage to

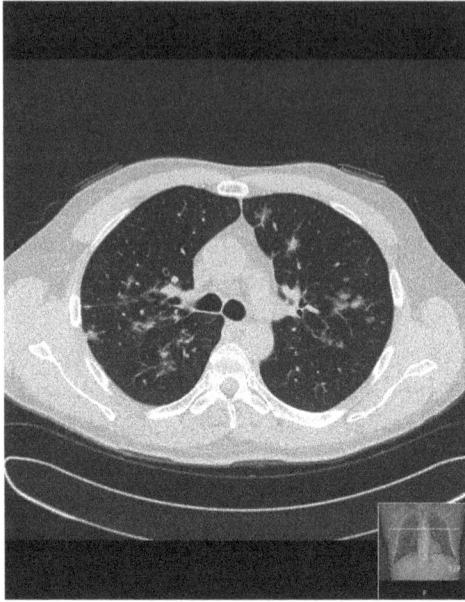

Figure 4. Computerized Tomography (CT) scan of a patient with sarcoidosis of the lung, stadium II. Diffuse peribronchial micronodular and diffuse infiltrates can be recognized, together with mediastinal lymph nodes.

the affected organs and systemic symptoms. Most of the patients in acute early stages do not need any form of treatment, thanks to the spontaneous resolution of the disease. Patients with advanced or symptomatic disease often need long-term treatment with oral steroids.[55,56] Interestingly, there is no evidence from large well-designed RCT on the dose and duration of the treatment with corticosteroids. Often the therapy is prescribed and continued based on local expertise and on the clinical response observed. Furthermore, it is not unusual to observe relapse of the disease when tapering down the dose or even after completion of a full treatment period.

Different strategies have been tested with steroid-sparing agents such as methotrexate,[57] azathioprine,[58] thalidomide,[59] cyclosporine A,[60] mycophenolate mofetil[61] and anti-malaria compounds such as hydroxychloroquine.[62] Even in these cases, only very small clinical trials have been performed with heterogeneous populations. Most of the data on safety and tolerability originates from clinical trials in rheumatological conditions.

Infliximab was also investigated in chronic sarcoidosis not responding to steroids in a few clinical trials, but heterogeneity of the population and of the inclusion criteria do not allow solid conclusions of the data.[63] Other anti-TNF agents such as adalimumab and etanercept have been used thanks to a more tolerable profile, but even with these drugs only anecdotal cases and limited case-series are available.[64,65] The same considerations are valid for rituximab.

Vasoactive intestinal peptide (VIP) via aerosol was tested in a small phase II study,[66] but despite a documented effect on the activation of alveolar macrophages its use cannot be recommended at the present time.

Critical Points with Clinical Trials and Orphan Drug Designation

The area of DPLD is undergoing an important expansion and development, mostly due to recent insights in the natural history and therapy of IPF, which are grabbing the attention of physicians and the market. Idiopathic pulmonary fibrosis has become the model for the development of new drugs in the field; the orphan drug designation offers today the possibility of a platform among industry, academics and patient societies, creating good conditions to solve unmet medical problems for patients with rare lung diseases. The development of new drugs is extremely expensive and qualified networks are necessary to allow randomized placebo-controlled clinical trials that are able to provide some evidence for new treatments. Multicentre international studies are necessary to reach a good sample-size and the study-design of trials is often complicated by the fact that the natural history of these conditions is not well known yet. Furthermore, any study with survival as endpoint would require a study-period of at least three years, with costs that are unbearable for industry and academic institutions; this has fuelled a debate on which endpoints could be considered as surrogates for survival and eventually included in the design of new studies.[67,68] Interestingly, decline of forced expiratory capacity (FVC) over time is the only marker able to predict mortality in IPF, and it is obtained with a technique, spirometry, that is more or less 150 years old. Therefore there is a huge need of empowering translational research in the field, to develop new biomarkers able to predict response to treatment and to simplify the medical management of this growing group of patients.

References

1. Travis, W.D., Costabel, U., Hansell, D.M., King, T.E., Lynch, D.A., Nicholson, A.G., *et al.* (2013). An official American Thoracic Society/European Respiratory Society statement: Update of the international multidisciplinary classification of the idiopathic interstitial pneumonias. *Am J Respir Crit Care Med*, **188**(6):733–748.

2. Goldstein, R.A., Rohatgi, P.K., Bergofsky, E.H., Block, E.R., Daniele, R.P., Dantzker, D.R. *et al.* (1990). Clinical role of bronchoalveolar lavage in adults with pulmonary disease. *Am Rev Respir Dis*, **142**(2):481–486.

3. Saltini, C., Spurzem, J.R., Lee, J.J., Pinkston, P., Crystal, R.G. (1986). Spontaneous release of interleukin 2 by lung T lymphocytes in active pulmonary sarcoidosis is primarily from the Leu3+DR+ T cell subset. *J Clin Invest*, **77**(6):1962–1970.

4. Venet, A., Hance, A.J., Saltini, C., Robinson, B.W., Crystal, R.G. (1985). Enhanced alveolar macrophage-mediated antigen-induced T-lymphocyte proliferation in sarcoidosis. *J Clin Invest*, **75**(1):293–301.

5. Saltini, C., Winestock, K., Kirby, M., Pinkston, P., Crystal, R.G. (1989). Maintenance of alveolitis in patients with chronic beryllium disease by beryllium-specific helper T cells. *N Engl J Med*, **320**(17):1103–1109.

6. (1995). Future directions for research on diseases of the lung. American Thoracic Society. Medical Section of the American Lung Association. This report was approved by the ATS Board of Directors in November 1994. *Am J Respir Crit Care Med*, **152**(5 Pt 1):1713–1735.

7. Richeldi, L., Sorrentino, R., Saltini, C. (1993). HLA-DPB1 glutamate 69: a genetic marker of beryllium disease. *Science*, **262**(5131):242–244.

8. Katzenstein, A.L., Myers, J.L. (1998). Idiopathic pulmonary fibrosis: clinical relevance of pathologic classification. *Am J Respir Crit Care Med*, **157**(4 Pt 1): 1301–1315.

9. Noble, P.W., Albera, C., Bradford, W.Z., Costabel, U., Glassberg, M.K., Kardatzke, D. *et al.* (2011). Pirfenidone in patients with idiopathic pulmonary fibrosis (CAPACITY): two randomised trials. *Lancet*, **377**(9779):1760–1769.

10. Raghu, G., Depaso, W.J., Cain, K., Hammar, S.P., Wetzel, C.E., Dreis, D.F. *et al.* (1991). Azathioprine combined with prednisone in the treatment of idiopathic pulmonary fibrosis: a prospective double-blind, randomized, placebo-controlled clinical trial. *Am Rev Respir Dis*, **144**(2):291–296.

11. Idiopathic Pulmonary Fibrosis Clinical Research Network, Raghu, G., Anstrom, K.J., King, T.E., Lasky, J.A., Martinez, F.J. (2012). Prednisone, azathioprine, and N-acetylcysteine for pulmonary fibrosis. *N Engl J Med*, **366**(21):1968–1977.

12. American Thoracic Society, European Respiratory Society. (2002). American Thoracic Society/European Respiratory Society International Multidisciplinary Consensus Classification of the Idiopathic Interstitial Pneumonias. This joint statement of the American Thoracic Society (ATS), and the European Respiratory Society (ERS) was adopted by the ATS board of directors, June 2001 and by the ERS Executive Committee, June 2001. *Am J Respir Crit Care Med*, **165**(2):277–304.

13. King, T.E., Albera, C., Bradford, W.Z., Costabel, U., Hormel, P., Lancaster, L. *et al*. Effect of interferon gamma-1b on survival in patients with idiopathic pulmonary fibrosis (INSPIRE): a multicentre, randomised, placebo-controlled trial. *Lancet*, **374**(9685):222–228.

14. Raghu, G., Collard, H.R., Egan, J.J., Martinez, F.J., Behr, J., Brown, K.K. *et al*. An official ATS/ERS/JRS/ALAT statement: idiopathic pulmonary fibrosis: evidence-based guidelines for diagnosis and management. *Am J Respir Crit Care Med*, **183**(6):788–824.

15. Raghu, G., Brown, K.K., Bradford, W.Z., Starko, K., Noble, P.W., Schwartz, D.A. *et al*. A placebo-controlled trial of interferon gamma-1b in patients with idiopathic pulmonary fibrosis. *N Engl J Med*, **350**(2):125–133.

16. Macías-Barragán, J., Sandoval-Rodríguez, A., Navarro-Partida, J., Armendáriz-Borunda, J. (2010). The multifaceted role of pirfenidone and its novel targets. *Fibrogenesis Tissue Repair*, **3**:16.

17. Schaefer, C.J., Ruhrmund, D.W., Pan, L., Seiwert, S.D., Kossen, K. (2011). Antifibrotic activities of pirfenidone in animal models. *Eur Respir Rev Off J Eur Respir Soc*, **20**(120):85–97.

18. Taniguchi, H., Ebina, M., Kondoh, Y., Ogura, T., Azuma, A., Suga, M. *et al*. (2010). Pirfenidone in idiopathic pulmonary fibrosis. *Eur Respir J*, **35**(4): 821–829.

19. King, T.E., Bradford, W.Z., Castro-Bernardini, S., Fagan, E.A., Glaspole, I., Glassberg, M.K. *et al*. (2014). A phase 3 trial of pirfenidone in patients with idiopathic pulmonary fibrosis. *N Engl J Med*, **370**(22):2083–2092.

20. Valeyre, D., Albera, C., Bradford, W.Z., Costabel, U., King, T.E., Leff, J.A. *et al*. (2014). Comprehensive assessment of the long-term safety of pirfenidone in patients with idiopathic pulmonary fibrosis. *Respirol Carlton Vic*, **19**(5):740–747.

21. Roth, G.J., Binder, R., Colbatzky, F., Dallinger, C., Schlenker-Herceg, R., Hilberg, F. *et al*. (2015). Nintedanib: From discovery to the clinic. *J Med Chem*, **58**(3):1053–1063.

22. Reck, M., Heigener, D., Reinmuth, N. (2014). Nintedanib for the treatment of patients with advanced non-small-cell lung cancer. *Expert Rev Clin Pharmacol*, **7**(5):579–590.

23. Reck, M., Kaiser, R., Mellemgaard, A., Douillard, J.-Y., Orlov, S., Krzakowski, M. *et al.* (2014). Docetaxel plus nintedanib versus docetaxel plus placebo in patients with previously treated non-small-cell lung cancer (LUME-Lung 1): a phase 3, double-blind, randomised controlled trial. *Lancet Oncol*, **15**(2):143–155.

24. Richeldi, L., Costabel, U., Selman, M., Kim, D.S., Hansell, D.M., Nicholson, A.G. *et al.* (2011). Efficacy of a tyrosine kinase inhibitor in idiopathic pulmonary fibrosis. *N Engl J Med*, **365**(12):1079–1087.

25. Richeldi, L., du Bois, R.M., Raghu, G., Azuma, A., Brown, K.K., Costabel, U. *et al.* (2014). Efficacy and safety of nintedanib in idiopathic pulmonary fibrosis. *N Engl J Med*, **370**(22):2071–2082.

26. Duffield, J.S., Lupher, M., Thannickal, V.J., Wynn, T.A. (2013). Host responses in tissue repair and fibrosis. *Annu Rev Pathol*, **8**:241–276.

27. Dellgren, G., Riise, G.C., Swärd, K., Gilljam, M., Rexius, H., Liden, H., Silverborn, M. (2015). Extracorporeal membrane oxygenation as a bridge to lung transplantation: a long-term study. *Cardiothorac Surg*, **47**(1):95–100.

28. Strizheva, G.D., Carsillo, T., Kruger, W.D., Sullivan, E.J., Ryu, J.H., Henske, E.P. (2001). The spectrum of mutations in TSC1 and TSC2 in women with tuberous sclerosis and lymphangiomyomatosis. *Am J Respir Crit Care Med*, **163**(1):253–258.

29. Henske, E.P., McCormack, F.X. (2012). Lymphangioleiomyomatosis — a wolf in sheep's clothing. *J Clin Invest*, **122**(11):3807–3816.

30. McCormack, F.X., Travis, W.D., Colby, T.V., Henske, E.P., Moss, J. (2012). Lymphangioleiomyomatosis: calling it what it is: a low-grade, destructive, metastasizing neoplasm. *Am J Respir Crit Care Med*, **186**(12):1210–1212.

31. Sehgal, S.N. (2003). Sirolimus: its discovery, biological properties, and mechanism of action. *Transplant Proc*, **35**(3 Suppl):7S–14S.

32. Glasgow, C.G., Steagall, W.K., Taveira-Dasilva, A., Pacheco-Rodriguez, G., Cai, X., El-Chemaly, S. *et al.* (2010). Lymphangioleiomyomatosis (LAM): molecular insights lead to targeted therapies. *Respir Med*, **104**(Suppl 1):S45–58.

33. Bissler, J.J., McCormack, F.X., Young, L.R., Elwing, J.M., Chuck, G., Leonard, J.M. *et al.* (2008). Sirolimus for angiomyolipoma in tuberous sclerosis complex or lymphangioleiomyomatosis. *N Engl J Med*, **358**(2):140–151.

34. McCormack, F.X., Inoue, Y., Moss, J., Singer, L.G., Strange, C., Nakata, K. *et al.* (2011). Efficacy and safety of sirolimus in lymphangioleiomyomatosis. *N Engl J Med*, **364**(17):1595–1606.

35. Sugimoto, R., Nakao, A., Yamane, M., Toyooka, S., Okazaki, M., Aoe, M. *et al.* (2008). Sirolimus amelioration of clinical symptoms of recurrent lymphangioleiomyomatosis after living-donor lobar lung transplantation. *J Heart Lung Transplant Off Publ Int Soc Heart Transplant*, **27**(8):921–924.

36. Ben-Dov, I., Segel, M.J. (2014). Autoimmune pulmonary alveolar proteinosis: clinical course and diagnostic criteria. *Autoimmun Rev*, **13**(4-5):513–517.

37. Patel, S.M., Sekiguchi, H., Reynolds, J.P., Krowka, M.J. (2012). Pulmonary alveolar proteinosis. *Can Respir J J Can Thorac Soc*, **19**(4):243–245.

38. Borie, R., Danel, C., Debray, M.-P., Taille, C., Dombret, M.-C., Aubier, M. *et al.* (2011). Pulmonary alveolar proteinosis. *Eur Respir Rev Off J Eur Respir Soc*, **20**(120):98–107.

39. Kavuru, M.S., Popovich, M. (2002). Therapeutic whole lung lavage: a stop-gap therapy for alveolar proteinosis. *Chest*, **122**(4):1123–1124.

40. Hasan, N., Bagga, S., Monteagudo, J., Hirose, H., Cavarocchi, N.C., Hehn, B.T. *et al.* (2013). Extracorporeal membrane oxygenation to support whole-lung lavage in pulmonary alveolar proteinosis: salvage of the drowned lungs. *J Bronchology Interv Pulmonol*, **20**(1):41–44.

41. Seymour, J.F., Presneill, J.J., Schoch, O.D., Downie, G.H., Moore, P.E., Doyle, I.R. *et al.* (2001). Therapeutic efficacy of granulocyte-macrophage colony-stimulating factor in patients with idiopathic acquired alveolar proteinosis. *Am J Respir Crit Care Med*, **163**(2):524–531.

42. Kavuru, M.S., Sullivan, E.J., Piccin, R., Thomassen, M.J., Stoller, J.K. (2000). Exogenous granulocyte-macrophage colony-stimulating factor administration for pulmonary alveolar proteinosis. *Am J Respir Crit Care Med*, **161**(4 Pt 1):1143–1148.

43. Tazawa, R., Inoue, Y., Arai, T., Takada, T., Kasahara, Y., Hojo, M. *et al.* (2014). Duration of benefit in patients with autoimmune pulmonary alveolar proteinosis after inhaled granulocyte-macrophage colony-stimulating factor therapy. *Chest*, **145**(4):729–737.

44. Kavuru, M.S., Malur, A., Marshall, I., Barna, B.P., Meziane, M., Huizar, I. *et al.* (2011). An open-label trial of rituximab therapy in pulmonary alveolar proteinosis. *Eur Respir J*, **38**(6):1361–1367.

45. Luisetti, M., Rodi, G., Perotti, C., Campo, I., Mariani, F., Pozzi, E. *et al.* (2009). Plasmapheresis for treatment of pulmonary alveolar proteinosis. *Eur Respir J*, **33**(5):1220–1222.

46. Leask, A. (2011). Possible strategies for anti-fibrotic drug intervention in scleroderma. *J Cell Commun Signal*, **5**(2):125–129.

47. Leask, A. (2012). Getting out of a sticky situation: targeting the myofibroblast in scleroderma. *Open Rheumatol J*, **6**:163–169.

48. Wells, A.U., Denton, C.P. (2014). Interstitial lung disease in connective tissue disease-mechanisms and management. *Nat Rev Rheumatol*, **10**(12): 728–739.

49. Tashkin, D.P., Elashoff, R., Clements, P.J., Goldin, J., Roth, M.D., Furst, D.E. *et al.* (2006). Cyclophosphamide versus placebo in scleroderma lung disease. *N Engl J Med*, **354**(25):2655–2666.

50. Tashkin, D.P., Elashoff, R., Clements, P.J., Roth, M.D., Furst, D.E., Silver, R.M. *et al.* (2007). Effects of 1-year treatment with cyclophosphamide on outcomes at 2 years in scleroderma lung disease. *Am J Respir Crit Care Med*, **176**(10):1026–1034.

51. Fischer, A., Brown, K.K., Du Bois, R.M., Frankel, S.K., Cosgrove, G.P., Fernandez-Perez, E.R. *et al.* (2013). Mycophenolate mofetil improves lung function in connective tissue disease-associated interstitial lung disease. *J Rheumatol*, **40**(5):640–646.

52. Burt, R.K., Shah, S.J., Dill, K., Grant, T., Gheorghiade, M., Schroeder, J. *et al.* (2011). Autologous non-myeloablative haemopoietic stem-cell transplantation compared with pulse cyclophosphamide once per month for systemic sclerosis (ASSIST): an open-label, randomised phase 2 trial. *Lancet*, **378**(9790):498–506.

53. Van Laar, J.M., Farge, D., Sont, J.K., Naraghi, K., Marjanovic, Z., Larghero, J. *et al.* (2014). Autologous hematopoietic stem cell transplantation vs intravenous pulse cyclophosphamide in diffuse cutaneous systemic sclerosis: a randomized clinical trial. *JAMA*, **311**(24):2490–2498.

54. Roberton, B.J., Hansell, D.M. (2011). Organizing pneumonia: a kaleidoscope of concepts and morphologies. *Eur Radiol*, **21**(11):2244–2254.

55. Israel, H.L., Fouts, D.W., Beggs, R.A. (1973). A controlled trial of prednisone treatment of sarcoidosis. *Am Rev Respir Dis*, **107**(4):609–614.

56. Gibson, G.J., Prescott, R.J., Muers, M.F., Middleton, W.G., Mitchell, D.N., Connolly, C.K. *et al.* (1996). British Thoracic Society Sarcoidosis study: effects of long term corticosteroid treatment. *Thorax*, **51**(3):238–247.

57. Baughman, R.P., Winget, D.B., Lower, E.E. (2000). Methotrexate is steroid sparing in acute sarcoidosis: results of a double blind, randomized trial. *Sarcoidosis Vasc Diffuse Lung Dis Off J Wasog World Assoc Sarcoidosis Granulomatous Disord*, **17**(1):60–66.

58. Müller-Quernheim, J., Kienast, K., Held, M., Pfeifer, S., Costabel, U. (1999). Treatment of chronic sarcoidosis with an azathioprine/prednisolone regimen. *Eur Respir J*, **14**(5):1117–1122.

59. Judson, M.A., Silvestri, J., Hartung, C., Byars, T., Cox, C.E. (2006). The effect of thalidomide on corticosteroid-dependent pulmonary sarcoidosis.

Sarcoidosis Vasc Diffuse Lung Dis Off J Wasog World Assoc Sarcoidosis Granulomatous Disord, **23**(1):51–57.

60. Wyser, C.P., van Schalkwyk, E.M., Alheit, B., Bardin, P.G., Joubert, J.R. (1997). Treatment of progressive pulmonary sarcoidosis with cyclosporin A. A randomized controlled trial. *Am J Respir Crit Care Med*, **156**(5):1371–1376.

61. Brill, A.-K., Ott, S.R., Geiser, T. (2013). Effect and safety of mycophenolate mofetil in chronic pulmonary sarcoidosis: a retrospective study. *Respir Int Rev Thorac Dis*, **86**(5):376–383.

62. Baltzan, M., Mehta, S., Kirkham, T.H., Cosio, M.G. (1999). Randomized trial of prolonged chloroquine therapy in advanced pulmonary sarcoidosis. *Am J Respir Crit Care Med*, **160**(1):192–197.

63. Rossman, M.D., Newman, L.S., Baughman, R.P., Teirstein, A., Weinberger, S.E., Miller, W. *et al.* (2006). A double-blinded, randomized, placebo-controlled trial of infliximab in subjects with active pulmonary sarcoidosis. *Sarcoidosis Vasc Diffuse Lung Dis Off J Wasog World Assoc Sarcoidosis Granulomatous Disord*, **23**(3):201–208.

64. Kamphuis, L.S., Lam-Tse, W.-K., Dik, W.A., van Daele, P.L., van Biezen, P., Kwekkeboom, D.J. *et al.* (2011). Efficacy of adalimumab in chronically active and symptomatic patients with sarcoidosis. *Am J Respir Crit Care Med*, **184**(10):1214–1216.

65. Erckens, R.J., Mostard, R.L.M., Wijnen, P.A., Schouten, J.S., Drent, M. (2012). Adalimumab successful in sarcoidosis patients with refractory chronic non-infectious uveitis. *Graefes Arch Clin Exp Ophthalmol Albrecht Von Graefes Arch Für Klin Exp Ophthalmol*, **250**(5):713–720.

66. Prasse, A., Zissel, G., Lützen, N., Schupp, J., Schmiedlin, R., Gonzalez-Rey, E. *et al.* (2010). Inhaled vasoactive intestinal peptide exerts immunoregulatory effects in sarcoidosis. *Am J Respir Crit Care Med*, **182**(4):540–548.

67. Wells, A.U., Behr, J., Costabel, U., Cottin, V., Poletti, V., Richeldi, L. *et al.* (2012). Hot of the breath: mortality as a primary end-point in IPF treatment trials: the best is the enemy of the good. *Thorax*, **67**(11):938–940.

68. Richeldi, L. (2012). Assessing the treatment effect from multiple trials in idiopathic pulmonary fibrosis. *Eur Respir Rev Off J Eur Respir Soc*, **21**(124): 147–151.

69. Azuma, A., Nukiwa, T., Tsuboi, E., Suga, M., Abe, S., Nakata, K. *et al.* (2005). Double-blind, placebo-controlled trial of pirfenidone in patients with idiopathic pulmonary fibrosis. *Am J Respir Crit Care Med*, **171**(9):1040–1047.

70. Demedts, M., Behr, J., Buhl, R., Costabel, U., Dekhuijzen, R., Jansen, H.M. *et al.* (2005). High-dose acetylcysteine in idiopathic pulmonary fibrosis. *N Engl J Med*, **353**(21):2229–2242.

71. Raghu, G., Brown, K.K., Costabel, U., Cottin, V., du Bois, R.M., Lasky, J.A. *et al.* (2008). Treatment of idiopathic pulmonary fibrosis with etanercept: an exploratory, placebo-controlled trial. *Am J Respir Crit Care Med*, **178**(9): 948–955.

72. King, T.E., Behr, J., Brown, K.K., du Bois, R.M., Lancaster, L., de Andrade, J.A. *et al.* (2008). BUILD-1: a randomized placebo-controlled trial of bosentan in idiopathic pulmonary fibrosis. *Am J Respir Crit Care Med*, **177**(1):75–81.

73. Idiopathic Pulmonary Fibrosis Clinical Research Network, Zisman, D.A., Schwarz, M., Anstrom, K.J., Collard, H.R., Flaherty, K.R. *et al.* (2010). A controlled trial of sildenafil in advanced idiopathic pulmonary fibrosis. *N Engl J Med*, **363**(7):620–628.

74. Daniels, C.E., Lasky, J.A., Limper, A.H., Mieras, K., Gabor, E., Schroeder, D.R. *et al.* (2010). Imatinib treatment for idiopathic pulmonary fibrosis: Randomized placebo-controlled trial results. *Am J Respir Crit Care Med*, **181**(6):604–610.

75. King, T.E., Brown, K.K., Raghu, G., du Bois, R.M., Lynch, D.A., Martinez, F. *et al.* (2011). BUILD-3: a randomized, controlled trial of bosentan in idiopathic pulmonary fibrosis. *Am J Respir Crit Care Med*, **184**(1):92–99.

76. Homma, S., Azuma, A., Taniguchi, H., Ogura, T., Mochiduki, Y., Sugiyama, Y. *et al.* (2012). Efficacy of inhaled N-acetylcysteine monotherapy in patients with early stage idiopathic pulmonary fibrosis. *Respirol Carlton Vic*, **17**(3):467–477.

77. Noth, I., Anstrom, K.J., Calvert, S.B., de Andrade, J., Flaherty, K.R., Glazer, C. *et al.* (2012). A placebo-controlled randomized trial of warfarin in idiopathic pulmonary fibrosis. *Am J Respir Crit Care Med*, **186**(1):88–95.

78. Raghu, G., Behr, J., Brown, K.K., Egan, J.J., Kawut, S.M., Flaherty, K.R. *et al.* (2013). Treatment of idiopathic pulmonary fibrosis with ambrisentan: a parallel, randomized trial. *Ann Intern Med*, **158**(9):641–649.

79. Idiopathic Pulmonary Fibrosis Clinical Research Network, Martinez, F.J., de Andrade, J.A., Anstrom, K.J., King, T.E., Raghu, G. (2014). Randomized trial of acetylcysteine in idiopathic pulmonary fibrosis. *N Engl J Med*, **370**(22):2093–2101.

80. Raghu, G., Million-Rousseau, R., Morganti, A., Perchenet, L., Behr, J., MUSIC Study Group. (2013). Macitentan for the treatment of idiopathic pulmonary fibrosis: the randomised controlled MUSIC trial. *Eur Respir J*, **42**(6):1622–1632.

CHAPTER 13

ADVANCES IN THERAPIES FOR MULTIPLE SCLEROSIS AND RELATED INFLAMMATORY DISEASES OF THE CNS

Fredrik Piehl

Introduction: Improved understanding of pathogenesis and disease mechanisms

In Multiple Sclerosis (MS) a presumed autoimmune disease process targets the central nervous system (CNS) leading to demyelination and oligodendrocyte loss, axonal damage and subsequent deterioration of neurological functions.[1] It is the most common non-traumatic cause of neurological disability among young adults, with an expected two million affected persons worldwide. As MS threatens personal autonomy, independency and future prospects, it has a significant impact on those affected and their families, and MS patients rate their health status low compared to other chronic diseases.[2] Disease onset is usually in the third and fourth decades of life and women are affected more than twice as often as men. MS usually presents with a relapsing-remitting (RRMS) disease course, in which there is a chronic tendency for immune cells from the peripheral compartment to enter the CNS and cause focal areas of inflammation. This is clinically reflected as worsening of any or a combination of a wide range of neuro-logical functions, but can also be sub-clinical as visualized with magnetic resonance imaging (MRI) (Fig. 1). A strong body of evidence links MS to aberrant adaptive immune system activation, with the strongest genetic linkage to the human leukocyte antigen (HLA) complex. Also many of the non-HLA risk genes are immune-related, some of which are shared with

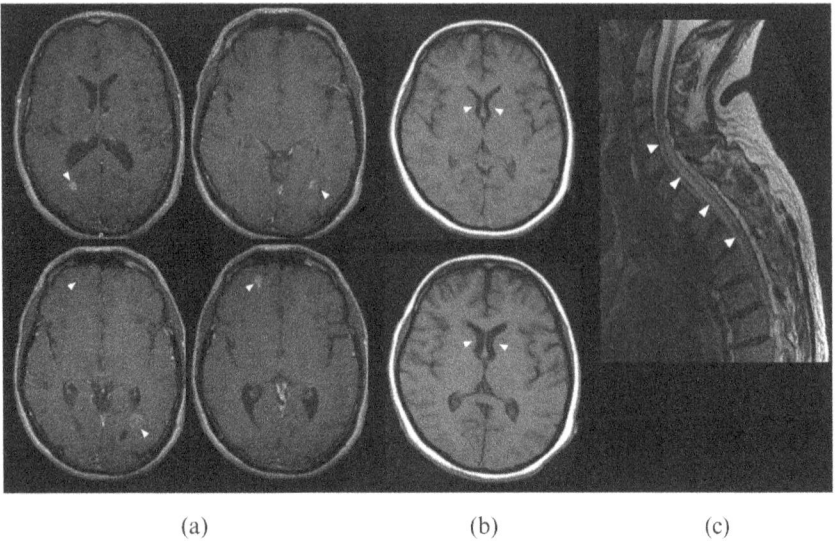

(a)   (b)   (c)

Figure 1. Magnetic resonance imaging (MRI) of the brain and spinal cord in multiple sclerosis (A), NMDA receptor encephalitis (B) and neuromyelitis optica (C). (A): Serial monthly brain MRIs show the appearance and evolution of contrast-enhancing inflamma-tory lesions (arrow heads) in the brain parenchyma of a patient with multiple sclerosis. In this case intense neuroradiological disease activity was not associated with clinical relapses, underscoring the value of MRI to assess inflammatory disease activity in this condition. (B): A patient with severe NMDA receptor encephalitis at initiation of disease (upper panel) and after five months of intensive care with invasive ventilation (lower panel). No focal pathologies are visible, but a generalized atrophy of the fronto-temporal brain parenchyma with increased ventricular volume (arrow heads) is evident. (C): A patient with neuromyelitis optica where a typical long extending myelitis is present in the lower cervical and thoracic spinal cord.

other autoimmune conditions.[3] As for other autoimmune diseases, environmental factors also play an important role. Among the most studied are common childhood infections, in particular with Epstein-Barr virus, and sunlight exposure/vitamin D deficiency.[4] More recently examples of gene-environment interactions have been demonstrated, *e.g.* between the main MS HLA risk haplotype DRB15*01 and smoking.[5] Based on current knowledge, it can be concluded that susceptibility to MS is determined by the combined effect of numerous genetic and environmental factors, some of which interact with each other. This is also the most likely explanation for the vast heterogeneity of MS in terms of clinical presentation, disease activity, disease severity and response to treatment.

With time a majority of patients with RRMS will experience an altered diseased course, with unrelenting progression of neurological deficits not explained by relapses; secondary progressive MS (SPMS).[1,6] Time to SPMS differs considerably, but at the group level a majority has converted to SPMS 20 years after disease onset.[7] In approximately 10% of patients, the disease course is progressive from onset: primary progressive MS (PPMS).[1,6] PPMS patients share similarities with SPMS such as more prominent spinal symptoms, onset after the fourth decade of life and a higher relative risk in men.[7] The current understanding of disease mechanisms and genetic and/or environmental determinants of progressive disease is much more limited than for RRMS. However, it is believed that the lack of recovery in the progressive phase is an accumulated effect of repeated attacks of inflammatory demyelination and inadequate remyelination, in turn leading to axonal damage, which now has been accepted as the major cause of irreversible disability in MS patients.[8] The fact that existing disease modifying therapies (DMTs) have such limited effects in progressive MS suggests that disease mechanisms other than adaptive inflammation might operate in SPMS, most likely predominately involving local tissue reactions.[9] A disputed issue has been whether inflammation and neurodegeneration are independent, parallel or sequential processes. However, accumulating evidence suggest that loss of axons in MS is initiated and maintained by complex inflammatory processes, whereas the inherent susceptibility to neurodegeneration may vary among individuals.[1]

From being a condition with limited treatment options, MS is now one of the most dynamic fields in clinical neurology, with a number of novel

DMTs already approved or in late stages of clinical testing. However, almost invariably these drugs target lymphocyte-mediated inflammation and are most effective in the early disease course, with more limited effects in more advanced disease states.[10,11,12] The fact that there is no approved drug with unequivocally proven efficacy in progressive MS has sparked an intense pharma industry interest in efforts to find targets amenable for drug therapy, such as enhancing remyelination. Since MS, especially in later disease stages, is a complex condition, there is an urgent need to find biomarkers that can reflect such disease processes.[13] In rheumatoid arthritis, the finding of anti-citrullinated protein antibodies has had great implications for the understanding of underlying disease processes and sub-phenotyping of patients. Considerable efforts have been made to elucidate antibody targets also in MS, but so far with mixed results. For example, antibodies recognising neurofascin, an antigen present on axons, have been suggested to mediate axonal pathology in MS,[14] but their relevance in a broader clinical context remains unclear. More recently the presence of antibodies recognising another neuronal antigen, KIR4.1, was described in a large proportion of MS patients.[15] However, subsequent studies have so far failed to replicate the finding,[16] casting doubts on the prospects of stratifying patients according to antibody profiling. In contrast, some progress has been made in the use of soluble non-antibody biomarkers. Thus, cerebrospinal fluid (CSF) biomarkers such as the B cell chemokine CXCL13 and matrix metalloprotein-9 (MMP-9), both markers of adaptive inflammation, are downregulated with increasing age and only partially correlate with nerve injury markers such as neurofilament-light (NF-L) and osteopontin.[17] NF-L is considered the best marker for ongoing nerve injury in MS and it has been convincingly shown that elevated levels of NF-L in RRMS are normalized upon start with natalizumab.[18,19]

Injectable Drugs, a First Step, but with Shortcomings

Recombinant interferon-β 1b (IFNβ-1b; Betaferon/Betaseron) became the first approved drug for RRMS in 1993, with the subsequent launch of two IFNβ-1a preparations (Avonex and Rebif).[11] The pivotal placebo-controlled phase III trials for the different IFNβs were conducted on 300–560 patients each and showed a 30–40% relative reduction in the annualized relapse rate (ARR) and an even stronger effects on different MRI measures (gadolinium enhancing lesions, new or enlarging T2 lesions), but with uncertain effects on permanent disability measures.[20–22] The next drug to be approved for RRMS was glatiramer acetate (GA; Copaxone), a mix of random oligomers of amino acids enriched in myelin proteins, with largely similar effects on clinical disease measures as IFN.[23] Very recently, a pegylated IFNβ-1a preparation with dosing every two weeks was approved.[24] Both IFNβ and GA are delivered by self-administered injections, varying in frequency from once per day to once every two weeks. Both IFNβ and GA delay conversion to definite MS in patients with a first clinical event.[25–28] According to current guidelines, IFNβ and GA are indicated as first-line drugs for the treatment of RRMS and in patients with a first clinical event and high risk of conversion to MS. More recent head-to-head studies of IFNβ and GA demonstrate a similar efficacy for reducing relapse frequency in RRMS.[29,30] However, long-term effects of these drugs are more uncertain, not least if they protect from permanent disability in RRMS or whether they delay conversion to a progressive disease course, even if some registry-based studies indicate this may be the case.[31,32] However, it is also clear that IFNβ and GA are not effective for all patients. Thus, delayed initiation of IFNβ by two years in patients with a first clinical event was not associated with worse outcome at five-year follow-up and half of the patients had developed MS, and a quarter of patients had progressed, in spite of being allocated to the active treatment arm in the first place.[33] In fact, if both clinical and neuroradiological evidence of continued disease activity is taken into account, more than half of the patients initiated on first-line drugs have an inadequate response (also called breakthrough disease) within the first two years.[34] Open long-term follow-up studies of participants in randomized controlled trials generally indicate that both IFNβ and GA display a favourable long-term safety profile; however, tolerability, especially in the real world context, is relatively poor. In a Canadian retrospective cohort study of patients initiating a first-line DMT, less than half of the patients remained on treatment after two years.[35] An important reason is drug-related side effects. For both GA and IFNβ irritation at the injection site, which may evolve into local destruction of fat tissue, is common. In addition, IFNβ gives influenza-like symptoms and some patients taking GA may experience a post-injection reaction manifested by chest tightness, heart palpitations and breathlessness. Another reason for poor treatment adherence is that it is difficult to perceive a beneficial treatment effect on an individual basis.[36]

Oral Drugs; Improved Tolerability and Efficacy

Fingolimod (Gilenya) became the first oral treatment approved for RRMS and is also first-in-class for drugs targeting sphingosine-1-phosphate receptors (S1PR). The drug is a derivate of the fungus Isaria sinclairii and a structural analog of sphingosine, acting as an S1PR antagonist. There are five known S1PR receptors, which are expressed on a number of different cell types. However, the main mechanism of action for fingolimod in MS is thought to be the sequestration of lymphocytes in lymph nodes due to blocking of S1PR1, present at variable levels on different immune cell populations.[37] Fingolimod causes a pronounced lymphopenia in peripheral blood, most pronounced for naive and central memory T cells (TCM), less so for peripheral effector memory T and B cells, while NK cells and monocytes are largely unaffected.[38] Notably, it reduces Th17 expressing TCMs, believed to be important for MS pathogenesis, without affecting T cell activation.[39] Thus, the drug mainly targets lymphocyte trafficking without affecting lymphocyte activation patterns. The half-life of fingolimod is around a week and it takes at least two months for lymphocyte counts to recover upon stopping drug dosing. The approval of fingolimod was based on three pivotal phase III studies; FREEDOMS I and II with fingolimod 1.25 mg or 0.5 mg vs placebo over two years,[40,41] and TRANSFORMS with fingolimod 1.25 mg or 0.5 mg vs weekly IFNβ over one year.[42] FREEDOMS I and TRANSFORMS largely included treatment naive patients and showed a reduction of annualized relapse frequency (ARR) with 53–60% compared to placebo and 38–52% compared to IFNβ. Secondary outcome measures were also significant and close to 90% of treated patients were free of gadolinium-enhancing MRI lesions compared to 65% in the placebo group. In FREEDOMS II, a majority of patients had previously been treated with IFNβ or GA. The study showed a 48% reduction in ARR and 87% of patients were free of gadolinium-enhancing MRI lesions.[41] The death of two study subjects in the 1.25 mg arm of the TRANSFORMS study, one due to herpes encephalitis and one due to a primary varicella zoster (VZV) infection, caused concerns over the risk for opportunistic infections. It is therefore recommended to check VZV immunity status before initiating therapy. Another safety concern is the fact that S1PR antagonists may lead to bradyarrhytmias and/or atrioventricular blocks, especially at first dosing, which requires close monitoring. Case reports of sudden death in MS patients on fingolimod have been reported, but the causal contribution of the drug is unknown.[43] A third safety concern is the risk of macular edema, which was detected in 0.5% of patients in the registration studies, although the frequency was lower with the approved 0.5 mg dose.[44] It is recommended that patients undergo ophthalmological examination after initiating therapy and fingolimod should only be used after carefully considering alternative DMTs in diabetic patients, since they incur increased risk. Fingolimod has been shown to mediate neuroprotective effects and to enhance remyelination in preclinical models of MS and is currently being tested in PPMS in the INFORMS trial.[45] Very recently, the sponsor communicated that the trial failed to meet its primary endpoint.[46] Several second-generation S1PR antagonists are now in clinical trials for MS.[47] The main advantage of these drugs is a higher selectivity for the S1PR1 subtype preferentially expressed on lymphocytes, thereby possibly reducing the risk of side effects, and shorter half-lives, enabling faster wash-out if therapy needs to be interrupted, such as in pregnancy or with a serious adverse event.

Teriflunomide (Aubagio) was recently approved for RRMS both in the US and EU. It is the active metabolite of leflunomide (Arava), a drug approved for rheumatoid arthritis, which blocks the mitochondrial enzyme dihydroorotate dehydrogenase (DHO-DH), an enzyme necessary for *de novo* pyrimidine synthesis in proliferating lymphocytes. Teriflunomide also appears to have additional effects independent of DHO-DH inhibition, with effects on cytokine production, expression of cell-surface molecules and cellular migration. The most commonly reported adverse events are upper respiratory and urinary tract infections, diarrhea, nausea, hair thinning and increases in liver enzymes. However, safety data pooled from several studies show a low incidence of serious infections, which was not different from placebo.[48] In the TEMSO trial, teriflunomide at 7 mg and 14 mg once daily doses were compared to placebo over two years in RRMS patients.[49] The results show a reduction of ARR with a third on both doses compared to placebo, while only the higher dose displayed an effect on disability progression. The proportion of patients free from gadolinium-enhancing lesions was 51% in the 7 mg group and 64% in the 14 mg group, compared with 39% in the placebo group. A similar study design was used in the TOWER study, where teriflunomide at 14 mg daily reduced both ARR and disability progression by a third compared with placebo.[50] A smaller phase III study, TENERE, comparing teriflunomide with three times weekly IFNβ, failed to meet its primary outcome measure; the proportion of patients experiencing treatment failure.[51]

Dimethylfumarate (DMF; Tecfidera) is the methyl ester of fumaric acid, an intermediate in the citric acid cycle. Different combinations of fumaric acid esters, including DMF, have since long been used for psoriasis, mainly in Germany. The phase III program in RRMS included two large placebo controlled studies with 240 mg DMF twice or three times daily. In DEFINE, ARR was reduced by 53% in the twice-daily DMF group.[52] The CONFIRM trial also included an active, open-label comparator arm with GA, and showed a 44% reduction in ARR for twice daily DMF and 29% for GA compared to placebo.[53] At two years, 93% of the patients in the twice-daily DMF arm were free from gadolinium-enhancing MRI lesions compared with 62% in the placebo group.[52] The relative risk of disability progression compared to placebo was reduced by a third in DEFINE, whereas the corresponding comparison in CONFIRM was not significant, perhaps due to a lower than expected proportion of patients displaying progression in the placebo group. DMF treatment was not associated with increased risk of serious adverse events compared to placebo. However, at least initially many patients starting DMF experience flushing and gastro-intestinal events, even if symptoms in most cases are mild to moderate. Low dose salicylic acid may be used to reduce gastrointestinal discomfort. The mode of action of DMF in MS has not been clarified in detail, but it is not a typical immunosuppressant drug, even if mild lymphopenia is common.[52,53] Preclinical data suggest that DMF mainly acts through activation of the nuclear factor (erythroid-derived 2)-like 2 (Nrf2) pathway, which is a cellular response pathway induced by stress that induces a number of different anti-oxidant genes.[54] In the animal model for MS, EAE, DMF reduces both the infiltration of immune cells in the CNS and affects their activation response to myelin antigen, and increases the preservation of myelin and axons.[55] Interestingly, DMF seems to mediate neuroprotective effects also in non-inflammatory preclinical models of neurodegeneration and a clinical trial in SPMS is planned.

Laquinimod (Nerventra) is a third oral drug in late stage clinical testing. It is a quinoline-3-carboxamide derivative of linomide (Roquinimex), a drug that was in late stage clinical trials for RRMS and SPMS in the late 90s, where the clinical development program was suspended due to several fatal cardiopulmonary adverse events.[56] Two large phase III trials in RRMS have been conducted; the two-year ALLEGRO study, comparing 0.6 mg daily oral laquinimod with placebo, and BRAVO in which 0.6 mg daily oral laquinimod was compared to both placebo and an active comparator, weekly IFNβ.[57,58] In ALLEGRO laquinimod displayed a relatively modest 23% reduction in ARR and a 37% relative reduction in gadolinium-enhancing MRI lesions.[57] Interestingly, the effect on confirmed disability was more robust, with a relative risk reduction of 29%. In the BRAVO study the effects on ARR and disability were not significant, however there was a significant effect on brain atrophy.[58] Tolerability was good and no serious safety concerns were raised, though a mild increase in liver enzymes was relatively common. In rodents increased malignancies have been noted, with unknown relevance for humans. In light of the mixed efficacy results and some worry of carcinogenic effects, regulatory authorities have so far declined to approve laquinimod for RRMS, but a third phase III study examining a higher 1.2 mg dose is ongoing as well as a trial in PPMS. The mode of action of laquinimod is not clarified in detail, but the effect is likely to be more immunomodulatory than immunosuppressive. In a study using both murine and human cells modulation of dendritic cell function, with reduced potential to induce CD4+ T cell proliferation and secretion of pro-inflammatory cytokines, possibly through inhibition of the NF-κB pathway, was noted.[59] Along the same line, laquinimod was shown to protect against toxic demyelination by modulating the NF-κB pathway in astrocytes.[60]

Biological Drugs: More Effective, but at the Price of Increased Risks

Natalizumab (Tysabri) was approved in 2006 for highly active RRMS and dramatically improved the management of breakthrough disease. Natalizumab is a humanized monoclonal antibody binding the α4-integrin of very late antigen-4 (VLA-4), a surface marker present on most immune cells, and is administered by monthly intravenous (IV) infusions. The binding to VLA-4 targets a non-redundant molecular pathway that almost entirely blocks the possibility of leukocytes to transmigrate across the blood-brain barrier.[61] Treatment with natalizumab does not alter the activation state of T-cells, which leads to sequestration of T cells with encephalitogenic potential in the peripheral compartment.[62] The approval of natalizumab was based on two pivotal phase III RRMS trials; AFFIRM with natalizumab in monotherapy compared to placebo and SENTINEL, with natalizumab as add-on to once weekly IFNβ.[63,64] Both were conducted in RRMS with a large proportion of treatment naive patients. Trial data demonstrated a reduction in ARR by two-thirds, a reduction of gadolinium-enhancing lesions by >90% and reduced progression of disability by 40%, a result much superior to then existing DMTs. This also led to a better understanding of disease mechanisms in MS, since it had been unclear to what degree immunomodulatory intervention can protect and retain axonal integrity.[19] Experiences in the post-marketing setting demonstrate that natalizumab generally is well-tolerated and shows beneficial effects on other treatment related outcome measures.[65] Unfortunately, follow-up studies also revealed that treatment with natalizumab increases the risk of progressive multifocal leukoencephalopathy (PML), a serious and potentially lethal opportunistic brain infection with JC virus. For this reason natalizumab is approved only as monotherapy, mainly in MS patients displaying breakthrough disease on first-line drugs. Other immunosuppressants have also been associated with PML, but with variable risk profiles.[66] Subsequently it was shown that the risk of natalizumab-associated PML can be assessed by serological testing for JC virus, where approximately half the population displays a positive test result.[67] Therefore natalizumab represents a good example of how the risk-benefit profile has to be determined at an individual level, where the drug represents an effective option with a good safety profile in JC virus serology negative patients with high disease activity. However, interruption of natalizumab treatment has to be managed carefully as disease activity will return upon cessation of drug dosing. In a review of close to 2000 patients that had participated in clinical trials, both relapses and neuroradiological disease activity increased shortly after natalizumab interruption and peaked between four and seven months after last dosing.[68] Smaller studies have also found evidence of rebound phenomena, with recurring disease activity over and beyond that of pretreatment levels, perhaps explained by the fact that patients treated in clinical practice generally have more active disease than patients recruited to the trials.[69] Currently there is no clear consensus on how to reduce the risk of a sometimes violent return of disease activity, but when switching to another therapy the wash out phase should be kept as short as possible while also considering the risk of a "carry over" subclinical PML, *i.e.* an emerging PML infection that becomes evident when natalizumab is stopped.

CD20-antagonists belong to a family of monoclonal drugs targeting a surface antigen present on B cells. Although none are currently approved, three different antibodies have been tested in MS; the mouse-human chimeric rituximab (Mabthera/Rituxan), humanized ocrelizumab and the fully human ofatumumab (Arzerra). The role of B cells in MS is not known in detail, but it has been suggested that B cells interacting with Epstein-Barr virus drives inflammation in the intrathecal compartment, especially in more advanced disease stages.[70] Treatment with rituximab has been shown to deplete B cells and also to reduce inflammatory mediators and T cells in cerebrospinal fluid.[71] In addition, the efficacy of B cell depleting therapies may depend on reduced presentation of autoantigens, in turn down-regulating T cell activation.[72]

Rituximab is approved for the treatment of B-cell lymphoma, rheumatoid arthritis and systemic vasculitis, but has also been used off-label for neuroimmunological conditions such as myasthenia gravis, neuromyelitis optica and antibody-mediated encephalitides. In HERMES, a phase II study in RRMS, two doses of 1000 mg rituximab led to a very robust drop in newly appearing gadolinium-enhancing lesions and a trend for reduction in relapse frequency over 48 weeks compared to placebo, in spite of a relatively small study population.[73] In a subsequent study, OLYMPUS, the effect of two 1000 mg rituximab or placebo infusions twice yearly on disease progression over two years in a much larger cohort of PPMS patients was examined.[74] Although the primary endpoint, time to confirmed progression, was not met, a subgroup analysis showed a significant effect in patients aged <51 years with one or more gadolinium enhancing lesions at randomization. Further clinical development of rituximab for MS has been stopped by the sponsor.

Ocrelizumab, similar to rituximab, exerted a very robust effect on gadolinium-enhancing MRI lesions in phase II testing, but in addition also had a significant effect on ARR.[75] The drug was generally well-tolerated, but one death occurred in the high dose ocrelizumab treatment arm due to disseminated intravascular coagulation. In the ongoing phase III program two studies, OPERA 1 and 2, examine the effect of 600 mg ocrelizumab twice yearly compared to thrice weekly IFNβ for RRMS and ORATORIO that examines the effect of 600 mg ocrelizumab twice yearly compared to placebo in PPMS.

Ofatumumab is the third CD20 antagonist tested in MS so far. It is approved for the treatment of chronic lymphocytic leukemia. A dose finding phase II study with 100, 300 or 700 mg has been completed, but not published in full. In another phase II study, subcutaneous delivery in RRMS patients will be investigated.

Alemtuzumab is a humanized monoclonal antibody binding CD52, a surface antigen expressed on various lymphocyte populations, and originally approved for hematological malignancies. The clinical development of alemtuzumab for MS has been tortuous, with the first study published already in 1999.[76] In a subsequent phase II study RRMS patients with high disease activity and very short disease duration where randomized to a yearly treatment course with 12 mg or 24 mg of alemtuzumab, or thrice weekly IFNβ.[77] The results demonstrated a quite remarkable superiority of alemtuzumab compared to the standard treatment in reducing the risk of disability over three years. However, a handful of patients developed autoimmune thrombocytopenia, and one of these died. Also, a high rate of thyroid disorders and a case of Goodpasture's syndrome were recorded in the alemtuzumab arms. Although further alemtuzumab treatment was suspended, the treatment displayed superiority over IFNβ even at five-year follow-up.[78] In two parallel phase III studies, CARE-MS I and II, the effect of alemtuzumab compared to IFNβ was examined over two years.[79,80] CARE-MS I included treatment naïve patients with less than five years of disease duration and demonstrated a 55% reduction of relapses and a non-significant reduction in risk of sustained progression.[79] In CARE-MS II also previously treated patients with up to ten years of disease duration were eligible and showed a similar reduction of relapses, 49%, as well as a 42% reduced risk of sustained disability relative to IFNβ.[80] Both studies confirmed a high rate of thyroid disorders, including two cases of thyroid papillary carcinoma, a low rate of autoimmune thrombocytopenia and an increased risk of herpes infections. Taken together alemtuzumab demonstrates a very good efficacy, but a high rate of adverse events requiring monthly blood and urine monitoring for at least four years after the last infusion. Alemtuzumab has been approved for treatment of RRMS in EU, and recently in the US, despite some concerns about the study design, since randomization to study drug or placebo was not blinded to the patients.

Daclizumab, a monoclonal antibody that targets the CD25 antigen (inter-leukin-2 receptor) has been approved for preventing transplant rejection and is in late-stage clinical development for MS. In a first phase II study, CHOICE, patients on IFNβ were randomized to receive add-on subcutaneous daclizumab 2 mg/kg every two weeks, daclizumab 1 mg/kg every four weeks or placebo, resulting in a 72% and 25% drop in gadolinium-enhancing MRI lesions in the high and low dose daclizumab treatment groups, respectively, compared to placebo.[81] A second phase II study, SELECT, studied the effect of 150 mg or 300 mg subcutaneous daclizumab monthly in monotherapy and showed a 50–54% reduction in ARR compared to placebo.[82] The treatment was generally well tolerated, but cutaneous events were more common in the daclizumab group, including one patient who first had a serious rash and later died of a psoas abscess. A two-year phase III study, DECIDE, comparing 150 mg subcutaneous daclizumab monthly in monotherapy compared to weekly IFNβ has recently been completed, but not published in full. The mechanism of daclizumab is not known, but the drug leads to a conspicuous expansion of CD56(bright) natural killer cells that may convey immunoregulatory effects.[83]

Treatment of Autoantibody-Mediated Inflammatory CNS Diseases

In contrast to MS, there are currently no approved DMTs for autoantibody mediated CNS diseases such as neuromyelitis optica (NMO) or the rapidly expanding list of antibody-mediated encephalitides, and treatments are mainly based on empirical data.

NMO is a condition where patients experience long extending myelitis and optic neuritis, and most patients display autoantibodies recognizing aquaporin-4, a surface water transport molecule present on astrocytes[84] (Fig 1). Oral immunosuppressants, such as azathioprine (AZA), cyclosporine-A or mycophenolate mofetil (MMF), alone or in combination with corticosteroids have long been used, but more recently biological drugs such as rituximab have been introduced. In a recent retrospective analysis of the response rate in a large single center cohort, rituximab and MMF proved more efficacious than AZA.[85] Interestingly, in contrast to MS, IFNβ may increase NMO disease activity and natalizumab is not effective for preventing relapses, underscoring the importance of a correct diagnostic work-up.[86,87] At least two monoclonal antibodies are currently in clinical development for NMO; eculizumab and tocilizumab. Eculizumab (Soliris) is a humanized monoclonal antibody binding complement protein C5 thereby blocking the terminal complement cascade. It is approved for the treatment of paroxysmal nocturnal hemoglobinuria. A smaller open-label study in NMO has been completed with encouraging results.[88] and a phase III trial is to be started. Tocilizumab (Actemra/RoActemra) is a humanized monoclonal antibody against the interleukin-6 receptor (IL-6R) that is approved for rheumatoid arthritis, and a small pilot study in NMO has shown promising effects.[89] Two phase III trials have recently been started.

NMDA receptor encephalitis (NMDAre) is likely the most common among an emerging family of conditions where autoantibodies target surface neurotransmitter receptors present in the CNS. The first larger cohort of NMDAre was reported in 2008 and described as a syndrome with neuropsychiatric symptoms mainly in young women in association with teratomas of the ovaries.[90] Many patients respond to first-line treatments such as plasmapheresis, corticosteroids or immunoglobulins, as well as tumor removal, if present. For those with more severe disease and insufficient response, a combination of cyclophosphamide and rituximab usually proves efficacious.[91] So far, no randomized trials have been conducted.

Cell-Based Therapies: Great Expectations, But Will They Deliver?

In addition to pharmacological treatments, different cell-based therapies are currently being explored in MS and other inflammatory conditions of the CNS.

Haematopoietic stem cell transplantation (HSCT) has been used empirically in MS since more than a decade. Clinical trial data are still limited, but promising results have been demonstrated in smaller case series.[92] Like existing DMTs this treatment seems to be most effective in the early, inflammatory phase of RRMS, rather than in progressive MS.[93,94] Due to a small, but non-negligible mortality risk with HSCT, this treatment is indicated only as a possible third-line option in carefully selected cases of severe and aggressive RRMS. More recently, smaller case series have been published also in NMO.[95]

Mesenchymal stem cell transplantation (MSCT) is a procedure where multipotent stromal cells that can differentiate into a variety of cell types are collected from individual patients and expanded *ex vivo* and finally given back by IV infusion. Preclinical data in experimental models of both inflammatory and neurodegenerative diseases show very promising effects, which has fuelled hopes for a treatment that may benefit patients also in more advanced disease states. Several trials are ongoing and a few pilot studies have been completed, mainly addressing safety aspects rather than efficacy.[96,97] Clearly, larger and controlled trials are needed to address the question of efficacy, and technical protocols that enable cell preparations at a larger scale need to be developed.

Conclusions and Further Directions: The Need to Define Pathways Related to the Neurodegenerative Aspects that can be Targeted Therapeutically

Recent years have seen a rapid expansion of treatment options for neuro-inflammatory conditions, especially MS. While new drugs clearly provide new opportunities for individualized treatment, they also create new chal-lenges, not least which drug should be given to a certain patient and at what stage of the disease. In the current treatment paradigm, IFNβ and GA are first-line drugs and fingolimod and natalizumab mainly second-line choices. Of the more recently approved DMTs, DMF and teriflunomide are likely to become first-line alternatives, while the monoclonal antibodies will mainly become second-line options based on safety data. A common dilemma in clinical practice is that treatments target inflammation rather than neurological symptoms. Many patients are in more advanced disease states, where inflammatory activity as reflected by relapse rates, MRI activity or CSF biomarker analyses has generally decreased. Along this line, it has been argued that MRI measures of inflammatory activity should be used rather than clinical outcome measures.[98] However, this would then require more intense MRI monitoring also in the clinical context. From a mechanistic perspective, drugs targeting T and/or B cells or lymphocyte migration have proven efficacy in RRMS. Their effect in progressive dis-ease is still uncertain, even if there is some support for the efficacy of B cell depletion, at least in younger patients with signs of inflammation on MRI. Further data will now come from the ongoing trials of fingolimod, siponimod, ocrelizumab and natalizumab in progressive MS. Of the drugs reviewed here, both laquinimod and DMF may have modes of action that make them interesting for progressive disease, at least on experimental grounds. However, there are inherent difficulties with studies in progressive disease, since the condition often evolves slowly over time and the natural disease course may include plateau phases with more stable function. Thus, there is a pressing need to refine and develop new disability outcome measures in MS, in particular for progressive disease.[99] One avenue that may prove fruitful is the development of biomarkers that better reflect relevant disease processes and to validate these against clinically relevant outcome measures.

Another common problem in the MS clinic is that many patients with active disease are women of child-bearing potential. Most of the drugs discussed here are given as a chronic treatment with potential adverse effects on the fetus and there is still limited information on safety aspects.[100] Careful post-marketing surveys are needed in order to collect important information on side effects and pregnancy outcomes that can guide clinical decisions on treatment choice.

With certain new drugs entering clinical practice, two different treatment strategies have become accessible; induction vs chronic treatment. Alemtuzumab and HSCT, and to some degree CD20-antagonists, are examples of the former strategy, while most of the remaining belong to the latter category. In current treatment paradigms, patients are expected to start on a first-line treatment that can be escalated or changed to a second-line therapy if signs of breakthrough disease become evident. Especially for younger patients with highly active disease, induction therapy may be preferable to effectively prevent further inflammation-induced nerve damage and the need for chronic treatment. Clearly, long-term data on safety and outcome in the real world use needs to be recorded also in this context.

Lastly, with increasing efficacy, but also perhaps increasing risk of long-term adverse effects, there is a great need of studies on how and when MS therapy can be de-escalated. From an ethical perspective, unnecessary long-term treatment of patients with costly drugs that may cause adverse effects should be avoided. However, this is an issue that is not prioritized by the drug industry and therefore academic initiatives and broader societal support are needed. Again, this underscores the importance of post-marketing follow-up studies and potentially also biomarker or MRI measures that can provide guidance for immunotherapy de-escalation.

In conclusion, in the last decade we have experienced an amazing development regarding knowledge of disease mechanisms, definition of new disease entities and development of novel therapeutic tools in clinical neuroimmunology. These successes have attracted additional interest and resources to the field that will help us to further refine our knowledge and therapeutic armamentarium in the coming years.

Table 1. Approved medications for MS.

	Mode of action	Side effects	Precautions
Alemtuzumab (Lemtrada) Two yearly cycles 12 mg IV daily x V first year 12 mg IV daily x III second year	Monoclonal antibody that eliminates CD52$^+$ immune cells	Thyroid disease Herpes infections Respiratory tract infections	Immune-mediated thrombocytopenia Goodpasture´s syndrome
Dimethylfumarate (Tecfidera) 240 mg PO twice daily	Nrf2 mediated anti-inflamma-tory and cytoprotective effects	Flushing, rash GI symptoms	Lymphopenia progressive multifocal leuko-encephalopathy (PML)?
Fingolimod (Gilenya) 0.5 mg PO daily	Blocks S1P-mediated recruit-ment of lymphocytes from secondary lymphoid organs	Bradyarrythmia Respiratory tract infections Elevated hepatic enzymes	Macular edema Herpes infections Teratogenic effects
Glatiramer acetate (Copaxone) 20 mg SC daily	Increased Th2, Treg cells, deletion myelin-reactive T cells	Injection site reactions Lipoatrophy Chest pain	
Interferon-β1a (Avonex, Rebif) 30 mcg IM weekly 22 or 44 mcg SC three timed weekly	Reduced Th1 responses, less trafficking across **BBB**, reduced antigen presentation, apoptosis of autoreactive T cells	Injection site reactions Flu-like symptoms Elevated hepatic enzymes	Depression Liver disease Lymphopenia
Interferon-β1a, pegylated (Plegridy) 30 mcg SC every two weeks	same as above	same as above	same as above

Interferon-β1b (Betferon/Betaseron, Extavia) 0.25 mg every other day	same as above	same as above	same as above
Natalizumab (Tysabri) 300 mg IV monthly	Monoclonal antibody that blocks α4-integrin on lymphocytes, which impedes transmigration of these cells to the CNS	Herpes infections Elevated hepatic enzymes	PML
Teriflunomide (Aubagio) 7 or 14 mg PO daily (US) 14 mg PO daily (EU)	Cytostatic effects on rapidly dividing lymphocytes through inhibition of pyrimidine synthesis	Elevated hepatic enzymes Hair thinning Neutropenia	Liver disease Peripheral neuropathy Teratogenic effects

References

1. Compston, A., Coles, A. (2008). Multiple sclerosis. *Lancet*, **372**, 1502–1517.
2. Sprangers, M.A., de Regt, E.B., Andries, F., *et al.* (2000). Which chronic conditions are associated with better or poorer quality of life? *J Clinical Epidemiol*, **53**, 895–907.
3. Sawcer, S., Hellenthal, G., Pirinen, M., *et al.* (2011). Genetic risk and a primary role for cell-mediated immune mechanisms in multiple sclerosis. *Nature*, **476**, 214–219.
4. Handel, A.E., Giovannoni, G., Ebers, G.C., Ramagopalan, SV. (2010). Environmental factors and their timing in adult-onset multiple sclerosis. *Nat Rev Neurol*, **6**, 156–166.
5. Hedstrom, A.K., Sundqvist, E., Baarnhielm, M., *et al.* (2011). Smoking and two human leukocyte antigen genes interact to increase the risk for multiple sclerosis. *Brain*, **134**, 653–664.
6. Lublin, F.D., Reingold, S.C., Cohen, J.A., *et al.* (2014). Defining the clinical course of multiple sclerosis: the 2013 revisions. *Neurology*, **83**, 278–286.
7. Confavreux, C., Vukusic, S. (2006). Natural history of multiple sclerosis: a unifying concept. *Brain*, **129**, 606–616.
8. Tallantyre, E.C., Bo, L., Al-Rawashdeh, O., Owens, T., Polman, C.H., Lowe, J.S., Evangelou, N. (2010). Clinico-pathological evidence that axonal loss underlies disability in progressive multiple sclerosis. *Mult Scler*, **16**, 406–411.
9. Lassmann, H., van Horssen, J., Mahad, D. (2012). Progressive multiple sclerosis: pathology and pathogenesis. *Nat Rev Neurol*, **8**, 647–656.
10. Matell, H., Lycke, J., Svenningsson, A., *et al.* (2014). Age-dependent effects on the treatment response of natalizumab in MS patients. *Mult Scler*.
11. Hutchinson, M., Kappos, L., Calabresi, P.A., *et al.* (2009). The efficacy of natalizumab in patients with relapsing multiple sclerosis: subgroup analyses of AFFIRM and SENTINEL. *J Neurol*, **256**, 405–415.
12. Piehl, F. (2014). A changing treatment landscape for multiple sclerosis: challenges and opportunities. *J Intern Med*.
13. Comabella, M., Montalban, X. (2014). Body fluid biomarkers in multiple sclerosis. *Lancet Neurol*, **13**, 113–126.
14. Mathey, E.K., Derfuss, T., Storch, M.K., *et al.* (2007). Neurofascin as a novel target for autoantibody-mediated axonal injury. *J Exp Med*, **204**, 2363–2372.
15. Srivastava, R., Aslam, M., Kalluri, S.R., *et al.* (2012). Potassium channel KIR4.1 as an immune target in multiple sclerosis. *N Engl J Med*, **367**, 115–123.

16. Brickshawana, A., Hinson, S.R., Romero, M.F., *et al.* (2014). Investigation of the KIR4.1 potassium channel as a putative antigen in patients with multiple sclerosis: a comparative study. *Lancet Neurol*, **13**, 795–806.

17. Khademi, M., Dring, A.M., Gilthorpe, J.D., *et al.* (2013). Intense inflammation and nerve damage in early multiple sclerosis subsides at older age: a reflection by cerebrospinal fluid biomarkers. *PLoS One*, **8**, e63172.

18. Teunissen, C.E., Khalil, M. (2012). Neurofilaments as biomarkers in multiple sclerosis. *Mult Scler*, **18**, 552–556.

19. Axelsson, M., Malmestrom, C., Gunnarsson, M., Zetterberg, H., Sundstrom, P., Lycke, J., Svenningsson, A. (2013). Immunosuppressive therapy reduces axonal damage in progressive multiple sclerosis. *Mult Scler*.

20. (1993). Interferon beta-1b is effective in relapsing-remitting multiple sclerosis. I. Clinical results of a multicenter, randomized, double-blind, placebo-controlled trial. The IFNB Multiple Sclerosis Study Group. *Neurology*, **43**, 655–661.

21. Jacobs, L.D., Cookfair, D.L., Rudick, R.A., *et al.* (1996). Intramuscular interferon beta-1a for disease progression in relapsing multiple sclerosis. The Multiple Sclerosis Collaborative Research Group (MSCRG). *Ann Neurol*, **39**, 285–294.

22. Randomised double-blind placebo-controlled study of interferon beta-1a in relapsing/remitting multiple sclerosis. PRISMS (Prevention of Relapses and Disability by Interferon beta-1a Subcutaneously in Multiple Sclerosis) Study Group. (1998). *Lancet*, **352**, 1498–1504.

23. Johnson, K.P., Brooks, B.R., Cohen, J.A., *et al.* (1995). Copolymer 1 reduces relapse rate and improves disability in relapsing-remitting multiple sclerosis: results of a phase III multicenter, double-blind placebo-controlled trial. The Copolymer 1 Multiple Sclerosis Study Group. *Neurology*, **45**, 1268–1276.

24. Calabresi, P.A., Kieseier, B.C., Arnold, D.L., *et al.* (2014). Pegylated interferon beta-1a for relapsing-remitting multiple sclerosis (ADVANCE): a randomised, phase 3, double-blind study. *Lancet Neurol*, **13**, 657–665.

25. Jacobs, L.D., Beck, R.W., Simon, J.H., *et al.* (2000). Intramuscular interferon beta-1a therapy initiated during a first demyelinating event in multiple sclerosis. CHAMPS Study Group. *N Engl J Med*, **343**, 898–904.

26. Comi, G., Filippi, M., Barkhof, F., *et al.* (2001). Effect of early interferon treatment on conversion to definite multiple sclerosis: a randomised study. *Lancet*, **357**, 1576–1582.

27. Kappos, L., Polman, C.H., Freedman, M.S., *et al.* (2006). Treatment with interferon beta-1b delays conversion to clinically definite and McDonald MS in patients with clinically isolated syndromes. *Neurology*, **67**, 1242–1249.

28. Comi, G., Martinelli, V., Rodegher, M., *et al.* (2009). Effect of glatiramer acetate on conversion to clinically definite multiple sclerosis in patients with clinically isolated syndrome (PreCISe study): a randomised, double-blind, placebo-controlled trial. *Lancet*, **374**, 1503–1511.
29. Mikol, D.D., Barkhof, F., Chang, P., *et al.* (2008). Comparison of subcutaneous interferon beta-1a with glatiramer acetate in patients with relapsing multiple sclerosis (the REbif vs Glatiramer Acetate in Relapsing MS Disease [REGARD] study): a multicentre, randomised, parallel, open-label trial. *Lancet Neurol*, **7**, 903–914.
30. O'Connor, P., Filippi, M., Arnason, B., *et al.* (2009). 250 microg or 500 microg interferon beta-1b versus 20 mg glatiramer acetate in relapsing-remitting multiple sclerosis: a prospective, randomised, multicentre study. *Lancet Neurol*, **8**, 889–897.
31. Bergamaschi, R., Quaglini, S., Tavazzi, E., *et al.* (2012). Immunomodulatory therapies delay disease progression in multiple sclerosis. *Mult Scler.*
32. Tedeholm, H., Lycke, J., Skoog, B., *et al.* (2012). Time to secondary progression in patients with multiple sclerosis who were treated with first generation immunomodulating drugs. *Mult Scler.*
33. Kappos, L., Freedman, M.S., Polman, C.H., *et al.* (2009). Long-term effect of early treatment with interferon beta-1b after a first clinical event suggestive of multiple sclerosis: 5-year active treatment extension of the phase 3 BENEFIT trial. *Lancet Neurol*, **8**, 987–997.
34. Rudick, R.A., Polman, C.H. (2009). Current approaches to the identification and management of breakthrough disease in patients with multiple sclerosis. *Lancet Neurol*, **8**, 545–559.
35. Wong, J., Gomes, T., Mamdani, M., Manno, M., O'Connor, P.W. (2011). Adherence to multiple sclerosis disease-modifying therapies in Ontario is low. *Can J Neurol Sci*, **38**, 429–433.
36. Tremlett, H.L., Oger, J. (2003). Interrupted therapy: stopping and switching of the beta-interferons prescribed for MS. *Neurology*, **61**, 551–554.
37. Matloubian, M., Lo, C.G., Cinamon, G., *et al.* (2004). Lymphocyte egress from thymus and peripheral lymphoid organs is dependent on S1P receptor 1. *Nature*, **427**, 355–360.
38. Mehling, M., Brinkmann, V., Antel, J., *et al.* (2008). FTY720 therapy exerts differential effects on T cell subsets in multiple sclerosis. *Neurology*, **71**, 1261–1267.
39. Mehling, M., Lindberg, R., Raulf, F., Kuhle, J., Hess, C., Kappos, L., Brinkmann, V. (2010). Th17 central memory T cells are reduced by FTY720 in patients with multiple sclerosis. *Neurology*, **75**, 403–410.

40. Kappos, L., Radue, E.W., O'Connor, P., *et al.* (2010). A placebo-controlled trial of oral fingolimod in relapsing multiple sclerosis. *N Engl J Med*, **362,** 387–401.

41. Calabresi, P.A., Radue, E.W., Goodin, D., *et al.* (2014). Safety and efficacy of fingolimod in patients with relapsing-remitting multiple sclerosis (FREEDOMS II): a double-blind, randomised, placebo-controlled, phase 3 trial. *Lancet Neurol*, **13,** 545–556.

42. Cohen, J.A., Barkhof, F., Comi, G., *et al.* (2010). Oral fingolimod or intra-muscular interferon for relapsing multiple sclerosis. *N Engl J Med*, **362,** 402–415.

43. Pelletier, D., Hafler, D.A. (2012). Fingolimod for multiple sclerosis. *N Engl J Med*, **366,** 339–347.

44. Jain, N., Bhatti, M.T. (2012). Fingolimod-associated macular edema: inci-dence, detection, and management. *Neurology*, **78,** 672–680.

45. Miller, D., Cree, B., Dalton, C., *et al.* (2013). Study design and baseline characteristics of the INFORMS study: fingolimod in patients with primary progressive multiple sclerosis. *Neurology*, **80,** P07.116.

46. http://www.novartis.com/newsroom/media-releases/en/2014/1875463.shtml.

47. Selmaj, K., Li, D.K., Hartung, H.P., *et al.* (2013). Siponimod for patients with relapsing-remitting multiple sclerosis (BOLD): an adaptive, dose-ranging, randomised, phase 2 study. *Lancet Neurol*, **12,** 756–767.

48. Barry Singer, G.C., Miller, A., Olsson, T., Wolinsky, J., Kappos, L., Confavreux, C., Freedman, M., Benzerdjeb, H., Li, H., Truffinet, P., and O'Connor, P. (2013). Frequency of infections during treatment with teriflu-nomide: pooled data from three placebo-controlled teriflunomide studies. *Neurology*, **80,** P01.171.

49. O'Connor, P., Wolinsky, J.S., Confavreux, C., *et al.* (2011). Randomized trial of oral teriflunomide for relapsing multiple sclerosis. *N Engl J Med*, **365,** 1293–1303.

50. Miller, A., Kappos, L., Comi, G., Confavreux, C,. Freedman, M., Olsson, T., Wolinsky, J., Bagulho, T., Delhay, J.-L., Zheng, Y., Truffinet P., and O'Connor, P. (2013). Teriflunomide efficacy and safety in patients with relapsing multiple sclerosis: results from TOWER, a second, pivotal, phase 3 placebo-controlled study. *Neurology*, **80,** S01.004.

51. Vermersch, P., Czlonkowska, A., Grimaldi, L.M., *et al.* (2014). Teriflunomide versus subcutaneous interferon beta-1a in patients with relapsing multiple sclerosis: a randomised, controlled phase 3 trial. *Mult Scler*, **20,** 705–716.

52. Gold, R., Kappos, L., Arnold, D.L., *et al.* (2012). Placebo-controlled phase 3 study of oral BG-12 for relapsing multiple sclerosis. *N Engl J Med*, **367,** 1098–1107.

53. Fox, R.J., Miller, D.H., Phillips, J.T., *et al.* (2012). Placebo-controlled phase 3 study of oral BG-12 or glatiramer in multiple sclerosis. *N Engl J Med*, **367**, 1087–1097.

54. Scannevin, R.H., Chollate, S., Jung, M.Y., *et al.* (2012). Fumarates promote cytoprotection of central nervous system cells against oxidative stress via the nuclear factor (erythroid-derived 2)-like 2 pathway. *J Pharmacol Exp Ther*, **341**, 274–284.

55. Linker, R.A., Lee, D.H., Ryan, S., *et al.* (2011). Fumaric acid esters exert neuroprotective effects in neuroinflammation via activation of the Nrf2 antioxidant pathway. *Brain*, **134**, 678–692.

56. Noseworthy, J.H., Wolinsky, J.S., Lublin, F.D., Whitaker, J.N., Linde, A., Gjorstrup, P., Sullivan, HC. (2000). Linomide in relapsing and secondary progressive MS: part I: trial design and clinical results. North American Linomide Investigators. *Neurology*, **54**, 1726–1733.

57. Comi, G., Jeffery, D., Kappos, L., Montalban, X., Boyko, A., Rocca, M.A., Filippi, M. (2012). Placebo-controlled trial of oral laquinimod for multiple sclerosis. *N Engl J Med*, **366**, 1000–1009.

58. Vollmer, T.L., Sorensen, P.S., Selmaj, K., *et al.* (2014). A randomized placebo-controlled phase III trial of oral laquinimod for multiple sclerosis. *J Neurol*, **261**, 773–783.

59. Jolivel, V., Luessi, F., Masri, J., *et al.* (2013). Modulation of dendritic cell properties by laquinimod as a mechanism for modulating multiple sclerosis. *Brain*, **136**, 1048–1066.

60. Bruck, W., Pfortner, R., Pham, T., *et al.* (2012). Reduced astrocytic NF-kappaB activation by laquinimod protects from cuprizone-induced demyelination. *Acta Neuropathol*, **124**, 411–424.

61. Yednock, T.A., Cannon, C., Fritz, L.C., Sanchez-Madrid, F., Steinman, L., Karin, N. (1992). Prevention of experimental autoimmune encephalomyelitis by antibodies against alpha 4 beta 1 integrin. *Nature*, **356**, 63–66.

62. Kivisakk, P., Healy, B.C., Viglietta, V., Quintana, F.J., Hootstein, M.A., Weiner, H.L., Khoury, SJ. (2009). Natalizumab treatment is associated with peripheral sequestration of proinflammatory T cells. *Neurology*, **72**, 1922–1930.

63. Polman, C.H., O'Connor, P.W., Havrdova, E., *et al.* (2006). A randomized, placebo-controlled trial of natalizumab for relapsing multiple sclerosis. *N Engl J Med*, **354**, 899–910.

64. Rudick, R.A., Stuart, W.H., Calabresi, P.A., *et al.* (2006). Natalizumab plus interferon beta-1a for relapsing multiple sclerosis. *N Engl J Med*, **354**, 911–923.

65. Holmen, C., Piehl, F., Hillert, J., *et al.* (2011). A Swedish national post-marketing surveillance study of natalizumab treatment in multiple sclerosis. *Mult Scler*, **17**, 708–719.

66. Tan, C.S., Koralnik, I.J. (2010). Progressive multifocal leukoencephalopathy and other disorders caused by JC virus: clinical features and pathogenesis. *Lancet Neurol*, **9**, 425–437.

67. Gorelik, L., Lerner, M., Bixler, S., *et al.* (2010). Anti-JC virus antibodies: implications for PML risk stratification. *Ann Neurol*, **68**, 295–303.

68. O'Connor, P.W., Goodman, A., Kappos, L., *et al.* (2011). Disease activity return during natalizumab treatment interruption in patients with multiple sclerosis. *Neurology*, **76**, 1858–1865.

69. West, T.W., Cree, B.A. (2010). Natalizumab dosage suspension: are we helping or hurting? *Ann Neurol*, **68**, 395–399.

70. Franciotta, D., Salvetti, M., Lolli, F., Serafini, B., Aloisi, F. (2008). B cells and multiple sclerosis. *Lancet Neurol*, **7**, 852–858.

71. Piccio, L., Naismith, R.T., Trinkaus, K., Klein, R.S., Parks, B.J., Lyons, J.A., Cross, A.H. (2010). Changes in B- and T-lymphocyte and chemokine levels with rituximab treatment in multiple sclerosis. *Arch Neurol*, **67**, 707–714.

72. Ireland, S.J., Blazek, M., Harp, C.T., Greenberg, B., Frohman, E.M., Davis, L.S., Monson, N.L. (2012). Antibody-independent B cell effector functions in relapsing remitting multiple sclerosis: clues to increased inflammatory and reduced regulatory B cell capacity. *Autoimmunity*, **45**, 400–414.

73. Hauser, S.L., Waubant, E., Arnold, D.L., *et al.* (2008). B-cell depletion with rituximab in relapsing-remitting multiple sclerosis. *N Engl J Med*, **358**, 676–688.

74. Hawker, K., O'Connor, P., Freedman, M.S., *et al.* (2009). Rituximab in patients with primary progressive multiple sclerosis: results of a randomized double-blind placebo-controlled multicenter trial. *Ann Neurol*, **66**, 460–471.

75. Kappos, L., Li, D., Calabresi, P.A., *et al.* (2011). Ocrelizumab in relapsing-remitting multiple sclerosis: a phase 2, randomised, placebo-controlled, multicentre trial. *Lancet*, **378**, 1779–1787.

76. Coles, A.J., Wing, M.G., Molyneux, P., *et al.* (1999). Monoclonal antibody treatment exposes three mechanisms underlying the clinical course of multiple sclerosis. *Ann Neurol*, **46**, 296–304.

77. Coles, A.J., Compston, D.A., Selmaj, K.W., *et al.* (2008). Alemtuzumab vs. interferon beta-1a in early multiple sclerosis. *N Engl J Med*, **359**, 1786–1801.

78. Coles, A.J., Fox, E., Vladic, A., *et al.* (2012). Alemtuzumab more effective than interferon beta-1a at 5-year follow-up of CAMMS223 clinical trial. *Neurology*, **78**, 1069–1078.

79. Cohen, J.A., Coles, A.J., Arnold, D.L., *et al.* (2012). Alemtuzumab versus interferon beta 1a as first-line treatment for patients with relapsing-remitting multiple sclerosis: a randomised controlled phase 3 trial. *Lancet*, **380,** 1819–1828.

80. Coles, A.J., Twyman, C.L., Arnold, D.L., *et al.* (2012). Alemtuzumab for patients with relapsing multiple sclerosis after disease-modifying therapy: a randomised controlled phase 3 trial. *Lancet*, **380,** 1829–1839.

81. Wynn, D., Kaufman, M., Montalban, X., *et al.* (2010). Daclizumab in active relapsing multiple sclerosis (CHOICE study): a phase 2, randomised, double-blind, placebo-controlled, add-on trial with interferon beta. *Lancet Neurol*, **9,** 381–390.

82. Gold, R., Giovannoni, G., Selmaj, K., *et al.* (2013). Daclizumab high-yield process in relapsing-remitting multiple sclerosis (SELECT): a randomised, double-blind, placebo-controlled trial. *Lancet*, **381,** 2167–2175.

83. Bielekova, B., Catalfamo, M., Reichert-Scrivner, S., *et al.* (2006). Regulatory CD56(bright) natural killer cells mediate immunomodulatory effects of IL-2Ralpha-targeted therapy (daclizumab) in multiple sclerosis. *Proc Natl Acad Sci U S A*, **103,** 5941–5946.

84. Lennon, V.A., Kryzer, T.J., Pittock, S.J., Verkman, A.S., Hinson, S.R. (2005). IgG marker of optic-spinal multiple sclerosis binds to the aquaporin-4 water channel. *J Exp Med*, **202,** 473–477.

85. Mealy, M.A., Wingerchuk, D.M., Palace, J., Greenberg, B.M., Levy, M. (2014). Comparison of relapse and treatment failure rates among patients with neuromyelitis optica: multicenter study of treatment efficacy. *JAMA Neurology*, **71,** 324–330.

86. Shimizu, J., Hatanaka, Y., Hasegawa, M., *et al.* (2010). IFNbeta-1b may severely exacerbate Japanese optic-spinal MS in neuromyelitis optica spectrum. *Neurology*, **75,** 1423–1427.

87. Kleiter, I., Hellwig, K., Berthele, A., *et al.* (2012). Failure of natalizumab to prevent relapses in neuromyelitis optica. *Arch Neurol*, **69,** 239–245.

88. Pittock, S.J., Lennon, V.A., McKeon, A., *et al.* (2013). Eculizumab in AQP4-IgG-positive relapsing neuromyelitis optica spectrum disorders: an open-label pilot study. *Lancet Neurol*, **12,** 554–562.

89. Araki, M., Matsuoka, T., Miyamoto, K., *et al.* (2014). Efficacy of the anti-IL-6 receptor antibody tocilizumab in neuromyelitis optica: a pilot study. *Neurology*, **82,** 1302–1306.

90. Dalmau, J., Gleichman, A.J., Hughes, E.G., *et al.* (2008). Anti-NMDA-receptor encephalitis: case series and analysis of the effects of antibodies. *Lancet Neurol*, **7,** 1091–1098.

91. Titulaer, M.J., McCracken, L., Gabilondo, I., *et al.* (2013). Treatment and prognostic factors for long-term outcome in patients with anti-NMDA receptor encephalitis: an observational cohort study. *Lancet Neurol*, **12**, 157–165.

92. Burt, R.K., Loh, Y., Cohen, B., *et al.* (2009). Autologous non-myeloablative haemopoietic stem cell transplantation in relapsing-remitting multiple sclerosis: a phase I/II study. *Lancet Neurol*, **8**, 244–253.

93. Samijn, J.P., te Boekhorst, P.A., Mondria, T., *et al.* (2006). Intense T cell depletion followed by autologous bone marrow transplantation for severe multiple sclerosis. *J Neurol Neurosurg Psychiatry*, **77**, 46–50.

94. Burman, J., Iacobaeus, E., Svenningsson, A., *et al.* (2014). Autologous haematopoietic stem cell transplantation for aggressive multiple sclerosis: the Swedish experience. *J Neurol Neurosurg Psychiatry*, **85**, 1116–1121.

95. Greco, R., Bondanza, A., Oliveira, M.C., *et al.* (2014). Autologous hematopoietic stem cell transplantation in neuromyelitis optica: A registry study of the EBMT Autoimmune Diseases Working Party. *Mult Scler.*

96. Karussis, D., Karageorgiou, C., Vaknin-Dembinsky, A., *et al.* (2010). Safety and immunological effects of mesenchymal stem cell transplantation in patients with multiple sclerosis and amyotrophic lateral sclerosis. *Arch Neurol*, **67**, 1187–1194.

97. Connick, P., Kolappan, M., Crawley, C., *et al.* (2012). Autologous mesenchymal stem cells for the treatment of secondary progressive multiple sclerosis: an open-label phase 2a proof-of-concept study. *Lancet Neurol*, **11**, 150–156.

98. Sormani, M.P., De Stefano, N. (2014). MRI measures should be a primary outcome endpoint in Phase III randomized, controlled trials in multiple sclerosis: yes. *Mult Scler*, **20**, 280–281.

99. Cohen, J.A., Reingold, S.C., Polman, C.H., Wolinsky, J.S. (2012). Disability outcome measures in multiple sclerosis clinical trials: current status and future prospects. *Lancet Neurol*, **11**, 467–476.

100. Lu, E., Wang, B.W., Guimond, C., Synnes, A., Sadovnick, D., Tremlett, H. (2012). Disease-modifying drugs for multiple sclerosis in pregnancy: a systematic review. *Neurology*, **79**, 1130–1135.

CHAPTER 14

CLINICAL THERAPY RESEARCH IN ALLERGIC DISEASES

Raffaela Campana, Rudolf Valenta, Jeanette Grundström,
Carl Hamsten, and Marianne van Hage

Introduction

Allergic diseases belong to the most common causes of chronic illnesses. They have become a public health concern of pandemic proportions, affecting more than 25% of the world population.[1,2] The diseases create a high burden of suffering not only due to life-threatening conditions such as anaphylaxis or asthma, but also due to the tremendous impairment in quality of life. If not properly diagnosed and treated, allergy tends to progress to a severe and chronic disabling disease.[3,4] The best treatment for allergic diseases is avoidance, but it is impractical for both indoor and outdoor allergens; and often unsatisfactory in clinical practice. Pharmacological treatments are recommended as first-line therapy which focus on controlling symptoms as well as reducing the allergic inflammation. However, pharmacological treatment does not change the chronic course of the disease. The only disease-modifying treatment with the ability of inducing long-lasting protection is allergen-specific immunotherapy (SIT).[5] The aim of SIT is to induce immune tolerance to the allergen[6] and has been used to treat allergic disease for over a century. In 1911, Noon started to inject patients suffering from hay fever with grass pollen-derived allergen extracts in increasing doses and showed that the treatment reduced allergic symptoms.[7] Current allergy vaccines for SIT are still prepared from relatively poorly defined allergen extracts which face problems related to efficacy and side effects. However, with the present knowledge of structures of the most common allergen molecules, IgE-mediated side effects of allergy vaccines can be overcome by engineering of vaccines based on recombinant and synthetic allergen molecules. In this chapter, we will describe the use of allergen components for improving treatment options for allergic patients, different approaches for new therapeutic vaccines, *e.g.*, unmodified or modified recombinant allergens, peptide-based vaccines, or allergens coupled or adsorbed to immunomodulatory components. Furthermore, novel routes aiming at enhanced safety and efficacy as well as possible prophylactic strategies for prevention of allergic diseases are discussed.

Allergic Disease

The most common type of allergic disease is mediated by IgE.[8,9] The IgE-mediated immune response may lead to several diseases, including allergic asthma, allergic rhinoconjunctivitis, anaphylaxis, urticaria and atopic dermatitis. It is a complex multiphase immune response that is characterized by an early and late phase reaction.[1] In the sensitization phase, IgE antibodies are produced against harmless substances, known as allergens, which bind to the high-affinity receptors for IgE (*i.e.* FcεRI) on the surface of mast cells and basophils. In the effector phase, a new encounter with the allergen causes cross-linking of IgE antibodies on sensitized mast cells and basophils, which are activated within a few minutes and release inflammatory mediators, proteases and pro-inflammatory cytokines and chemokines.[10,11] These potent substances are responsible for the immediate allergic reaction. The second phase of the allergic response constitutes the activation of allergen-specific T cells, which produce pro-inflammatory cytokines that can lead to late-phase reactions and the more chronic forms of allergic inflammation. This phase may be strongly enhanced by IgE-facilitated allergen presentation,[12] but can also occur without the presence of IgE epitopes.

Today a variety of medications are utilized for symptomatic therapy, such as antihistamines and anti-leukotrienes which inhibit key mediators of inflammation. Glucocorticosteroids act by blocking cytokines that enhance and sustain the airway inflammation. In asthma, the use of bronchodilators helps to open up the airways by relaxing the tightened bronchial smooth muscles.

Subcutaneous injection immunotherapy (SCIT) is the most common form of allergy vaccination. It is based on repeated injections of the clinical relevant allergen over the course of several months, building up to monthly injections over a period of 3–5 years.[13] It has been shown to be effective for, above all, seasonal allergens and hymenoptera venom. SCIT has been demonstrated to reduce the risk of developing clinical asthma in patients with allergic rhinoconjunctivitis and to prevent new allergen sensitization.[14] Thus, it should be considered as a treatment strategy in those with early-onset and/or mild airway disease.

From Allergen Extracts to Allergenic Molecules and Improved Diagnosis for SIT

Allergens can be derived from various allergen sources (*e.g.*, pollen, pets, moulds, house dust mites, food and insects) and are mainly proteins or glycoproteins.[15] Traditional allergy diagnostics, such as skin prick tests or *in vitro* IgE tests, are based on crude allergen extracts that are composed of allergenic and non-allergenic molecules. Unfortunately, the content and the quality of such allergen extracts have shown great variability. Advances in molecular biology during the last decades have enabled the generation of allergenic molecules with well-defined molecular, immunological and biological characteristics. Today, allergenic molecules from the most important allergen sources are available either as recombinantly expressed proteins or as native molecules purified from natural sources. The availability of these allergenic molecules (allergen components) has led to a new phase in diagnostics, termed molecular-based allergy (MA) diagnostics. MA diagnostics has enabled the identification of the relevant allergen(s) for SIT as it may distinguish genuine sensitizations from cross-reactions in poly-sensitized patients.[16] For instance, a patient who is primarily sensitized to grasses (*e.g.*, the major *Phleum pratense* allergens Phl p 1 and/

or Phl p 5) may also have IgE antibodies to birch as birch extract contains profilins (*e.g.*, *Betula verucosa* Bet v 2), which are largely similar to those in grasses (*e.g.*, Phl p 12) but seldom give rise to symptoms. Thus in poly-sensitized allergic patients, the relevant sensitizing allergens for which SIT should be prescribed can now be clearly identified. Furthermore, MA diag-nostics also improves the selection of patients, *e.g.*, for hymenoptera venom SIT. Sensitization to the major allergens of honeybee, *Apis mellifera*, Api m 1, and of yellow jackets, *Vespula spp.*, Ves v 5 and/or Ves v 1, may be helpful in discriminating true double bee and wasp sensitization from cross-reactivity caused by cross-reactive carbohydrates found in extracts from both bee and wasp. In addition, patients with sensitization to minor allergens alone will likely not receive sufficient amounts of specific allergen to achieve a successful outcome by SIT with allergen extracts. Companion diagnostic tools for MA testing are available as single or multiplex (microarray) platforms.

Mechanisms of Allergen-Specific Immunotherapy

Although SIT has been carried out for more than a century, the mecha-nisms of the treatment are not yet fully understood. The aim of SIT is to induce tolerance to the allergen, change the course of allergic disease and reduce the allergic symptoms. The mechanisms involve basophil and mast cell desensitization and effects on T cell reactivity. During therapy, an early increase in allergen-specific IgE is noted, which is followed by a gradual decrease usually after 3–6 months.[17] However, the changes in IgE levels do not correlate with clinical improvement. The changes in IgE levels are followed by an increase in allergen-specific IgG antibodies, particularly IgG_4 and IgG_1 which are considered to be the major blocking antibody isotypes.[18–20] These antibodies block the binding of IgE to the allergen[21] and thus inhibit IgE-mediated release of inflammatory media-tors from basophils and mast cells[22] as well as IgE facilitated antigen presentation to T cells.[23] It has been demonstrated that long-term SIT (>1 year) induces blocking antibodies to a much higher degree than short-term SIT[24] and clinical improvement after SIT is associated with increases in allergen-specific IgG.

SIT also alters the T cell response with a shift in the allergen-specific T-helper (Th) cell response, from a Th2 to a Th1/Treg profile.[25–28] Generation of allergen-specific Treg cells is another mechanism in the induction of allergen tolerance. Patients who have gone through SIT may produce Treg cells that secrete the regulatory cytokine IL-10.[18,29] Both IL-10 and Treg cells may suppress total and allergen-specific IgE and, at the same time, increase IgG_4 production.[13]

New Molecular Approaches for Allergen-Specific Immunotherapy

Even though SIT is currently well established, there are major problems that need to be overcome.

First, therapeutic allergy vaccines are prepared from poorly defined allergen extracts containing mixtures of allergenic as well as non-allergenic compounds and/or unwanted materials such as bacterial endotoxins.[30] Second, the systemic administration of allergens during the course of SIT may lead to side effects that can range from local reactions at the site of allergen injection to systemic and potentially life-threatening anaphylactic reactions. Another major problem is that the available commercial extracts may lack important allergens resulting in poor immunogenicity of the vaccines.[31–34] Moreover, because of the poor characterization of the extracts and the risk of adverse reactions, it is difficult to reach therapeutically effective doses.[35–37] The variability in clinical efficacy and safety together with the time-consuming treatment leading to low patient adherence are problems that limit the broad application of SIT.

The first attempts of reducing therapy-induced side effects included adsorption of the extracts to adjuvants which makes the allergen remain at the injection site, thus reducing systemic side effects. Furthermore, chemical modification of allergen extracts have been carried out to reduce their allergenic activity. In the last decade, the growing knowledge on mechanisms of SIT in combination with technological developments has generated novel treatment strategies to improve the current problems of the therapy. These approaches are based on recombinant allergen-based vaccines containing only well-characterized clinically relevant allergen molecules or

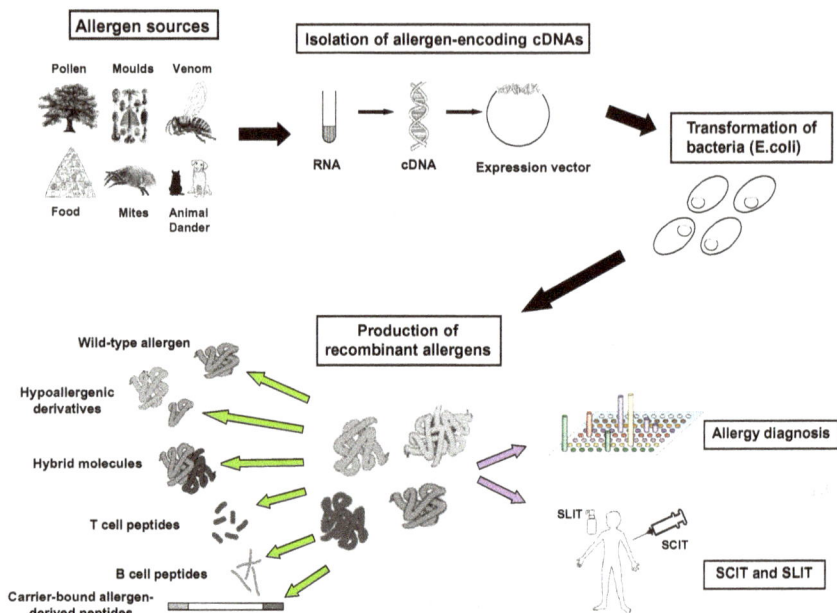

Figure 1.   From allergen sources to new approaches for SIT.

modification of these (*e.g.*, hypoallergenic allergen derivatives, allergen hybrid molecules, T cell peptides) (Fig. 1). All of these new molecular approaches for vaccines against allergic diseases aim to bring SIT to a less dangerous (reduction of side-effects), arduous (decrease number of injections), and time-consuming treatment. Table 1 provides an overview of new molecular approaches for SIT which will be described in the following paragraphs. A number of these approaches have been applied into clinical trials (Table 1) and several are under current investigation (Table 2). The outcomes of representative allergen-SIT trials are shown in Table 3.

Recombinant allergens for SIT

The introduction of defined recombinant allergens using gene technology approaches was a significant step in the history of allergy diagnosis and therapy since wild-type recombinant molecules were shown to be comparable to their natural counterparts regarding IgE binding, skin reactivity and *in vitro* diagnostics.[35] Moreover, standardization problems associated with using natural allergen extracts can be overcome.

Table 1. Novel allergy vaccine approaches tested for allergen-SIT.

Type of the vaccine/approach	Mechanism					References
	IgE reactivity	T cell reactivity	Induction of protective IgG antibodies	Possible IgE-mediated side effects	Possible T cell mediated side effects	
Recombinant wild-type allergens	+	+	+	+	+	38, 39, 40, 86
						Klimek L *et al.*, 2012
						NCT00671268 *
						NCT01353755 *
						NCT01449786 *
Recombinant hypoallergenic modified allergen derivatives	+/−	+	+	−	+	43, 47, 45, 49
						Reisinger J et al., 2005
						Gafvelin G et al., 2005
						Pree I *et al.*, 2007
						Wood RA *et al.*, 2013
						NCT02098551*
						NCT01353924*
						NCT00309062*
						NCT00554983*
						NCT02017626*
						NCT00309036*
T cell epitope containing peptides	−	+	−	−	+	64, 69, 35, 66, 68
						Litwin A *et al.*, 1991
						Maguire P *et al.*, 1999

(Continued)

Table 1. (*Continued*)

Type of the vaccine/approach	IgE reactivity	T cell reactivity	Mechanism			References
			Induction of protective IgG antibodies	Possible IgE-mediated side effects	Possible T cell mediated side effects	
						Fellrath JM *et al.*, 2003
						Worm M *et al.*, 2011
						Spertini F *et al.*, 2014
						NCT01620762*
						NCT00685711*
						NCT00867906*
						NCT00729508*
						NCT02311413*
						NCT00813046*
						NCT00833066*
						NCT01166061*
						NCT01385800*
						NCT01923779*
						NCT02292875*
						NCT01447784*
						NCT01008332*
						NCT01198613*
						NCT00878774*
Carrier-bound B cell epitope containing peptides	–	–	+	–	–	NTC01350635*
						NCT01445002*
						NTC01538979*

* Clinical trials under investigation (Table 2)

Table 2. Registered clinical trials for allergen-SIT under current investigation.

Type of approach	Intervention	Purpose	Trial registration (Clinical Trials.gov Identifier)
Recombinant wild-type allergens in SIT trials	AL0704rP; Placebo	Efficacy and safety of high-dosed SCIT with recombinant major allergens of timothy grass in patients suffering from allergic rhinoconjunctivitis and/or controlled asthma	NCT00671268
	rPhleum; Placebo	Efficacy and safety of SCIT with rPhleum in adults and adolescents suffering from rhinoconjunctivitis and/or controlled asthma	NCT01353755
	rMald 1; rBet v 1; Placebo	Clinical and immunological effects of SLIT of birch pollen associated apple allergy	NCT01449786
Recombinant hypoallergenic modified allergen derivatives in SIT trials	rBet v 1; rBet v 1 F1; rBet v 1 F2	Novel route approach study: SPT and APT with hypoallergenic rBet v 1 fragments to investigate the contribution of IgE versus non-IgE-mediated mechanisms in chronic skin inflammation in AD patients	NCT02098551
	rBet v 1 F1-Alum; rBet v 1 F2-Alum; Placebo	Prophylactic approach study: Immune response of non-allergic individuals	NCT01353924
	Hypoallergenic rBet v 1 derivative	Safety and efficacy of SIT with Alum-adsorbed hypoallergenic rBet v 1 derivative for the treatment of allergic rhinoconjunctivitis	NCT00309062
	rBet v 1-FV	Safety and efficacy of SIT with Alum-adsorbed rBet v 1-FV	NCT00554983
	mCyp c 1	Safety and tolerability of SCIT treatment with incremental doses of modified recombinant fish parvalbumin (mCyp c 1)	NCT02017626
	Recombinant grass pollen allergens	Efficacy and safety of SIT with Alum-adsorbed cocktail of recombinant derivatives of major allergens of timothy grass	NCT00309036

(Continued)

Table 2.   (*Continued*)

Type of approach	Intervention	Purpose	Trial registration (Clinical Trials.gov Identifier)
T cell epitope containing peptides in SIT trials	Cat-PAD; Placebo	Phase III Cat-PAD Study	NCT01620762
		Safety of Cat-PAD in cat allergic subjects	NCT00685711
		Safety of Cat-PAD in cat allergic patients with controlled asthma	NCT00867906
		Effectiveness of Cat-PAD	NCT00729508
		Effect of Fel d 1 peptide immunotherapy on allergen-specific T cells	NCT02311413
	gpASIT+TM; Placebo	Safety and tolerability of grass pollen-derived peptides for oral use in SIT	NCT00813046
		Safety and immunogenicity of grass pollen-derived peptides for oral use in SIT os seasonal allergic rhinoconjunctivitis	NCT00833066
	ToleroMune Grass; Placebo	Safety and tolerability of multiple rising doses of synthetic allergen-derived peptide desensitising vaccine (ToleroMune Grass) for treatment of grass allergy	NCT01166061
		Efficacy, safety and tolerability of ToleroMune Grass in grass pollen allergic subjects following challenge with grass allergen in an EEU	NCT01385800
		Follow-up studies: Evaluation of continue efficacy of ToleroMune Grass in grass pollen allergic subjects following challenge with grass allergen in an EEU	NCT01923779 NCT02292875
	ToleroMune HDM; Placebo	Safety and tolerability of 3 doses of synthetic allergen-derived peptide desensitising vaccine (ToleroMune HDM) for treatment of house dust mite allergy following challenge with HDM allergen in an EEC	NCT01447784

(*Continued*)

Table 2. *(Continued)*

Type of approach	Intervention	Purpose	Trial registration (Clinical Trials.gov Identifier)
		Safety and tolerability of multiple rising doses of ToleroMune HDM in HDM allergic subjects with rhinoconjunctivitis and Efficacy of intradermal injection of ToleroMune HDM	NCT01008332
	ToleroMune Ragweed; Placebo	Safety and tolerability of 2 doses of synthetic allergen-derived peptide desensitising vaccine (ToleroMune Ragweed) for treatment of ragweed allergy following challenge with ragweed in an EEC	NCT01198613
		Safety of intradermal injection of ToleroMune Ragweed in rag weed allergic subjects with rhinoconjunctivitis	NCT00878774
Carrier-bound B cell epitope containing peptides in SIT trials	BM32; Placebo	Skin test study of BM32	NCT01350635
		Safety and dose finding trial of BM32, a recombinant hypoallergenic grass pollen vaccine, in grass pollen allergic patients	NCT01445002
		Phase II study of grass pollen allergy vaccine BM32	NCT01538979

SCIT: Subcutaneous immunotherapy, SLIT: Sublingual immunotherapy
SPT: Skin prick test; APT: Atopy patch test
EEU: Environmental Exposure Unit,
EEC: Environmental Exposure Chamber

Table 3. Outcomes of representative allergen-SIT trials.

Type of approach	Treatment	Allergen	Outcome	References
Recombinant wild-type allergens in SIT trials	SCIT	Mixture of recombinant grass pollen allergens (Phl p 1, Phl p 2, Phl p 5, and Phl p 6)	Improvment of symptom medication score with reduction in symptoms and medication usage; Induction of allergen-specific IgG_1 and IgG_4	Jutel M et al., 2005
	SCIT	Recombinant Bet v 1	Reduction of rhinoconjuctivitis symptoms, rescue medication and skin sensitivities; Increased Bet v 1-specific IgG	Pauli G et al., 2008
	SLIT	Recombinant Bet v 1	Tolerability of rBet v 1 in SLIT	Winther LPL et al., 2009
	ILIT	Recombinant Fel d 1	Increased nasal tolerance; Induction of regulatory T cell responses; Increased IgG_4	Senti G et al., 2012
Recombinant hypoallergenic modified allergen derivatives in SIT trials	SCIT	Recombinant Bet v 1, rBet v 1 trimer, rBet v 1 fragments	Induction of protective IgG; Reduction of cutaneous sensitivity and improvment of symptoms; Reduction of allergen-specific IgE by seasonal birch pollen exposure	Niederberger V et al., 2004*
	SCIT	Recombinant Bet v 1, rBet v 1 trimer, rBet v 1 fragments	Induction of allergen-specific IgG_1, IgG_2, and IgG_4 associated with reduced nasal sensitivity	Reisinger J et al., 2005

SCIT	Recombinant Bet v 1, rBet v 1 trimer, rBet v 1 fragments	Reduction in skin and nasal sensitivity; Induction of allergen-specific IgG_1 and IgG_4	Purohit A et al., 2008
SCIT	Recombinant Bet v 1-FV	Improvement in symptom scores; Induction of IgG_1	Meyer W et al., 2013
T cell epitope containing peptides in SIT trials			
SCIT	Amb a I-derived peptic fragments	Reduced symptom-medication scores; Increased preseasonal specific IgG	Litwin A et al., 1991
SCIT	Fel d 1-derived peptides	Reduced baseline nasal and lung scores; Improved allergic responses to cats	Norman PS et al., 1996
SCIT	Short T cell peptides of PLA (major honeybee venom)	Induction of epitope-specific anergy in peripheral T cells; Inhibition of Th1 and Th2 cytokines	Mueller U et al., 1998
Intradermal IT	Fel d 1-derived peptides	Induction of T cell-dependent late asthmatic reactions	Haselden BM et al., 1999
SCIT	Fel d 1-derived peptides	Improved tolerance to cats; Improved pulmonary function	Maguire P et al., 1999
SCIT	Fel d 1-derived peptides	Reduction in size of late reaction to whole cat dander; Reduction in size of early reaction to Fel d 1; Decreased IFN-γ, IL-4, IL13 and proliferation; Increased IL-10	Oldfield WL et al., 2002
SCIT	Long T cell peptides of PLA2	Induction of Th1-type immuno deviation; Induction of IL-10; T cell hyporesponsiveness	Fellrath JM et al., 2003

(Continued)

Table 3. *(Continued)*

Type of approach	Treatment	Allergen	Outcome	References
	SCIT	Fel d 1-derived peptides	Improvement in ocular and nasal rhinoconjunctivitis symptoms	Patel D *et al.,* 2013
	SCIT	Bet v 1-derived peptides	T cell hyporesponsiveness; Induction of IFN-γ and IL-10: Increased levels of IL-5 and IL-13; Improvment in rhinoconjunctivitis-related scores and total quality-of-life; Increased serum Bet v 1-specific IgG$_4$; Indication of long-term memory	Spertini F *et al.,* 2014

SCIT: Subcutaneous immunotherapy, SLIT: Sublingual immunotherapy, ILIT: Intralymphatic immunotherapy

* main outcome is shown in Figure 2

Vaccines Using Unmodified Recombinant Allergens

The term wild-type recombinant allergen is used to describe natural unmodified recombinant allergens that mimic the fold and contain the relevant IgE- and T cell epitopes of the natural allergens. They can induce similar side effects as natural allergens, but have the advantage that they can be produced in large quantities of well-defined pure proteins allowing the formulation of vaccine batches consistent in properties and potencies.

The first immunotherapy trial with unmodified recombinant allergens was published in 2005 by Jutel *et al.*[38] In a randomized, double-blind, placebo controlled trial, patients with grass pollen-induced rhinoconjunctivitis, with or without asthma, were treated by subcutaneous injections with an equimolar mixture of the major recombinant grass pollen allergens (Phl p 1, Phl p 2, Phl p 5a, Phl p 5b, and Phl p 6) or placebo adsorbed to aluminium hydroxide. The treatment was continued for 18 months. Significant improvement in combined symptoms and medication scores, thus improvement in quality-of-life, was observed in patients receiving recombinant allergens. Active treatment induced statistically significant increases in serum allergen-specific IgG_1 and IgG_4 antibodies. The second SIT trial with recombinant wild-type allergens was performed in 2006 using recombinant Bet v 1, the major birch pollen allergen.[39] This randomized, double-blind, placebo-controlled trial treated patients suffering from birch pollen-induced rhinitis with either commercial birch pollen extract, purified natural Bet v 1, recombinant Bet v 1 or placebo. The treatment was continued for two years. All three actively treated groups showed significant reductions in rhinoconjunctivitis symptoms, rescue medication scores, and skin-sensitivity in both treatment years. Such reductions were associated with significant increases in Bet v 1-specific IgG_1, IgG_2, and IgG_4 antibodies. The levels of IgG antibodies were higher in the rBet v 1-treated group than in the birch and natural Bet v 1-treated groups. No development of specific-IgE against new birch pollen allergens were induced in the rBet v 1-treated patients. No severe IgE-mediated systemic side effects were observed in all actively treated groups. The safety and tolerability of the wild-type recombinant Bet v 1 has also been reported for tablet-based sublingual immunotherapy.[40]

Currently, cDNAs coding for the most important allergens have been isolated, enabling expression of recombinant allergens that can be used for basic research, and diagnostic and therapeutic purposes.[41]

Vaccines Using Modified Recombinant Allergens

Since unmodified recombinant allergens are immunologically equivalent to their natural counterpart, they bear the risk of IgE- and T cell-mediated side effects. To address these issues of immunogenicity and allergenicity, modified recombinant allergens have been developed (Fig. 1) and a number of them have been applied into clinical trials (Table 3) or are under current investigations (Table 2).

Hypoallergenic recombinant allergens

IgE-binding epitopes are either linear (continuous epitopes) or conformational (discontinuous epitopes) in nature. Disruption of the IgE binding epitopes modifies the ability of an allergen to elicit a reaction. Hypoallergenic recombinant allergens are designed to affect the IgE-binding sites (reduce IgE reactivity) but retain T cell epitopes and are produced by manipulation of the amino acid sequence of important allergens (*i.e.*, mutations in the allergen sequence, fragmentation, reassembly of sequences, oligomerization and deletion of sequences).[42] Hypoallergenic vaccines may induce the production of allergen-specific IgG antibodies that block the binding of IgE to the allergen and/or compete with nonspecific IgE for mast cell FcεRI, whereby IgE-mediated allergic reactions are largely avoided.

Several recombinant allergen-derivatives suitable for immunotherapy have been developed and a number of successful studies have been conducted with genetically modified versions of the major birch pollen allergen, Bet v 1.

The first immunotherapy trial with recombinant hypoallergenic derivatives was performed with two recombinant Bet v 1 fragments comprising the entire sequence of the allergen and a recombinant trimer of Bet v 1 adsorbed to aluminium hydroxide.[43] The study was carried out as a pre-seasonal treatment of eight weekly increasing doses. Active treatment

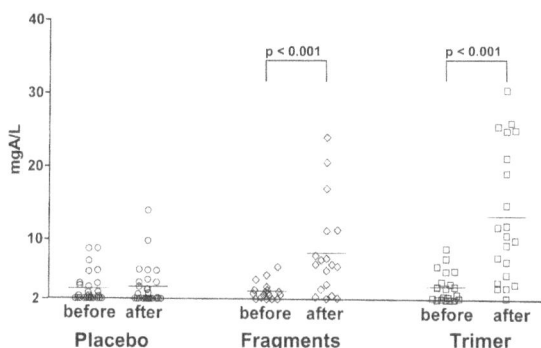

Figure 2. Bet v 1-specific IgG Ab levels [y axis, mg of antigen per liter (mgA/L)] (placebo, $n = 27$; fragments, $n = 18$; or trimer, $n = 21$) before and after treatment. Statistically significant differences are indicated.

led to significant induction of protective IgG_1, IgG_2, and IgG_4 antibody responses against natural Bet v 1 in serum (Fig. 2) and nasal secretions. These IgG antibodies inhibited Bet v 1-induced basophil degranulation and allergic patients' IgE binding to Bet v 1 as well as reduced IgE-facilitated allergen presentation to T cells and thus, reduced T cell activation.[43,12,44,42] The treatment improved Bet v 1-related allergic symptoms. Low rates of adverse side effects were noted and if present, they were more frequently associated with rBet v 1 trimer and mainly appeared several hours after injection, a sign for non-IgE mediated type reactions.[43,45] Based on the encouraging results, a hypoallergenic folding variant of Bet v 1 has been developed through chemical rearrangement of the protein structure (rBet v 1-FV).[46] This fold/variant molecule has been evaluated in clinical immunotherapy trials up to phase III studies, showing it to be safe and significant in increasing Bet v 1-specific IgG_1 and IgG_4 levels.[47–49]

Recombinant allergen hybrids

Recombinant hybrid molecules consist of the most important epitopes or peptides of two or more unrelated allergens into a single molecule. The hybrid approach has the advantage that only one molecule, containing primarily the major allergens of an allergen source, needs to be produced and purified instead of many single recombinant allergens. The conformational changes in such molecules may disrupt the 3D structure compared to the natural allergens and thus reduce IgE binding capacity, whereas T cell epitopes are conserved and can induce protective response after allergen challenge.[36]

Bee venom allergy has been addressed by the construction of two hybrid molecules: one containing two major bee venom allergens Api m 1 and Api m 2,[50] and one containing three major bee venom allergens Api m 1, Api m 2 and Api m 3.[51] Both molecules strongly reduced skin prick test reactivity and prevented allergic sensitization to native bee venom protein in a prophylactic mouse model of immunotherapy.

A number of hybrid grass allergens suitable for immunotherapy have been generated by the combination of two different grass pollen allergens or the combination of the four most frequently recognized timothy grass pollen allergens (*i.e.*, Phl p 1, Phl p 2, Phl p 5 and Phl p 6).[52–54] Immunization with these hybrids demonstrated the increased immunogenicity of these molecules by induction of protective IgG antibodies which block allergen-induced basophil degranulation. In addition, the utility of hybrid allergen proteins for immunotherapy of house dust mite and pollen allergy (*Chenopodium album* pollen and *Parietaria* pollen) has also been reported.[55–58]

Hypoallergenic mosaic allergens

The different strategies used for the construction of recombinant hypoallergenic allergens (*i.e.*, fragmentation, mutations, molecular inversion, and random gene shuffling) have demonstrated clinical efficacy but there are disadvantages. The fragmentation approach carries the disadvantage of generating small protein fragments that may induce low levels of blocking IgG. Deletion/mutation strategies may lack important portions of the protein or T cell epitopes that are important in the induction of protective IgG antibodies. Randomly shuffled allergens can be a time-consuming approach during the selection step of mutants with the most advantageous properties.[59] To overcome these limitations, mosaic strategies were developed. For the construction of mosaic proteins, two steps are necessary: (1) the allergen is split into different parts and the IgE reactivity is determined; (2) different segments of the allergens which have no detectable IgE reactivity are combined in a different order from that of the naturally occurring allergen. Hypoallergenic mosaics of the major pollen allergens of grass Phl p 1 and Phl p 2,[59,60] of birch Bet v 1,[61] and of cat dander Fel d 1[62] have been produced. All of them showed reduced IgE reactivity and allergenic activity. Preclinical characterization of hypoallergenic mosaic allergens supports the idea of this approach for improvement of future allergy vaccines.

Peptide-Based Vaccines

T cell epitope-containing peptides

Another approach designed to overcome the negative effects of SIT is based on the administration of allergen-derived synthetic peptides containing T cell epitopes. These peptides represent short linear allergen fragments that target allergen-specific CD4+ T cells but do not bind IgE. The mechanism behind this approach is the ability of the peptides to induce tolerance and/or anergy in allergen-specific T cells with markedly reduced IgE-mediated side effects[63] (Table 1).

The first T cell-based epitope vaccine study, performed in the 1990s, evaluated the safety and clinical efficacy of two T cell peptides (27-amino acids sequences) of the major cat allergen Fel d 1[64] (Table 3). The Fel d 1 peptides showed variable improvement of immediate allergic responses to cats. Moreover, the treatment was associated with symptoms of rhinitis, asthma, and pruritus, which were reported several hours after peptide injection.[65] These issues were solved by the use of short peptides of Fel d 1 administered intradermally to cat-asthmatic patients.[66] Related studies using lower doses of peptides could show a significant reduction on the magnitude of cutaneous late phase reaction.[67] Interestingly, studies focusing on the mechanisms have reported that tolerance induced by the treatment peptides could extend to other peptide sequences within the Fel d 1 molecule.[63] In a recent study, a mixture of seven immunodominant peptides selected on the basis of MHC-binding was evaluated in patients with cat-induced allergic rhinoconjunctivitis who were exposed to cat allergen in an environmental exposure chamber before and after therapy. The treatment had apparent effects on nasal and ocular symptoms which persisted nine months later without any further treatment.[68]

T cell-based epitope vaccines have also been evaluated for bee venom allergy. Three T cell epitope peptides of phospholipase A2 (PLA2) have been administered to bee sting venom-allergic individuals. All patients tolerated subcutaneous challenge with PLA2, and a live bee sting was tolerated in three of the five treated subjects.[69] In a second double-blind, placebo-controlled phase I clinical trial, venom-allergic subjects were treated with a mixture of three Api m 1-derived long synthetic overlapping peptides. The peptide-based immunotherapy induced IFN-γ and IL-10, and T cell hyporesponsiveness but not Th2 cytokines.[70] Similar results were obtained in an open-label, single-blind study.[71]

B cell epitope-containing peptides

An alternative peptide-based approach for improvement of therapy of IgE-mediated allergy is the use of B cell epitope-derived synthetic peptides without allergenic activity but with the potential to induce protective IgG antibodies.[72] Such peptides are selected from B cell epitopes, which are determined from IgE-binding epitope-mapping data and from the three-dimensional structure of the allergen. Recombinant B cell epitope-containing peptides of the major grass pollen allergen, Phlp 1, have been produced and evaluated for grass pollen allergy vaccination.[73,74] *In vitro* and *in vivo* evaluation showed the lack of IgE-binding capacity and allergenic activity as demonstrated by basophil histamine release and skin prick testing. Moreover, immunization in mice and rabbits was able to induce protective IgG responses against the complete Phl p 1 wild-type allergen and related allergens, as well as inhibit human IgE binding to the wild-type allergen. Since then, candidate vaccines based on the peptide carrier approach have been developed for many important allergen sources such as grass pollen, birch pollen, cat, *Alternaria* and olive pollen.[74–78] Importantly, a vaccine for grass pollen allergy has advanced into phase IIb clinical trials (NCT01538979) (Table 2). Thus, synthetic hypoallergenic peptides derived from B cell epitopes may present as potential candidates for treatment of IgE-mediated allergies.

Novel Routes of Administration

One approach to improve SIT, such as increasing the convenience of administration and eventually allowing self-administration, reducing side effects and targeting different immune mechanisms (*e.g.*, mucosal tolerance), has been to vary the route of administration. In recent years, the mucosal routes in particular have been tested.

Sublingual route

Sublingual immunotherapy (SLIT) is based on sublingual administration of tablets or drops and is proposed as an alternative to SCIT. The treatment is in clinical practice and SLIT is considered more patient friendly with a more favourable safety profile. The treatment period is still several years and typically requires daily dosing. SLIT seems to have effects on antigen-presenting cells and T cells and induces elevated allergen-specific IgG_4 and IgA responses.[79] In double-blind, placebo-controlled trials, the treatment benefit of SLIT seems to be slightly less than subcutaneous SIT[80] and changes in immunological markers are modest. Recently, three years of SLIT treatment for grass pollen allergy was shown to be associated with clinical improvement that was maintained two years after treatment.[81] The clinical efficacy was associated with sustained increases in serum grass pollen allergen-specific IgG_4 antibodies. A concern with SLIT is the requirement of high-dose allergen administration over years. At present, there are several allergen extract-based preparations on the market for SLIT. However, SLIT is still based on poorly defined allergen extract and safer and more effective strategies are needed.

Oral route

The oral route, oral immunotherapy (OIT), has been evaluated for treatment of food allergy in young children. The food allergen is mixed in a food vehicle and ingested by the patient in gradual increasing doses, starting with extremely small amounts. Preliminary data for peanut and egg OIT are encouraging and have shown that OIT can be effective in inducing tolerance against the allergen.[82] The findings were associated with favourable immunological changes, *e.g.*, decreased skin prick test size and Th2 cytokine levels as well as increased peanut specific-IgG_4 levels and Treg cell numbers. Today, OIT is still for research purposes only. Adverse reactions to OIT are common and data regarding long-term safety and efficacy are lacking. Thus, further research and double-blind, placebo-controlled clinical trials are needed before OIT can be used in clinical practice.

Intralymphatic route

Intralymphatic SIT (ILIT), where the allergen is delivered directly into the lymph node of the inguinal area, has been investigated as a possible route for therapy. ILIT was originally tested for cancer immunotherapy.[83] As intra lymph node injection delivers the allergen directly to dendritic cells and T and B cells, much lower allergen doses can be used.[84] The treatment was shown to be clinically effective after three injections only and induces allergen-specific IgG similarly to SCIT.[85] In an attempt to further improve ILIT, the major cat allergen Fel d 1 was fused to a HIV-derived translocation peptide TAT and part of the human invariant chain, generating a modular antigen transporter vaccine (MAT) to enhance presentation through the MHC class II pathway. In a double-blind, placebo-controlled clinical trial, cat allergic patients received three injections with the MAT-Fel d 1 vaccine at 4-week intervals.[86] The treatment induced robust regulatory T cell responses correlating with IgG_4 responses and nasal tolerance to cat dander as well as allergen-specific peripheral T cell tolerance.[86,87] The safety profile of ILIT has been shown to be very good. However, the long-term efficacy of ILIT needs to be demonstrated as well as its efficacy compared to SCIT.

Epicutaneous route

Several attempts have also been made to administer allergens via the skin. Epicutaneous immunotherapy (EPIT) is based on administration of allergens using patches that are mounted onto tape stripped skin.[88] The treatment activates skin Langerhans cells, with subsequent migration to lymph nodes and down regulation of effector cell responses.[89] EPIT is convenient and has shown to ameliorate symptoms after a few patch applications. Placebo-controlled trials for grass pollen allergy, where grass pollen extract was administered by application of a patch to the skin, have demonstrated significant symptom amelioration over placebo after a few patch applications. EPIT may also be effective in the treatment of food allergies.[90] Transcutaneous delivery of CpG-adjuvanted allergen via laser-generated micropores has been evaluated in a murine model and shown to increase the safety of the therapy by abrogating the Th2 polarizing potential of skin immunization.[91] However, further data regarding the immunological mechanisms of the epicutaneous route and objective clinical parameters are needed.

New Adjuvants

The most widely used adjuvant for SIT today is aluminium hydroxide (alum), which induces a slower release of the allergen through a depot effect. However, alum-based allergy vaccines may also induce granuloma formation at the site of injection. Thus, another way of increasing the efficacy of SIT is to develop more efficient adjuvants that stimulate various aspects of the immune system.

Monophosphoryl lipid A (MPL) is a detoxified derivative of LPS found on the gram-negative bacteria *Salmonella Minnesota* and is used as an adjuvant that binds to Toll like receptor 4. In a randomized placebo-controlled study, more than 1000 patients were given four pre-seasonal injections in increasing doses with a chemically modified grass pollen extract adjuvanted with MPL.[92] The ultrashort course was well tolerated and provided a significant benefit over placebo in relieving allergy symptoms. The treatment was able to inhibit the seasonal rise in allergen-specific IgE, and significantly increase the allergen-specific IgG levels. The MPL-adjuvanted vaccine is available in Europe.

Immunostimulatory CpG motifs as adjuvants conjugated to allergens have also been evaluated in SIT. The CpG interacts with Toll-like receptor 9, which can skew the immune response towards a Th1 response. Coupling the major ragweed allergen Amb 1 to CpG motifs has been tested in a placebo-controlled SIT trial for ragweed allergy. The treatment induced allergen-specific blocking IgG antibodies, reduced the seasonal boost in IgE production and decreased rhinitis symptoms during both the first and second pollen season.[93] However, a later clinical trial was discontinued as no significant differences were found between the actively and placebo-treated patients.

Virus like particles (VLP) consisting of the bacteriophage Qbeta coat protein associated with CpGs (QbG10) have been evaluated as adjuvant.[94] The association with VLPs stabilizes the CpGs. A SIT trial using QbG10 together with house dust mite allergen extract has been tested as treatment for house dust mite allergy.[94] The therapy led to an increase in allergen-specific IgG antibodies, a transient increase in allergen-specific IgE levels and a significant reduction of allergic symptoms. Furthermore, peptides from the major house dust mite allergen Der p 1 have been conjugated to VLPs (Qbeta-Der p 1). Immunization of healthy subjects induced a strong IgG antibody response against Der p 1 and the treatment was well tolerated.[95] Moreover, the major cat allergen Fel d 1 has been covalently linked to VLPs and one single injection was shown to be sufficient in preventing IgE-mediated allergic reactions in a mouse model of cat allergy.[96]

Carbohydrate-based particles (CBPs) as allergen carriers have been evaluated in murine models. Mice that had been sensitized with Fel d 1 and treated with Fel d 1 covalently linked to CBPs before airway challenges showed reduced airway hyperreactivity and a reduction in inflammatory cells in bronchoalveolar lavage compared to untreated mice, a finding which was not noted in mice treated with Fel d 1 alone.[97] In a similar mouse model of cat allergy, it was shown that treatment with Fel d 1 covalently coupled to $1\alpha,25$-dihydroxyvitamin D3, the active form of vitamin D3 (VD3) was effective at a suboptimal treatment dose, whereas Fel d 1 alone was not.[98] It seems that coupling or co-administration of VD3 is necessary for inducing the beneficial adjuvant properties. In a recent study where children received SIT for mite allergy, one study group also obtained an oral supplement of vitamin D but the supplement did not have any significant impact on the effect of SIT.[99]

Prophylactic SIT Approaches

At present, the new approaches for allergen-specific immunotherapy aim to improve therapeutic allergy vaccines. As allergic diseases are a major health threat, resulting in a high burden of suffering and socioeconomic costs, prophylactic vaccines would offer a major step forward in handling the allergy epidemic. However, three major challenges should be addressed (Fig. 3).

First, the clinically relevant allergens need to be defined. The idea is to have a prophylactic vaccine that comprises allergens which are most frequently recognized and responsible for the most common allergic symptoms. Allergen-microarray technology allows population-wide screening for IgE reactivities towards a large number of allergens using small volumes of serum and thus enables identification of frequently recognized allergens at the population level.[100,20,101] Recently, an allergen-chip (*i.e.* MeDALL allergen-chip) has been developed for more than 170 allergen molecules and sera collected in European birth cohorts were screened to identify the key allergens.[101]

The second aspect is the safety of the vaccine. Currently, allergy vaccines are based on the administration of natural allergen extracts that can induce IgE sensitization to new allergens and increase the allergen-specific IgE response in allergic patients. Therefore, prophylactic treatment with these extracts would bear a considerable risk of sensitizing non-allergic individuals. For this reason, modified allergen derivatives lacking IgE-binding sites and/or capacity to degranulate effector cells would be preferred for prophylactic vaccination. The concept behind prophylactic allergy vaccines is the induction of allergen-specific protective IgG responses, which should bind to the allergen and thus prevent stimulation of the immune system. Another useful approach is tolerance induction. Modified allergens, such as carrier-bound B cell epitopes-containing peptides with the capacity to induce robust allergen-specific IgG antibodies and/or allergen-derived T cell epitope containing peptides and recombinant hypoallergenic allergen, which can be used for induction of selective T cell tolerance, would be ideally suitable for prophylactic vaccination.[20]

A third very important aspect is the time point for intervention. It has been shown that IgE sensitizations, initially directed to food proteins and then to respiratory forms of allergens, occurs in the first months and years of life, respectively.[20] Analyzing sera from adult allergic patients collected retrospectively over a 10-year period by allergen-micro array showed that *de novo* sensitization does not occur in adults.[102] In this context, it seems that prophylactic vaccination would be suitable for pre-natal and/or early

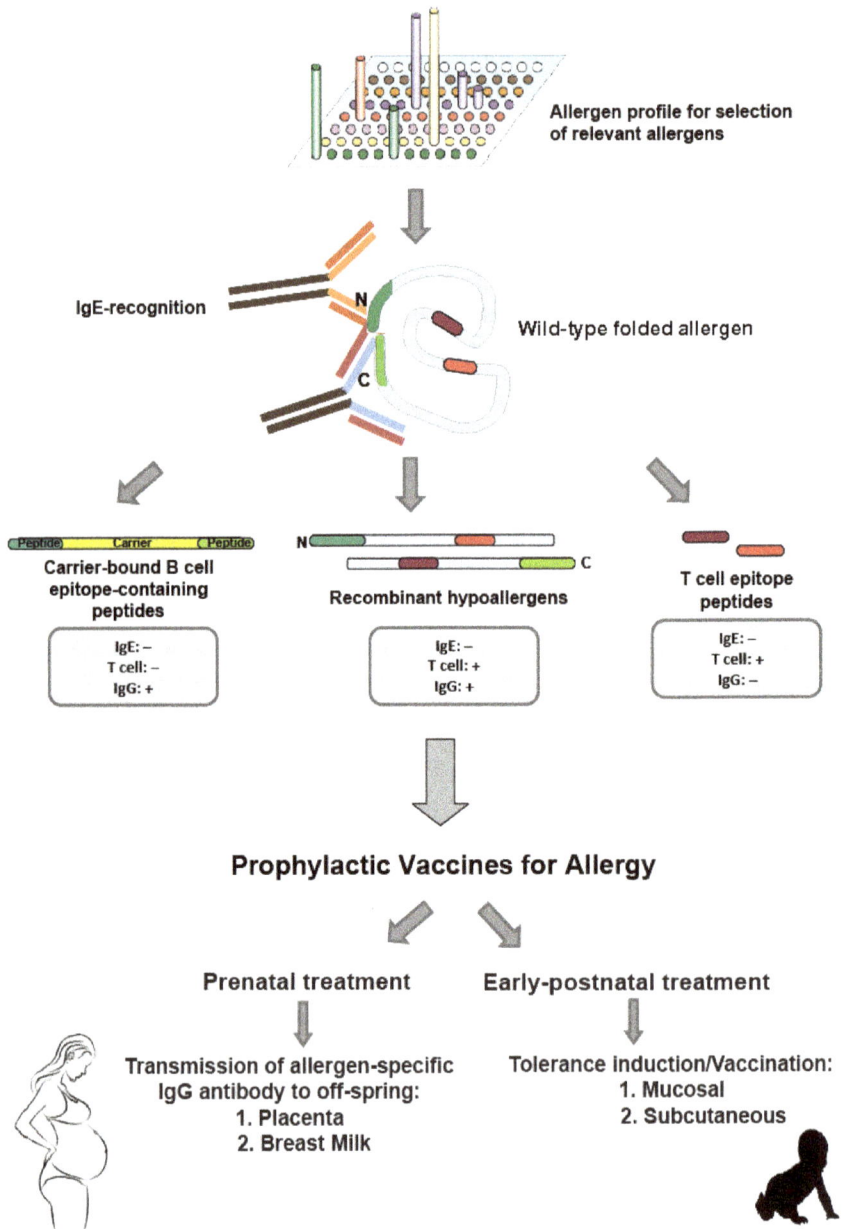

Figure 3. Strategies for prophylactic allergy vaccines.

postnatal treatment. Pre-natal therapy would involve active vaccination or passive immunization of the pregnant allergic mother (Fig. 3). Active vaccination of pregnant mothers is a possible approach as IgG antibodies are transmitted through the placenta to the child.[103,104] Likewise, passive immunization through application of allergen-specific protective IgG antibodies to mothers would be an alternative pre-natal therapy approach.[20] The induction of protective IgG by early postnatal vaccination with non-allergenic allergen derivatives may be a possibility for prophylaxis (Fig. 3). Another strategy would involve induction of early T cell tolerance, preventing the development of allergic immune response.[20] First steps towards prophylactic allergy vaccines have been made in experimental animal models. For instance, a clinical study has been conducted in which two hypoallergenic fragments of the major birch pollen allergen, Bet v 1, were injected in non-allergic adults to determine safety, immunological effects and lack of allergenicity (NCT01353924).

Acknowledgements

Supported by the Swedish Research Council, the Stockholm County Council, the Swedish Asthma and Allergy Association's Research Foundation, the King Gustaf V 80th Birthday Foundation, the Swedish Heart-Lung Foundation, the Hesselman Foundation, the Konsul Th C Bergh Foundation, the Center for Inflammatory Diseases, the Swedish Cancer and Allergy Foundation, the Magnus Bergvall foundation, Karolinska Institutet and project F4605 of the Austrian Science Fund (FWF).

References

1. Kay, A.B. (2008). *Allergy and Allergic Diseases* (2nd ed.). Chichester, West Sussex, UK; Hoboken, NJ: Wiley-Blackwell.

2. Ring, J., Akdis, C., Lauener, R., Schappi, G., Traidl-Hoffmann, C., Akdis, M., *et al.* (2014). Global Allergy Forum and Second Davos Declaration 2013 Allergy: Barriers to cure--challenges and actions to be taken. *Allergy,* **69**(8), 978–982.

3. Bousquet, J., Anto, J.M., Bachert, C., Bousquet, P.J., Colombo, P., Crameri, R., *et al.* (2006). Factors responsible for differences between asymptomatic

subjects and patients presenting an IgE sensitization to allergens. A GA2LEN project. *Allergy,* **61**(6), 671–680.

4. Van Cauwenberge, P., Watelet, J.B., Van Zele, T., Wang, D.Y., Toskala, E., Durham, S., *et al.* (2007). Does rhinitis lead to asthma? *Rhinology,* **45**(2), 112–121.

5. Durham, S.R., Emminger, W., Kapp, A., Colombo, G., de Monchy, J.G., Rak, S., *et al.* (2010). Long-term clinical efficacy in grass pollen-induced rhinoconjunctivitis after treatment with SQ-standardized grass allergy immunotherapy tablet. *J Allergy Clin Immunol,* **125**(1), 131–138, e131–137.

6. Akdis, C.A. (2012). Therapies for allergic inflammation: refining strategies to induce tolerance. *Nat Med,* **18**(5), 736–749.

7. Noon, L. (1911). Prophylactic inoculation against hay fever. *The Lancet,* **177**(4580), 1572–1573.

8. Ishizaka, K., & Ishizaka, T. (1967). Identification of gamma-E-antibodies as a carrier of reaginic activity. *J Immunol,* **99**(6), 1187–1198.

9. Johansson, S.G., & Bennich, H. (1967). Immunological studies of an atypical (myeloma) immunoglobulin. *Immunology,* **13**(4), 381–394.

10. Bischoff, S.C. (2007). Role of mast cells in allergic and non-allergic immune responses: comparison of human and murine data. *Nat Rev Immunol,* **7**(2), 93–104.

11. Kalesnikoff, J., & Galli, S.J. (2008). New developments in mast cell biology. *Nat Immunol,* **9**(11), 1215–1223.

12. van Neerven, R.J., Knol, E.F., Ejrnaes, A., & Wurtzen, P.A. (2006). IgE-mediated allergen presentation and blocking antibodies: regulation of T-cell activation in allergy. *Int Arch Allergy Immunol,* **141**(2), 119–129.

13. Burks, A.W., Calderon, M.A., Casale, T., Cox, L., Demoly, P., Jutel, M., *et al.* (2013). Update on allergy immunotherapy: American Academy of Allergy, Asthma & Immunology/European Academy of Allergy and Clinical Immunology/PRACTALL consensus report. *J Allergy Clin Immunol,* **131**(5), 1288–1296 e1283.

14. Jacobsen, L., Niggemann, B., Dreborg, S., Ferdousi, H.A., Halken, S., Host, A., *et al.* (2007). Specific immunotherapy has long-term preventive effect of seasonal and perennial asthma: 10-year follow-up on the PAT study. *Allergy,* **62**(8), 943–948.

15. Valenta, R. (2008). Biochemistry of Allergens and Recombinant Allergens In A.B. Kay (Ed.), *Allergy and Allergic Diseases* (pp. 895–912). Chichester, West Sussex, UK ; Hoboken, NJ: Wiley-Blackwell.

16. Canonica, G.W., Ansotegui, I.J., Pawankar, R., Schmid-Grendelmeier, P., van Hage, M., Baena-Cagnani, C.E., *et al.* (2013). A WAO — ARIA —

GA(2)LEN consensus document on molecular-based allergy diagnostics. *World Allergy Organ J, 6*(1), 17.

17. Van Ree, R., Van Leeuwen, W.A., Dieges, P.H., Van Wijk, R.G., De Jong, N., Brewczyski, P.Z., *et al.* (1997). Measurement of IgE antibodies against purified grass pollen allergens (Lol p 1, 2, 3 and 5) during immunotherapy. *Clin Exp Allergy, 27*(1), 68–74.

18. Nouri-Aria, K.T., Wachholz, P.A., Francis, J.N., Jacobson, M.R., Walker, S.M., Wilcock, L.K., *et al.* (2004). Grass pollen immunotherapy induces mucosal and peripheral IL-10 responses and blocking IgG activity. *J Immunol, 172*(5), 3252–3259.

19. Gadermaier, E., Staikuniene, J., Scheiblhofer, S., Thalhamer, J., Kundi, M., Westritschnig, K., *et al.* (2011). Recombinant allergen-based monitoring of antibody responses during injection grass pollen immunotherapy and after 5 years of discontinuation. *Allergy, 66*(9), 1174–1182.

20. Valenta, R., Campana, R., Marth, K., & van Hage, M. (2012). Allergen-specific immunotherapy: from therapeutic vaccines to prophylactic approaches. *J Intern Med, 272*(2), 144–157.

21. Loveless, M. (1940). Immunological studies of pollinosis: I. The presence of two antibodies related to the same pollen-antigen in the serum of treated hay-fever patients. *J Immunol, 38*(1), 25–50.

22. Jutel, M., Muller, U.R., Fricker, M., Rihs, S., Pichler, W.J., & Dahinden, C. (1996). Influence of bee venom immunotherapy on degranulation and leukotriene generation in human blood basophils. *Clin Exp Allergy, 26*(10), 1112–1118.

23. van Neerven, R.J., Wikborg, T., Lund, G., Jacobsen, B., Brinch-Nielsen, A., Arnved, J., *et al.* (1999). Blocking antibodies induced by specific allergy vaccination prevent the activation of CD4+ T cells by inhibiting serum-IgE-facilitated allergen presentation. *J Immunol, 163*(5), 2944–2952.

24. Gadermaier, E., Flicker, S., Aberer, W., Egger, C., Reider, N., Focke, M., *et al.* (2010). Analysis of the antibody responses induced by subcutaneous injection immunotherapy with birch and Fagales pollen extracts adsorbed onto aluminum hydroxide. *Int Arch Allergy Immunol, 151*(1), 17–27.

25. Ebner, C., Siemann, U., Bohle, B., Willheim, M., Wiedermann, U., Schenk, S., *et al.* (1997). Immunological changes during specific immunotherapy of grass pollen allergy: reduced lymphoproliferative responses to allergen and shift from TH2 to TH1 in T-cell clones specific for Phl p 1, a major grass pollen allergen. *Clin Exp Allergy, 27*(9), 1007–1015.

26. Bohle, B., Kinaciyan, T., Gerstmayr, M., Radakovics, A., Jahn-Schmid, B., & Ebner, C. (2007). Sublingual immunotherapy induces IL-10-producing

T regulatory cells, allergen-specific T-cell tolerance, and immune deviation. *J Allergy Clin Immunol*, **120**(3), 707–713.

27. Akdis, C.A., & Akdis, M. (2011). Mechanisms of allergen-specific immunotherapy. *J Allergy Clin Immunol*, **127**(1), 18–27; quiz 28–19.

28. Deifl, S., & Bohle, B. (2011). Factors influencing the allergenicity and adjuvanticity of allergens. *Immunotherapy*, **3**(7), 881–893.

29. Jutel, M., Akdis, M., Budak, F., Aebischer-Casaulta, C., Wrzyszcz, M., Blaser, K., *et al.* (2003). IL-10 and TGF-beta cooperate in the regulatory T cell response to mucosal allergens in normal immunity and specific immunotherapy. *Eur J Immunol*, **33**(5), 1205–1214.

30. Chapman, M.D., Smith, A.M., Vailes, L.D., Arruda, L.K., Dhanaraj, V., & Pomes, A. (2000). Recombinant allergens for diagnosis and therapy of allergic disease. *J Allergy Clin Immunol*, **106**(3), 409–418.

31. Focke, M., Marth, K., & Valenta, R. (2009). Molecular composition and biological activity of commercial birch pollen allergen extracts. *Eur J Clin Invest*, **39**(5), 429–436.

32. Brunetto, B., Tinghino, R., Braschi, M.C., Antonicelli, L., Pini, C., & Iacovacci, P. (2010). Characterization and comparison of commercially available mite extracts for in vivo diagnosis. *Allergy*, **65**(2), 184–190.

33. Curin, M., Reininger, R., Swoboda, I., Focke, M., Valenta, R., & Spitzauer, S. (2011). Skin prick test extracts for dog allergy diagnosis show considerable variations regarding the content of major and minor dog allergens. *Int Arch Allergy Immunol*, **154**(3), 258–263.

34. Casset, A., Valenta, R., & Vrtala, S. (2013). Allergen content and in vivo allergenic activity of house dust mite extracts. *Int Arch Allergy Immunol*, **161**(3), 287–288.

35. Valenta, R., Vrtala, S., Focke-Tejkl, M., Twardosz, A., Swoboda, I., Bugajska-Schretter, A., *et al.* (2002). Synthetic and genetically engineered allergen derivatives for specific immunotherapy of type I allergy. *Clin Allergy Immunol*, **16**, 495–517.

36. Larche, M., Akdis, C.A., & Valenta, R. (2006). Immunological mechanisms of allergen-specific immunotherapy. *Nat Rev Immunol*, **6**(10), 761–771.

37. Winther, L., Arnved, J., Malling, H.J., Nolte, H., & Mosbech, H. (2006). Side-effects of allergen-specific immunotherapy: a prospective multi-centre study. *Clin Exp Allergy*, **36**(3), 254–260.

38. Jutel, M., Jaeger, L., Suck, R., Meyer, H., Fiebig, H., & Cromwell, O. (2005). Allergen-specific immunotherapy with recombinant grass pollen allergens. *J Allergy Clin Immunol*, **116**(3), 608–613.

39. Pauli, G., Larsen, T.H., Rak, S., Horak, F., Pastorello, E., Valenta, R., *et al.* (2008). Efficacy of recombinant birch pollen vaccine for the treatment of birch-allergic rhinoconjunctivitis. *J Allergy Clin Immunol,* **122**(5), 951–960.

40. Winther, L., Poulsen, L.K., Robin, B., Mélac, M., & Malling, H. (2009). Safety and tolerability of recombinant Bet v 1 (rBet v 1) tablets in sublingual immunotherapy (SLIT). *J Allergy Clin Immunol,* **123**(2, Supplement), S215.

41. Valenta, R., Ferreira, F., Focke-Tejkl, M., Linhart, B., Niederberger, V., Swoboda, I., *et al.* (2010). From allergen genes to allergy vaccines. *Annu Rev Immunol,* **28**, 211–241.

42. Valenta, R., Niespodziana, K., Focke-Tejkl, M., Marth, K., Huber, H., Neubauer, A., *et al.* (2011). Recombinant allergens: what does the future hold? *J Allergy Clin Immunol,* **127**(4), 860–864.

43. Niederberger, V., Horak, F., Vrtala, S., Spitzauer, S., Krauth, M.T., Valent, P., *et al.* (2004). Vaccination with genetically engineered allergens prevents progression of allergic disease. *Proc Natl Acad Sci U S A,* **101 Suppl 2**, 14677–14682.

44. Pree, I., Shamji, M.H., Kimber, I., Valenta, R., Durham, S.R., & Niederberger, V. (2010). Inhibition of CD23-dependent facilitated allergen binding to B cells following vaccination with genetically modified hypoallergenic Bet v 1 molecules. *Clin Exp Allergy,* **40**(9), 1346–1352.

45. Purohit, A., Niederberger, V., Kronqvist, M., Horak, F., Gronneberg, R., Suck, R., *et al.* (2008). Clinical effects of immunotherapy with genetically modified recombinant birch pollen Bet v 1 derivatives. *Clin Exp Allergy,* **38**(9), 1514–1525.

46. Kahlert, H., Suck, R., Weber, B., Nandy, A., Wald, M., Keller, W., *et al.* (2008). Characterization of a hypoallergenic recombinant Bet v 1 variant as a candidate for allergen-specific immunotherapy. *Int Arch Allergy Immunol,* **145**(3), 193–206.

47. Klimek, L., Bachert, C., Doemer, C., Meyer, H., & Narkus, A. (2005). Specific immunotherapy with recombinant birch pollen allergen rBet v 1-FV is clinically efficacious. *Allergy Clin Immunol Int,* Suppl. 1:15.

48. Rak, S. (2009). *Clinical results with a hypoallergenic recombinant birch pollen allergen derivative.* Paper presented at the The 27th Congress of the European Academy for Allergology and Clinical Immunology, Warsaw, Poland.

49. Meyer, W., Narkus, A., Salapatek, A.M., & Hafner, D. (2013). Double-blind, placebo-controlled, dose-ranging study of new recombinant hypoallergenic Bet v 1 in an environmental exposure chamber. *Allergy,* **68**(6), 724–731.

50. Kussebi, F., Karamloo, F., Rhyner, C., Schmid-Grendelmeier, P., Salagianni, M., Mannhart, C., *et al.* (2005). A major allergen gene-fusion protein for potential usage in allergen-specific immunotherapy. *J Allergy Clin Immunol,* **115**(2), 323–329.

51. Karamloo, F., Schmid-Grendelmeier, P., Kussebi, F., Akdis, M., Salagianni, M., von Beust, B.R., *et al.* (2005). Prevention of allergy by a recombinant multi-allergen vaccine with reduced IgE binding and preserved T cell epitopes. *Eur J Immunol,* **35**(11), 3268–3276.

52. Linhart, B., Jahn-Schmid, B., Verdino, P., Keller, W., Ebner, C., Kraft, D., *et al.* (2002). Combination vaccines for the treatment of grass pollen allergy consisting of genetically engineered hybrid molecules with increased immunogenicity. *FASEB J,* **16**(10), 1301–1303.

53. Linhart, B., Hartl, A., Jahn-Schmid, B., Verdino, P., Keller, W., Krauth, M.T., *et al.* (2005). A hybrid molecule resembling the epitope spectrum of grass pollen for allergy vaccination. *J Allergy Clin Immunol,* **115**(5), 1010–1016.

54. Linhart, B., Mothes-Luksch, N., Vrtala, S., Kneidinger, M., Valent, P., & Valenta, R. (2008). A hypoallergenic hybrid molecule with increased immunogenicity consisting of derivatives of the major grass pollen allergens, Phl p 2 and Phl p 6. *Biol Chem,* **389**(7), 925–933.

55. Asturias, J.A., Ibarrola, I., Arilla, M.C., Vidal, C., Ferrer, A., Gamboa, P.M., *et al.* (2009). Engineering of major house dust mite allergens Der p 1 and Der p 2 for allergen-specific immunotherapy. *Clin Exp Allergy,* **39**(7), 1088–1098.

56. Bonura, A., Passantino, R., Costa, M.A., Montana, G., Melis, M., Bondi, M.L., *et al.* (2012). Characterization of a Par j 1/Par j 2 mutant hybrid with reduced allergenicity for immunotherapy of Parietaria allergy. *Clin Exp Allergy,* **42**(3), 471–480.

57. Chen, K.W., Blatt, K., Thomas, W.R., Swoboda, I., Valent, P., Valenta, R., *et al.* (2012). Hypoallergenic Der p 1/Der p 2 combination vaccines for immunotherapy of house dust mite allergy. *J Allergy Clin Immunol,* **130**(2), 435–443, e434.

58. Nouri, H.R., Varasteh, A., Vahedi, F., Chamani, J., Afsharzadeh, D., & Sankian, M. (2012). Constructing a hybrid molecule with low capacity of IgE binding from Chenopodium album pollen allergens. *Immunol Lett,* **144**(1–2), 67–77.

59. Mothes-Luksch, N., Stumvoll, S., Linhart, B., Focke, M., Krauth, M.T., Hauswirth, A., *et al.* (2008). Disruption of allergenic activity of the major grass pollen allergen Phl p 2 by reassembly as a mosaic protein. *J Immunol,* **181**(7), 4864–4873.

60. Ball, T., Linhart, B., Sonneck, K., Blatt, K., Herrmann, H., Valent, P., *et al.* (2009). Reducing allergenicity by altering allergen fold: a mosaic protein of Phl p 1 for allergy vaccination. *Allergy,* **64**(4), 569–580.

61. Campana, R., Vrtala, S., Maderegger, B., Jertschin, P., Stegfellner, G., Swoboda, I., *et al.* (2010). Hypoallergenic derivatives of the major birch pollen allergen Bet v 1 obtained by rational sequence reassembly. *J Allergy Clin Immunol,* **126**(5), 1024–1031, 1031, e1021–1028.

62. Curin, M., Weber, M., Thalhamer, T., Swoboda, I., Focke-Tejkl, M., Blatt, K., *et al.* (2014). Hypoallergenic derivatives of Fel d 1 obtained by rational reassembly for allergy vaccination and tolerance induction. *Clin Exp Allergy,* **44**(6), 882–894.

63. Campbell, J.D., Buckland, K.F., McMillan, S.J., Kearley, J., Oldfield, W.L., Stern, L.J., *et al.* (2009). Peptide immunotherapy in allergic asthma generates IL-10-dependent immunological tolerance associated with linked epitope suppression. *J Exp Med,* **206**(7), 1535–1547.

64. Norman, P.S., Ohman, J.L., Jr., Long, A.A., Creticos, P.S., Gefter, M.A., Shaked, Z., *et al.* (1996). Treatment of cat allergy with T-cell reactive peptides. *Am J Respir Crit Care Med,* **154**(6 Pt 1), 1623–1628.

65. Haselden, B.M., Larche, M., Meng, Q., Shirley, K., Dworski, R., Kaplan, A.P., *et al.* (2001). Late asthmatic reactions provoked by intradermal injection of T-cell peptide epitopes are not associated with bronchial mucosal infiltration of eosinophils or T(H)2-type cells or with elevated concentrations of histamine or eicosanoids in bronchoalveolar fluid. *J Allergy Clin Immunol,* **108**(3), 394–401.

66. Oldfield, W.L., Larche, M., & Kay, A.B. (2002). Effect of T-cell peptides derived from Fel d 1 on allergic reactions and cytokine production in patients sensitive to cats: a randomised controlled trial. *Lancet,* **360**(9326), 47–53.

67. Alexander, C., Tarzi, M., Larche, M., & Kay, A.B. (2005). The effect of Fel d 1-derived T-cell peptides on upper and lower airway outcome measurements in cat-allergic subjects. *Allergy,* **60**(10), 1269–1274.

68. Patel, D., Couroux, P., Hickey, P., Salapatek, A.M., Laidler, P., Larche, M., *et al.* (2013). Fel d 1-derived peptide antigen desensitization shows a persistent treatment effect 1 year after the start of dosing: a randomized, placebo-controlled study. *J Allergy Clin Immunol,* **131**(1), 103–109 e101–107.

69. Muller, U., Akdis, C.A., Fricker, M., Akdis, M., Blesken, T., Bettens, F., *et al.* (1998). Successful immunotherapy with T-cell epitope peptides of bee venom phospholipase A2 induces specific T-cell anergy in patients allergic to bee venom. *J Allergy Clin Immunol,* **101**(6 Pt 1), 747–754.

70. Fellrath, J.M., Kettner, A., Dufour, N., Frigerio, C., Schneeberger, D., Leimgruber, A., *et al.* (2003). Allergen-specific T-cell tolerance induction with allergen-derived long synthetic peptides: results of a phase I trial. *J Allergy Clin Immunol,* **111**(4), 854–861.

71. Tarzi, M., Klunker, S., Texier, C., Verhoef, A., Stapel, S.O., Akdis, C.A., *et al.* (2006). Induction of interleukin-10 and suppressor of cytokine signalling-3 gene expression following peptide immunotherapy. *Clin Exp Allergy,* **36**(4), 465–474.

72. Focke, M., Swoboda, I., Marth, K., & Valenta, R. (2010). Developments in allergen-specific immunotherapy: from allergen extracts to allergy vaccines bypassing allergen-specific immunoglobulin E and T cell reactivity. *Clin Exp Allergy,* **40**(3), 385–397.

73. Ball, T., Fuchs, T., Sperr, W.R., Valent, P., Vangelista, L., Kraft, D., *et al.* (1999). B cell epitopes of the major timothy grass pollen allergen, phl p 1, revealed by gene fragmentation as candidates for immunotherapy. *FASEB J,* **13**(11), 1277–1290.

74. Focke, M., Mahler, V., Ball, T., Sperr, W.R., Majlesi, Y., Valent, P., *et al.* (2001). Nonanaphylactic synthetic peptides derived from B cell epitopes of the major grass pollen allergen, Phl p 1, for allergy vaccination. *FASEB J,* **15**(11), 2042–2044.

75. Focke, M., Linhart, B., Hartl, A., Wiedermann, U., Sperr, W.R., Valent, P., *et al.* (2004). Non-anaphylactic surface-exposed peptides of the major birch pollen allergen, Bet v 1, for preventive vaccination. *Clin Exp Allergy,* **34**(10), 1525–1533.

76. Twaroch, T.E., Focke, M., Civaj, V., Weber, M., Balic, N., Mari, A., *et al.* (2011). Carrier-bound, nonallergenic Ole e 1 peptides for vaccination against olive pollen allergy. *J Allergy Clin Immunol,* **128**(1), 178–184, e177.

77. Twaroch, T.E., Focke, M., Fleischmann, K., Balic, N., Lupinek, C., Blatt, K., *et al.* (2012). Carrier-bound Alt a 1 peptides without allergenic activity for vaccination against Alternaria alternata allergy. *Clin Exp Allergy,* **42**(6), 966–975.

78. Focke-Tejkl, M., Campana, R., Reininger, R., Lupinek, C., Blatt, K., Valent, P., *et al.* (2014). Dissection of the IgE and T-cell recognition of the major group 5 grass pollen allergen Phl p 5. *J Allergy Clin Immunol,* **133**(3), 836–845, e811.

79. Scadding, G.W., Shamji, M.H., Jacobson, M.R., Lee, D.I., Wilson, D., Lima, M.T., *et al.* (2010). Sublingual grass pollen immunotherapy is associated with increases in sublingual Foxp3-expressing cells and elevated allergen-specific immunoglobulin G4, immunoglobulin A and serum inhibi-

tory activity for immunoglobulin E-facilitated allergen binding to B cells. *Clin Exp Allergy,* **40**(4), 598–606.

80. Wilson, D.R., Lima, M.T., & Durham, S.R. (2005). Sublingual immunotherapy for allergic rhinitis: systematic review and meta-analysis. *Allergy,* **60**(1), 4–12.

81. Durham, S.R., Emminger, W., Kapp, A., de Monchy, J.G., Rak, S., Scadding, G.K., *et al.* (2012). SQ-standardized sublingual grass immunotherapy: confirmation of disease modification 2 years after 3 years of treatment in a randomized trial. *J Allergy Clin Immunol,* **129**(3), 717–725, e715.

82. Jones, S.M., Burks, A.W., & Dupont, C. (2014). State of the art on food allergen immunotherapy: oral, sublingual, and epicutaneous. *J Allergy Clin Immunol,* **133**(2), 318–323.

83. Juillard, G.J., Boyer, P.J., & Yamashiro, C.H. (1978). A phase I study of active specific intralymphatic immunotherapy (ASILI). *Cancer,* **41**(6), 2215–2225.

84. Senti, G., Johansen, P., & Kundig, T.M. (2011). Intralymphatic immunotherapy: from the rationale to human applications. *Curr Top Microbiol Immunol,* **352**, 71–84.

85. Senti, G., Prinz Vavricka, B.M., Erdmann, I., Diaz, M.I., Markus, R., McCormack, S.J., *et al.* (2008). Intralymphatic allergen administration renders specific immunotherapy faster and safer: a randomized controlled trial. *Proc Natl Acad Sci U S A,* **105**(46), 17908–17912.

86. Senti, G., Crameri, R., Kuster, D., Johansen, P., Martinez-Gomez, J.M., Graf, N., *et al.* (2012). Intralymphatic immunotherapy for cat allergy induces tolerance after only 3 injections. *J Allergy Clin Immunol,* **129**(5), 1290–1296.

87. Zaleska, A., Eiwegger, T., Soyer, O., van de Veen, W., Rhyner, C., Soyka, M.B., *et al.* (2014). Immune regulation by intralymphatic immunotherapy with modular allergen translocation MAT vaccine. *Allergy,* **69**(9), 1162–1170.

88. Senti, G., Graf, N., Haug, S., Ruedi, N., von Moos, S., Sonderegger, T., *et al.* (2009). Epicutaneous allergen administration as a novel method of allergen-specific immunotherapy. *J Allergy Clin Immunol,* **124**(5), 997–1002.

89. Dioszeghy, V., Mondoulet, L., Dhelft, V., Ligouis, M., Puteaux, E., Benhamou, P.H., *et al.* (2011). Epicutaneous immunotherapy results in rapid allergen uptake by dendritic cells through intact skin and downregulates the allergen-specific response in sensitized mice. *J Immunol,* **186**(10), 5629–5637.

90. Dupont, C., Kalach, N., Soulaines, P., Legoue-Morillon, S., Piloquet, H., & Benhamou, P.H. (2010). Cow's milk epicutaneous immunotherapy in children: a pilot trial of safety, acceptability, and impact on allergic reactivity. *J Allergy Clin Immunol,* **125**(5), 1165–1167.

91. Hessenberger, M., Weiss, R., Weinberger, E.E., Boehler, C., Thalhamer, J., & Scheiblhofer, S. (2013). Transcutaneous delivery of CpG-adjuvanted allergen via laser-generated micropores. *Vaccine,* **31**(34), 3427–3434.

92. DuBuske, L.M., Frew, A.J., Horak, F., Keith, P.K., Corrigan, C.J., Aberer, W., *et al.* (2011). Ultrashort-specific immunotherapy successfully treats seasonal allergic rhinoconjunctivitis to grass pollen. *Allergy Asthma Proc,* **32**(3), 239–247.

93. Creticos, P.S., Schroeder, J.T., Hamilton, R.G., Balcer-Whaley, S.L., Khattignavong, A.P., Lindblad, R., *et al.* (2006). Immunotherapy with a ragweed-toll-like receptor 9 agonist vaccine for allergic rhinitis. *N Engl J Med,* **355**(14), 1445–1455.

94. Senti, G., Johansen, P., Haug, S., Bull, C., Gottschaller, C., Muller, P., *et al.* (2009). Use of A-type CpG oligodeoxynucleotides as an adjuvant in allergen-specific immunotherapy in humans: a phase I/IIa clinical trial. *Clin Exp Allergy,* **39**(4), 562–570.

95. Kundig, T.M., Senti, G., Schnetzler, G., Wolf, C., Prinz Vavricka, B.M., Fulurija, A., *et al.* (2006). Der p 1 peptide on virus-like particles is safe and highly immunogenic in healthy adults. *J Allergy Clin Immunol,* **117**(6), 1470–1476.

96. Schmitz, N., Dietmeier, K., Bauer, M., Maudrich, M., Utzinger, S., Muntwiler, S., *et al.* (2009). Displaying Fel d1 on virus-like particles prevents reactogenicity despite greatly enhanced immunogenicity: a novel therapy for cat allergy. *J Exp Med,* **206**(9), 1941–1955.

97. Neimert-Andersson, T., Thunberg, S., Swedin, L., Wiedermann, U., Jacobsson-Ekman, G., Dahlen, S.E., *et al.* (2008). Carbohydrate-based particles reduce allergic inflammation in a mouse model for cat allergy. *Allergy,* **63**(5), 518–526.

98. Grundstrom, J., Neimert-Andersson, T., Kemi, C., Nilsson, O.B., Saarne, T., Andersson, M., *et al.* (2012). Covalent coupling of vitamin D3 to the major cat allergen Fel d 1 improves the effects of allergen-specific immunotherapy in a mouse model for cat allergy. *Int Arch Allergy Immunol,* **157**(2), 136–146.

99. Baris, S., Kiykim, A., Ozen, A., Tulunay, A., Karakoc-Aydiner, E., & Barlan, I.B. (2014). Vitamin D as an adjunct to subcutaneous allergen immu-

notherapy in asthmatic children sensitized to house dust mite. *Allergy,* **69**(2), 246–253.

100. Hiller, R., Laffer, S., Harwanegg, C., Huber, M., Schmidt, W.M., Twardosz, A., *et al.* (2002). Microarrayed allergen molecules: diagnostic gatekeepers for allergy treatment. *FASEB J,* **16**(3), 414–416.

101. Lupinek, C., Wollmann, E., Baar, A., Banerjee, S., Breiteneder, H., Broecker, B.M., *et al.* (2014). Advances in allergen-microarray technology for diagnosis and monitoring of allergy: the MeDALL allergen-chip. *Methods,* **66**(1), 106–119.

102. Lupinek, C., Marth, K., Niederberger, V., & Valenta, R. (2012). Analysis of serum IgE reactivity profiles with microarrayed allergens indicates absence of *de novo* IgE sensitizations in adults. *J Allergy Clin Immunol,* **130**(6), 1418–1420, e1414.

103. Glovsky, M.M., Ghekiere, L., & Rejzek, E. (1991). Effect of maternal immunotherapy on immediate skin test reactivity, specific rye I IgG and IgE antibody, and total IgE of the children. *Ann Allergy,* **67**(1), 21–24.

104. Flicker, S., Marth, K., Kofler, H., & Valenta, R. (2009). Placental transfer of allergen-specific IgG but not IgE from a specific immunotherapy-treated mother. *J Allergy Clin Immunol,* **124**(6), 1358–1360, e1351.

CHAPTER 15

FUTURE PROSPECTS FOR THE THERAPIES OF INFLAMMATORY DISEASES

Ronald F. van Vollenhoven

Introduction

Developments over the past twenty years in the therapeutic field of the inflammatory diseases have been nothing but breathtaking. The combination of enhanced understanding of the immunological and inflammatory mechanisms behind these diseases and the advent of biotechnology which made it possible to capitalize on these learnings in a manner that directly translates to therapeutics has resulted in dramatic changes in our ability to alleviate the suffering of patients affected by inflammatory diseases. In some cases, treatment has progressed from very limited palliative possibilities to achieving such outstanding disease control that discussions on possible cure have begun.[1]

Although all this may seem very obvious from today's perspective, it would not necessarily have been easy to predict in 1990. When confronted with the very first encouraging results of TNF blockade in rheumatoid arthritis,[2] many potential risks and practical difficulties were considered. Would this type of treatment be too strongly immunosuppressive? Would it be associated with increasing rates of infections or malignancies?

Would immune deviation lead to the development of other autoimmune diseases? And in terms of practicalities, was it reasonable to presume that patients with a chronic disease could be treated long term with parenterally administered monoclonal antibodies and other biologicals?

Today just as it was then, it may be a tall order to attempt to predict the future for the field of therapeutics in inflammatory diseases. Certainly many ongoing developments will lead to additional treatment options, and some of these could be considered extensions of the current treatment paradigms: additional refinements in cytokine antagonism, targeting of other cell-surface molecules, etc. However, completely different approaches are also being considered and some will hopefully result in additional advances in therapeutics (Table 1). Among these approaches could be the activation of naturally occurring regulatory T cells (Tregs), neuro-immunomodulatory approaches, cell-based therapies and others. And importantly, the reevaluation and reassessment of treatment *strategies* for many diseases will continue and lead to new treatment paradigms.

Additional Cytokine Targets

While the number of anti-cytokine biologics that are in clinical use today is quite substantial, there are obviously many more cytokines that could be targeted. Indeed, selective inhibitors of the IL-17 pathway are in late-stage development for the treatment of psoriasis,[3–6] Crohn's disease,[7] rheumatoid arthritis,[8] psoriatic arthritis,[9,10] and spondyloarthropathies[11] and the first of these, secukinumab has been approved for the treatment of psoriasis by both the US and European regulatory authorities; the anti-IL4 monoclonal antibody dupilumab has shown excellent results in phase II/III trials in asthma[12,13] and atopic dermatitis;[14] the monoclonal antibody mavrilimumab that targets the granulocyte-monocyte colony stimulating factor (which has important immunoregulatory functions) showed efficacy in a trial in RA;[15] and other examples have been presented in the preceding chapters in this book.

A more novel approach to cytokine antagonism is represented by "kinoids", vaccines engineered based on modified cytokines.[16,17] The underlying idea is that the patient who suffers from an autoimmune inflammatory disease that is clearly linked to a certain cytokine could be

Table 1. Future approaches to inflammatory diseases.

Approach	Examples	Promises	Challenges
Additional anti-cytokine therapies	Anti-IL4, anti-IL17, anti-GMCSF, "kinoids"	Novel therapies for new disease areas; additional options where some already exist	Difficulties to predict "fit" between molecular target and disease; challenging for industry to enter competitive field with new product
Additional cell-surface targeting therapies	Anti-CD22	Novel therapies for new disease areas; additional options where some already exist	Difficulties to predict "fit" between molecular target and disease; challenging for industry to enter competitive field with new product
Activation of regulatory T cells	Tregalizumab	Completely new approach to autoimmunity might find wide applications across many diseases	Difficulties in translating from lab to clinic; disastrous experience with TGN1412 in phase I; uncertainties on efficacy and safety for this entirely new approach
Neuroimmuno-modulatory approaches	Implantable vagus nerve stimulator	Completely new approach to autoimmunity; wide lay appeal for neuro-immunology concept	Practical issues with implantable device; uncertainties on efficacy and safety for this entirely new approach
Cell-based therapies and related procedures	Mesenchymal stromal cell infusions	Combines tissue selectivity with specific regulatory functions that can in principle be pre-programmed	Practical aspects; uncertainties on efficacy and safety for this entirely new approach

"vaccinated" against the cytokine, that is, a polyclonal antibody response against the cytokine could be induced intended to down-regulate the disease. Early trials with kinoids containing interferon-α[18] and TNF[19] showed biological efficacy, and further trials with these two kinoids in SLE and RA, respectively, are ongoing.

In addition, the number of novel anti-cytokine approaches currently under investigation at the pre-clinical level or in very early-phase human trials is large. Unfortunately, it has become clear that our ability to predict therapeutic benefits on the basis of *in vitro* or animal experimental data has remained rather limited, and it remains to be seen which approaches will make it to the clinic while others fall by the way-side.

There are also many non-scientific aspects to these questions. For biotech or pharma industry it is mostly realistic, for business reasons, to develop a drug for one particular indication or a small number at most, rather than the dozens of possibilities that could reasonably be suggested based on scientific data. Other factors also need to be considered in these decisions, such as the remaining medical need, the competitive landscape, patent issues, and so forth. Clearly, for the more prevalent inflammatory diseases — including psoriasis, inflammatory bowel disease, and RA — many agents are now available, making the business proposition of developing an additional one all the more difficult. For uncommon and rare diseases, regulatory mechanisms do exist that make development of specific treatments a bit less burdensome; but for such diseases, the trials themselves are often hard to conduct. All things told, one could predict that although some development of additional cytokine-targeting biologic agents will continue, the rapid pace of innovation seen in the past two decades will not be sustained.

Novel Cellular Targets

In the treatment of systemic inflammatory diseases, monoclonal antibodies and other biologics targeting cellular markers have not been as successful as many had originally hoped. Approaches using anti-CD4 (targeting helper T cells) were ineffective,[20,21] and although alemtuzumab (Campath-1H), an anti-CD52 monoclonal that targets all T cells, can be used with efficacy in multiple sclerosis[22] and RA,[22,23] it is generally felt to be too toxic for general use in inflammatory conditions. Abatacept which targets the B7-CD28 interaction has demonstrated efficacy in RA[24] and possibly psoriasis[25] but not in other inflammatory diseases. B cell depleting anti-CD20 antibodies are effective in some inflammatory diseases including RA,[26–28] vasculitis,[29,30] and possibly SLE[31] while the B cell down-regulatory monoclonal epratuzumab (anti-CD22) has shown promise in SLE.[32,33]

Activation of Regulatory T Cells

An entirely different conceptual approach to autoimmunity would be the activation of regulatory T cells (Tregs). Extensive animal experience suggests the feasibility of this approach, but human trials have encountered difficulties. The activating anti-CD28 monoclonal TGN1412 caused severe side effects in its first-in-man trial, which were clearly caused by the widespread activation of inflammatory pathways. This episode delayed further developments in this direction by many years. However, more recently the monoclonal antibody tregalizumab which is directed against a specific epitope on the CD4 molecule was shown to activate Tregs only[34] (Fig. 1) and was safe in phase I trials in healthy volunteers. A small trial in RA suggested possible efficacy and a large trial in RA was recently completed; a press release from the sponsoring company announced that the trial had not achieved its primary outcome. Nonetheless, an approach that would harness the regulatory T cells would have potential applications in many other diseases characterized by excessive immunological activity.

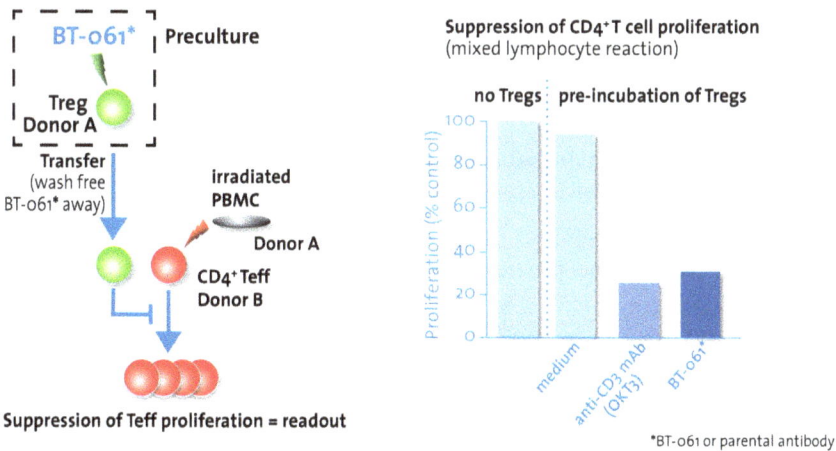

Figure 1. Tregalizumab (BT-061) selective down-regulates proliferation through activation of regulatory T-cells. Reproduced, with permission, from Kubach J., Rharbaoui F., König M., Schüttrumpf J., Aigner S., Dälken B., Jonuleit H. (2014). The Effect of a Proinflammatory Milieu on Tregalizumab (BT-061)-Induced Regulatory T-cell Activity. Presented at the ACR 2014 national congress.

Neuroimmunomodulatory Approaches

While the field of "neuroimmunology" — studying the effects that the neurological system has on immunity and inflammation and vice versa — has been a subject of considerable interest not in the least from lay audiences, practical therapeutic approaches based on such interactions have not been forthcoming. An important new development in this field has been the clarification of the "inflammatory reflex".[35] It was shown that in mice, immune responses in the spleen are "monitored" in the central nervous system through afferent vagal pathways and, perhaps even more importantly, regulated through efferent vagal pathways acting through macrophages upon T cells[36–38] (Fig. 2). It has been suggested that similar mechanisms might occur in humans and a small pilot study was recently initiated in which subjects with RA received an implantable device in the chest/neck region that electrically stimulates the vagus nerve, in the hopes of down-regulating systemic inflammation in this manner. In this very small group of patients some improvements were noted, but complications with the procedure did occur and it would seem that considerable hurdles, both practical and scientific, would need to be overcome before this approach can reach clinical application.

Cell-Based Therapies

Treatment approaches based on the infusion of modified autologous or allogeneic cells were discussed in Chapter 4 by Marits *et al.* The advantages of cell-based therapies could, in theory, be very significant but tremendous technical and practical issues must also be overcome. Perhaps the most interesting approach that is currently in early-phase trials is the use of mesenchymal stromal cells. These cells, which can be engineered to develop into cells belonging to various tissue types, exhibit anti-inflammatory and immunosuppressive properties that make them attractive for the treatment of inflammatory diseases by virtue of the combined benefits of this general regulatory effect and the tissue- or organ-tropism that would be conferred by their particular cellular differentiation in relationship to the disease under study.

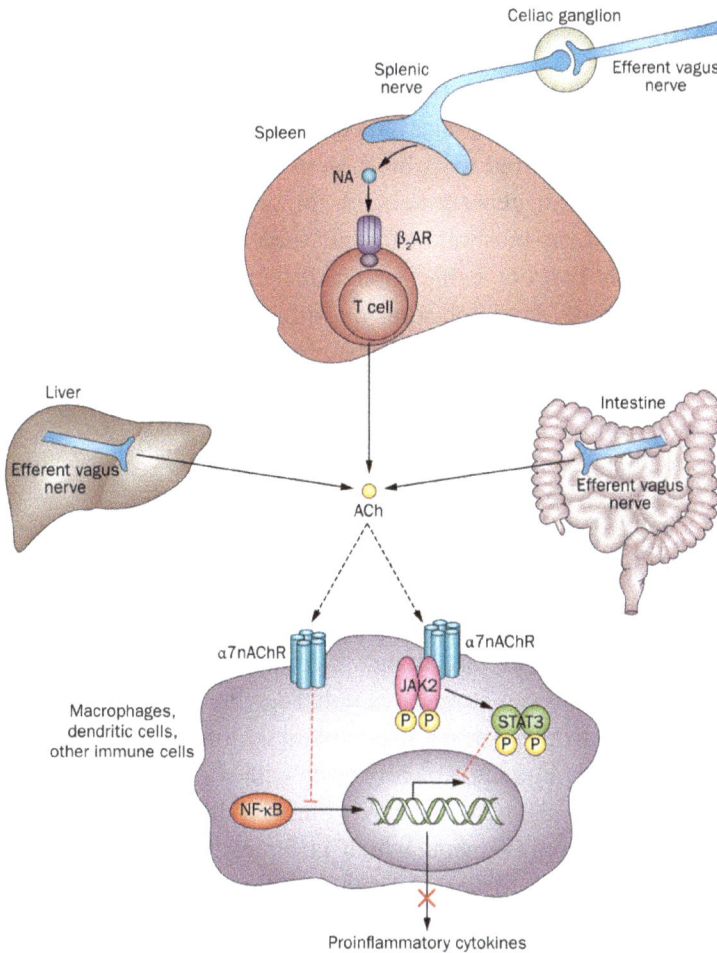

Figure 2. Molecular mechanisms of cholinergic control of inflammation. Efferent vagus nerve activity is translated into catecholamine-mediated activation of T cell-derived acetylcholine release in the spleen and into direct acetylcholine release from efferent vagus nerve endings in other organs. Inhibition of NF-κB nuclear translocation and activation of a JAK2-STAT3-mediated signalling cascade in macrophages and other immune cells are implicated in cholinergic α7nAChR-mediated control of proinflammatory cytokine production. Abbreviations: ACh, acetylcholine; β_2AR, β_2 adrenergic receptor; JAK2, Janus kinase 2; α7nAChR, α 7 nicotinic acetylcholine receptor; NA, noradrenaline; NF-κB, nuclear factor κB; STAT3, signal transducer and activator of transcription 3.

Reproduced, with permission, from Pavlov V.A., Tracey K.J. (2014). The vagus nerve and the inflammatory reflex — linking immunity and metabolism. *Nat Rev Endocrinol*, **8**(12), 743–754.

Biosimilars

As the first biologics to enter the clinic are losing patent protection, many companies are developing similar molecules. As proteins cannot be entirely identical, they are referred to as biosimilars and they are regulated somewhat differently than generic versions of conventional pharmaceutical products. The first two biosimilars for infliximab (being the same substance but marketed by two companies under different names) have now been approved in Europe. Although some questions continue to be asked about the interchangeability of these biologic products, the economic pressures to lower costs are such that there is little doubt that biosimilars will play an increasing role in the treatment of inflammatory diseases.

Future Prospects for Treatment *Strategies* in the Inflammatory Diseases

The most important inflammatory diseases are those that are chronic or frequently recurring and that impart significant consequences onto the patients on account of symptoms, functional decline over time, or late organ dysfunction due to the disease itself or its treatment. Because of these characteristics, the clinician typically deals with similar demands in establishing the most optimal treatments over time: he/she must balance the need for symptomatic improvement, which is typically needed on relatively short time frames (days to weeks), while avoiding long-term complications from the disease and toxicities from the medications, which typically emerge over the course of months, years, or decades. Glucocorticoids represent one of the main conundrums in the treatment of inflammatory diseases: while exceptionally and almost uniformly effective in the short term, they are associated with numerous long-term toxicities and detrimental consequences. Many conventional immunosuppressives, on the other hand, combine relatively good long-term safety with a slow onset of action and uncertain efficacy at the individual patient level. Moreover, biologics add their own particular dimension to these complex balances by adding the aspect of costs. In this context, it is useful to refer to the conceptual framework for treating chronic diseases by Fries *et al.*[39] expressed as the five D's that must be avoided or minimized: death, discomfort, disability, drug side effects, and dollar costs.

Faced with these challenges, the clinician needs to employ a long-term treatment strategy. While the development and assessment of individual drugs have been intense and productive over the past two decades, there have been more modest inroads in improving optimal treatment *strategies*. Nevertheless, some important concepts have emerged in multiple disease areas and are increasingly being implemented in clinical care (Table 2).

Table 2.   Novel treatment strategies for the inflammatory diseases.

Strategy	Example	Promises	Challenges
Early treatment	Immunosuppressives as first-line treatment in rheumatoid arthritis	Well established in several diseases; achieves better disease control, reduces risk for complications, prevents long-term damage	Not (yet) proven effective for other diseases; may unnecessarily expose patients to toxicities; may be more costly
Induction-maintenance	Early aggressive treatment followed by continued treatment with simpler medications in IBD, RA, and SLE	Strong evidence in some and emerging evidence in other diseases; promise to achieve rapid disease control without the need for indefinite "heavy" medication	Not (yet) proven effective for other diseases; may unnecessarily expose patients to toxicities; unclear how to deal with partial responses
Treat to target	T2T guidance for RA and other rheumatic diseases	Strong evidence for RA; compelling arguments; may "fit" with modern medical organization	No evidence for other inflammatory diseases; requires large changes in approach to patient; may require significant investments in time and money from the healthcare system

Early treatment

In many inflammatory diseases, older treatment paradigms based on clinical experience with limited therapeutic options could be summarized as "go slow" approaches. Simple symptom-relieving therapies, local or topical therapies, and low-doses of anti-inflammatory drugs — both steroidal and non-steroidal — were used and cautiously escalated, while more powerful immunosuppressives were reserved for refractory cases, often in quite late stages of the disease.

However, based on theoretical considerations, animal models, and increasingly on clinical studies, it has become clear that this approach, while sparing many patients the toxicities of more effective treatment, allows irreversible organ damage to accrue over time in many others. Thus, *early treatment* has increasingly been advocated, for example, in rheumatoid arthritis, inflammatory bowel disease, and lupus nephritis.

Induction-maintenance

A further development of early treatment is the employment of *induction-maintenance* strategies. Patients diagnosed with an inflammatory disease can, in many instances, be managed with moderately strong immunomodulatory agents as the first-line treatment, but the option of starting treatment at a more intensive level could in theory be considered. One key question is whether such early intensive treatment can be shown to be sufficiently more effective than standard therapy to warrant the additional side-effects and risks. For many diseases this has, in principle, been proven — lupus nephritis,[40] rheumatoid arthritis,[41] and IBD.[42] However, the prospect of continuing such more aggressive interventions indefinitely is not attractive, from the patient's perspective (more medications to take or receive, more controls etc.), the physician's perspective (more risks to monitor, more side effects to deal with) but also increasingly from the societal perspective, given the high costs of treatments. This balance has propelled a major renewed interest in induction-maintenance approaches, where more intensive treatments are administered initially in order to achieve a favorable disease state, followed by de-escalation leading to maintenance of the favorable disease state with simpler means. For some diseases, it has clearly been demonstrated that this approach is both effective and applicable in clinical practice. Thus, for lupus nephritis an initial induction with the rather toxic agent cyclophosphamide can be used for six months, followed by less toxic long-term treatment with azathioprine[43] or mycophenolate.[44] In RA, a number of studies have investigated the possibility of initiating treatment with both methotrexate (MTX) and a TNF-antagonist — this combination is generally considered the most effective therapy for RA today — and then continuing with MTX only in patients who respond favorably after 3–12 months. Thus, Quinn *et al.*[45] noted very good results with this approach in a group of 10 patients, and in the BeSt trial, the majority of patients with an initial good response were able to maintain it with MTX monotherapy.[46] The Optima trial investigated this possibility more formally in a complex study design where the *discontinuation* of anti-TNF was also randomized and controlled[47] (Fig. 3). In various analyses it was found that the difference between the patients who did and who did not continue anti-TNF was quite small, for example, only about 10% fewer patients with low-disease activity and around 20% difference in sustained remission. Taken together, these results and others provide sufficient evidence that *if* treatment is started with MTX + anti-TNF and *if* the combination achieves remission or low disease activity, *then* the treatment can in most cases be continued with MTX alone. However, two big questions remain before this approach can be widely implemented. First, the clinical problem will be to decide what to do for patients who do not achieve the targeted outcome with the combination therapy but, nonetheless, have a good therapeutic response. It would seem wrong to try to reduce the intensity of their therapy, but the prospect of staying on combination therapy indefinitely or of switching therapies to other biologics is clinically unappealing and unattractive from a health-economic perspective. The second major question is whether this early "induction" approach provides a lasting benefit. Could the same end result be achieved by simpler means? The answer to this question is still not completely clear. Some studies, including the aforementioned Optima trial and the much smaller French study Guépard,[48] suggest that the early intensive treatment makes it somewhat more likely that the disease can later be controlled by MTX alone; however other trials, such as the German Hit-Hard trial[49] and the Danish Opera trial[50] did not support this possibility. A somewhat similar

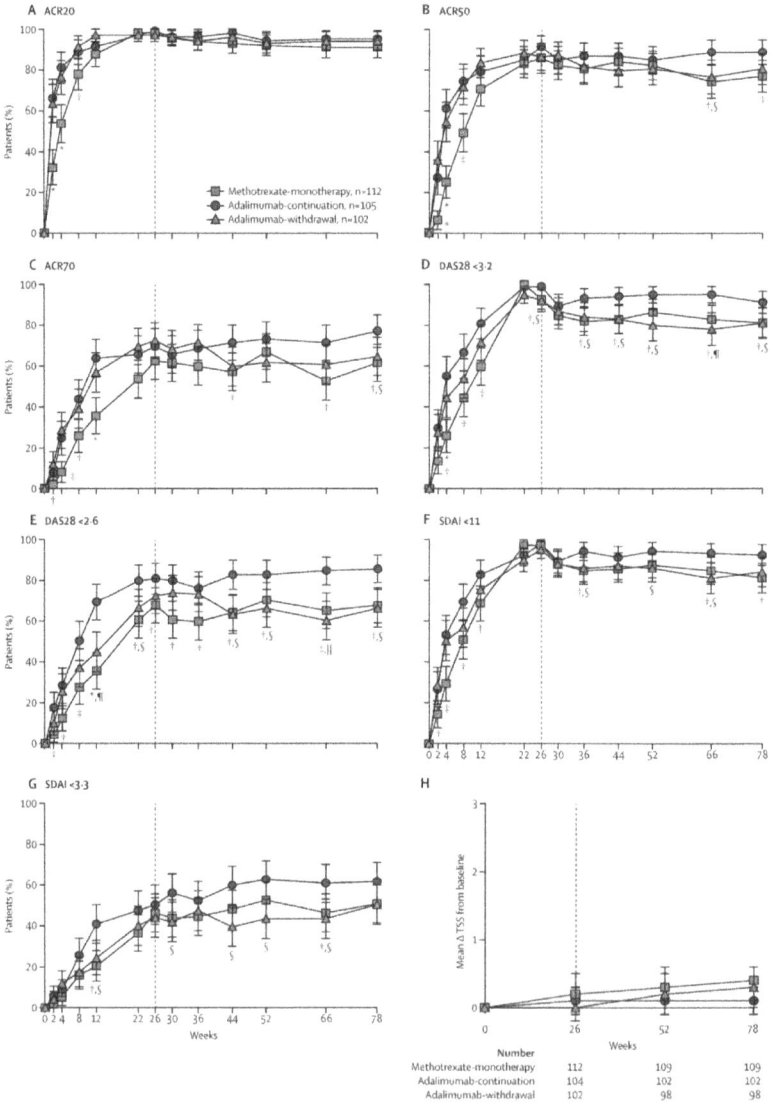

Figure 3. Clinical and radiographic outcomes in patients who achieved the target of DAS of less than 3·2 at weeks 22 and 26. The proportions of patients who achieved ACR response criteria (A–C), favorable DAS28 (D–E) and SDAI levels (F–G), and radiographic progression (H) are shown. Reproduced, with permission, from Smolen J.S., Emery P., Fleischmann R., van Vollenhoven R.F., Pavelka K., Durez P. *et al.* (2014). Adjustment of therapy in rheumatoid arthritis on the basis of achievement of stable low disease activity with adalimumab plus methotrexate or methotrexate alone: the randomised controlled OPTIMA trial. *Lancet*, **383**(9914), 321–332.

study design to the above mentioned trials was employed for the combination of MTX plus abatacept, the T cell co-stimulation modulator. It was found that if an excellent initial response (remission) was achieved with the combination, then it could be maintained in most patients with MTX alone, and a small minority of patients would even maintain remission without any treatment[51].

Thus, in early RA, induction-maintenance approaches are being investigated intensively and for the time being at least some of the available evidence supports the principle. In contrast, in established RA, an induction-maintenance approach of the same type is generally not possible: when biologics are discontinued, the risk of a disease flare is quite big. However, several studies now suggest that in many patients, the disease can be controlled in the long run with a lower dose of the biologic than is used for the initial treatment and this would be attractive from the patients' and also certainly from the societies' perspective.[52,53]

Treat-to-target

The principle of treating to target was originally derived from diseases such as hypertension, where trials demonstrated that long-term outcomes were better if clinicians clearly identified the blood pressure that they wanted to achieve and took action to achieve it. For rheumatoid arthritis, at least two randomized trials also provided direct evidence that such an approach, based on targeting a certain level of the disease activity score (DAS), yielded better long-term results[54,55] (Fig. 4). Formal Treat-to-Target (T2T) guidance for RA was published several years ago and the principle has increasingly been implemented.[56] Similar recommendations have also been developed for several other rheumatic diseases.[57,58] It should be emphasized that T2T is not only about choosing a target, but also about deciding on how and when to measure that target and about the principle that failure to achieve the target should lead to a therapeutic change in most cases.

In summary, the progress of therapeutics and of therapy research for the inflammatory disease has been remarkable, but many challenges still exist. The challenge for the researcher in clinical therapeutics for inflammatory diseases is not only to find new potential treatments but also to ensure that the available treatments are used in an optimal manner and that

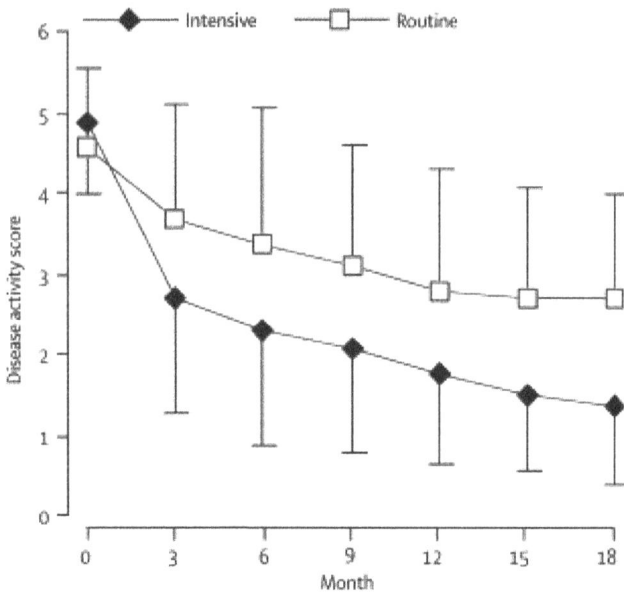

Figure 4. Routine versus intensive care ("tight-control", "treat-to-target") in rheumatoid arthritis.
Mean disease activity score Student's t-test used. Intensive vs routine after month 3, $p < 0.0001$. Error bars show SD.
Reproduced, with permission, from Grigor C., Capell H., Stirling A., McMahon A.D., Lock P., Vallance R. *et al.* (2014). Effect of a treatment strategy of tight control for rheumatoid arthritis (the TICORA study): a single-blind randomised controlled trial. *Lancet*, **364**(9430), 263–269.

the patients suffering from inflammatory conditions receive the best possible care today, even as new developments make it virtually certain that ever better therapies will become available for the treatment of these important diseases.

References

1. Brooks, P.M. (1998). The Heberden Oration 1997. Treatment of rheumatoid arthritis: from symptomatic relief to potential cure. *Br J Rheumatol*, **37**(12), 1265–1271.

2. Elliott, M.J., Maini, R.N., Feldmann, M., Long-Fox, A., Charles, P., Katsikis, P., *et al.* (1993). Treatment of rheumatoid arthritis with chimeric monoclonal antibodies to tumor necrosis factor alpha. *Arthritis Rheum*, **36**(12), 1681–1690.
3. Paul, C., Reich, K., Gottlieb, A.B., Mrowietz, U., Philipp, S., Nakayama, J., *et al.* (2014). Secukinumab improves hand, foot and nail lesions in moderate-to-severe plaque psoriasis: subanalysis of a randomized, double-blind, placebo-controlled, regimen-finding phase 2 trial. *J Eur Acad Dermatol Venereol*, **28**(12), 1670–1675.
4. Gordon, K.B., Leonardi, C.L., Lebwohl, M., Blauvelt, A., Cameron, G.S., Braun, D., *et al.* (2014). A 52-week, open-label study of the efficacy and safety of ixekizumab, an anti-interleukin-17A monoclonal antibody, in patients with chronic plaque psoriasis. *J Am Acad Dermatol*, **71**(6), 1176–1182.
5. Leonardi, C., Matheson, R., Zachariae, C., Cameron, G., Li, L., Edson-Heredia, E., *et al.* (2012). Anti-interleukin-17 monoclonal antibody ixekizumab in chronic plaque psoriasis. *N Engl J Med*, **366**(13), 1190–1199.
6. Wu, J.J. (2012). Anti-interleukin-17 monoclonal antibody ixekizumab in psoriasis. *N Engl J Med*, **367**(3), 274–275; author reply 5.
7. Hueber, W., Sands, B.E., Lewitzky, S., Vandemeulebroecke, M., Reinisch, W., Higgins, P.D., *et al.* (2012). Secukinumab, a human anti-IL-17A monoclonal antibody, for moderate to severe Crohn's disease: unexpected results of a randomised, double-blind placebo-controlled trial. *Gut*, **61**(12), 1693–1700.
8. Genovese, M.C., Greenwald, M., Cho, C.S., Berman, A., Jin, L., Cameron, G.S., *et al.* (2012). A phase II randomized study of subcutaneous ixekizumab, an anti-interleukin-17 monoclonal antibody, in rheumatoid arthritis patients who were naive to biologic agents or had an inadequate response to tumor necrosis factor inhibitors. *Arthritis Rheumatol*, **66**(7), 1693–1704.
9. McInnes, I.B., Sieper, J., Braun, J., Emery, P., van der Heijde, D., Isaacs, J.D., *et al.* (2014). Efficacy and safety of secukinumab, a fully human anti-interleukin-17A monoclonal antibody, in patients with moderate-to-severe psoriatic arthritis: a 24-week, randomised, double-blind, placebo-controlled, phase II proof-of-concept trial. *Ann Rheum Dis*, **73**(2), 349–356.
10. Mease, P.J., Genovese, M.C., Greenwald, M.W., Ritchlin, C.T., Beaulieu, A.D., Deodhar, A., *et al.* (2014). Brodalumab, an anti-IL17RA monoclonal antibody, in psoriatic arthritis. *N Engl J Med*, **370**(24), 2295–2306.
11. Baeten, D., Baraliakos, X., Braun, J., Sieper, J., Emery, P., van der Heijde, D., *et al.* (2013). Anti-interleukin-17A monoclonal antibody secukinumab in treatment of ankylosing spondylitis: a randomised, double-blind, placebo-controlled trial. *Lancet*, **382**(9906), 1705–1713.

12. Wenzel, S.E., Wang, L., Pirozzi, G. (2013) Dupilumab in persistent asthma. *N Engl J Med*, **369**(13), 1276.

13. Wenzel, S., Ford, L., Pearlman, D., Spector, S., Sher, L., Skobieranda, F., *et al.* (2013). Dupilumab in persistent asthma with elevated eosinophil levels. *N Engl J Med*, **368**(26), 2455–2466.

14. Beck, L.A., Thaci, D., Hamilton, J.D., Graham, N.M., Bieber, T., Rocklin, R., *et al.* (2014). Dupilumab treatment in adults with moderate-to-severe atopic dermatitis. *N Engl J Med*, **371**(2), 130–139.

15. Burmester, G.R., Feist, E., Sleeman, M.A., Wang, B., White, B., Magrini, F. (2011). Mavrilimumab, a human monoclonal antibody targeting GM-CSF receptor-alpha, in subjects with rheumatoid arthritis: a randomised, double-blind, placebo-controlled, phase I, first-in-human study. *Ann Rheum Dis*, **70**(9), 1542–1549.

16. Bizzini, B., Achour, A. (1995). "Kinoids": the basis for anticytokine immunization and their use in HIV infection. *Cell Mol Biol (Noisy-le-grand)*, **41**(3), 351–356.

17. Bizzini, B., Drouet, B., Zagury, D., Abitbol, M., Burny, A., Boissier, M.C. (2010). Kinoids: a family of immunogens for active anticytokine immunotherapy applied to autoimmune diseases and cancer. *Immunotherapy*, **2**(3), 347–365.

18. Lauwerys, B.R., Hachulla, E., Spertini, F., Lazaro, E., Jorgensen, C., Mariette, X., *et al.* (2013). Down-regulation of interferon signature in systemic lupus erythematosus patients by active immunization with interferon alpha-kinoid. *Arthritis Rheum*, **65**(2), 447–456.

19. Durez, P., Vandepapeliere, P., Miranda, P., Toncheva, A., Berman, A., Kehler, T., *et al.* (2014). Therapeutic vaccination with TNF-kinoid in TNF antagonist-resistant rheumatoid arthritis: a phase II randomized, controlled clinical trial. *PLoS One*, **9**(12), e113465.

20. van der Lubbe, P.A., Dijkmans, B.A., Markusse, H.M., Nassander, U., Breedveld, F.C. (1995). A randomized, double-blind, placebo-controlled study of CD4 monoclonal antibody therapy in early rheumatoid arthritis. *Arthritis Rheum*, **38**(8), 1097–1106.

21. Moreland, L.W., Pratt, P.W., Mayes, M.D., Postlethwaite, A., Weisman, M.H., Schnitzer, T., *et al.* (1995). Double-blind, placebo-controlled multicenter trial using chimeric monoclonal anti-CD4 antibody, cM-T412, in rheumatoid arthritis patients receiving concomitant methotrexate. *Arthritis Rheum*, **38**(11), 1581–1588.

22. Cohen, J.A., Coles, A.J., Arnold, D.L., Confavreux, C., Fox, E.J., Hartung, H.P., *et al.* (2012). Alemtuzumab versus interferon beta 1a as first-line treatment

for patients with relapsing-remitting multiple sclerosis: a randomised controlled phase 3 trial. *Lancet*, **380**(9856), 1819–1828.

23. Isaacs, J.D., Manna, V.K., Rapson, N., Bulpitt, K.J., Hazleman, B.L., Matteson, E.L., *et al.* (1996). CAMPATH-1H in rheumatoid arthritis — an intravenous dose-ranging study. *Br J Rheumatol*, **35**(3), 231–240.

24. Kremer, J.M., Genant, H.K., Moreland, L.W., Russell, A.S., Emery, P., Abud-Mendoza, C., *et al.* (2006). Effects of abatacept in patients with methotrexate-resistant active rheumatoid arthritis: a randomized trial. *Ann Intern Med*, **144**(12), 865–876.

25. Abrams, J.R., Lebwohl, M.G., Guzzo, C.A., Jegasothy, B.V., Goldfarb, M.T., Goffe, B.S., *et al.* (1999). CTLA4Ig-mediated blockade of T-cell costimulation in patients with psoriasis vulgaris. *J Clin Invest*, **103**(9), 1243–1252.

26. Emery, P., Fleischmann, R., Filipowicz-Sosnowska, A., Schechtman, J., Szczepanski, L., Kavanaugh, A., *et al.* (2006). The efficacy and safety of rituximab in patients with active rheumatoid arthritis despite methotrexate treatment: results of a phase IIB randomized, double-blind, placebo-controlled, dose-ranging trial. *Arthritis Rheum*, **54**(5), 1390–1400.

27. Edwards, J.C., Szczepanski, L., Szechinski, J., Filipowicz-Sosnowska, A., Emery, P., Close, D.R., *et al.* (2004). Efficacy of B-cell-targeted therapy with rituximab in patients with rheumatoid arthritis. *N Engl J Med*, **350**(25), 2572–2581.

28. Cohen, S.B., Emery, P., Greenwald, M.W., Dougados, M., Furie, R.A., Genovese, M.C., *et al.* (2006). Rituximab for rheumatoid arthritis refractory to anti-tumor necrosis factor therapy: Results of a multicenter, randomized, double-blind, placebo-controlled, phase III trial evaluating primary efficacy and safety at twenty-four weeks. *Arthritis Rheum*, **54**(9), 2793–2806.

29. Jones, R.B., Tervaert, J.W., Hauser, T., Luqmani, R., Morgan, M.D., Peh, C.A., *et al.* (2010). Rituximab versus cyclophosphamide in ANCA-associated renal vasculitis. *N Engl J Med*, **363**(3), 211–220.

30. Stone, J.H., Merkel, P.A., Spiera, R., Seo, P., Langford, C.A., Hoffman, G.S., *et al.* (2010). Rituximab versus cyclophosphamide for ANCA-associated vasculitis. *N Engl J Med*, **363**(3), 221–232.

31. Gunnarsson, I., Sundelin, B., Jonsdottir, T., Jacobson, S.H., Henriksson, E.W., van Vollenhoven, R.F. (2007). Histopathologic and clinical outcome of rituximab treatment in patients with cyclophosphamide-resistant proliferative lupus nephritis. *Arthritis Rheum*, **56**(4), 1263–1272.

32. Wallace, D.J., Gordon, C., Strand, V., Hobbs, K., Petri, M., Kalunian, K., *et al.* (2013). Efficacy and safety of epratuzumab in patients with moderate/severe flaring systemic lupus erythematosus: results from two randomized, double-blind,

placebo-controlled, multicentre studies (ALLEVIATE) and follow-up. *Rheumatology (Oxford)*, **52**(7), 1313–1322.

33. Wallace, D.J., Kalunian, K., Petri, M.A., Strand, V., Houssiau, F.A., Pike, M., *et al.* (2014). Efficacy and safety of epratuzumab in patients with moderate/severe active systemic lupus erythematosus: results from EMBLEM, a phase IIb, randomised, double-blind, placebo-controlled, multicentre study. *Ann Rheum Dis*, **73**(1), 183–190.

34. Helling, B., Konig, M., Dalken, B., Engling, A., Kromer, W., Heim, K., *et al.* (2014). A specific CD4 epitope bound by tregalizumab mediates activation of regulatory T cells by a unique signaling pathway. *Immunol Cell Biol.*

35. Tracey, K.J. (2002). The inflammatory reflex. *Nature*, **420**(6917), 853–859.

36. Oke, S.L., Tracey, K.J. (2008). From CNI-1493 to the immunological homunculus: physiology of the inflammatory reflex. *J Leukoc Biol*, **83**(3), 512–517.

37. Olofsson, P.S., Katz, D.A., Rosas-Ballina, M., Levine, Y.A., Ochani, M., Valdes-Ferrer, S.I., *et al.* (2011). alpha7 nicotinic acetylcholine receptor (alpha7nAChR) expression in bone marrow-derived non-T cells is required for the inflammatory reflex. *Mol Med*, **18**: 539–543.

38. Pavlov, V.A., Tracey, K.J. (2012). The vagus nerve and the inflammatory reflex — linking immunity and metabolism. *Nat Rev Endocrinol*, **8**(12), 743–754.

39. Fries, J.F., Spitz, P., Kraines, R.G., Holman, H.R. (1980). Measurement of patient outcome in arthritis. *Arthritis Rheum*, **23**(2), 137–145.

40. Boumpas, D.T., Austin, H.A., 3rd Vaughn, E.M., Klippel, J.H., Steinberg, A.D., Yarboro, C.H., *et al.* (1992). Controlled trial of pulse methylprednisolone versus two regimens of pulse cyclophosphamide in severe lupus nephritis. *Lancet*, **340**(8822), 741–745.

41. Goekoop-Ruiterman, Y.P., de Vries-Bouwstra, J.K., Allaart, C.F., van Zeben, D., Kerstens, P.J., Hazes, J.M., *et al.* (2005). Clinical and radiographic outcomes of four different treatment strategies in patients with early rheumatoid arthritis (the BeSt study): a randomized, controlled trial. *Arthritis Rheum*, **52**(11), 3381–3390.

42. Colombel, J.F., Sandborn, W.J., Reinisch, W., Mantzaris, G.J., Kornbluth, A., Rachmilewitz, D., *et al.* (2010). Infliximab, azathioprine, or combination therapy for Crohn's disease. *N Engl J Med*, **362**(15), 1383–1395.

43. Houssiau, F.A., Vasconcelos, C., D'Cruz, D., Sebastiani, G.D., Garrido Ed Ede, R., Danieli, M.G., *et al.* (2002). Immunosuppressive therapy in lupus nephritis: the Euro-Lupus Nephritis Trial, a randomized trial of low-dose versus high-dose intravenous cyclophosphamide. *Arthritis Rheum*, **46**(8), 2121–2131.

44. Houssiau, F.A., D'Cruz, D., Sangle, S., Remy, P., Vasconcelos, C., Petrovic, R., *et al.* (2010). Azathioprine versus mycophenolate mofetil for long-term immunosuppression in lupus nephritis: results from the MAINTAIN Nephritis Trial. *Ann Rheum Dis*, **69**(12), 2083–2089.

45. Quinn, M.A., Conaghan, P.G., O'Connor, P.J., Karim, Z., Greenstein, A., Brown, A., *et al.* (2005). Very early treatment with infliximab in addition to methotrexate in early, poor-prognosis rheumatoid arthritis reduces magnetic resonance imaging evidence of synovitis and damage, with sustained benefit after infliximab withdrawal: results from a twelve-month randomized, double-blind, placebo-controlled trial. *Arthritis Rheum*, **52**(1), 27–35.

46. van der Kooij, S.M., Goekoop-Ruiterman, Y.P., de Vries-Bouwstra, J.K., Guler-Yuksel, M., Zwinderman, A.H., Kerstens, P.J., *et al.* (2009). Drug-free remission, functioning and radiographic damage after 4 years of response-driven treatment in patients with recent-onset rheumatoid arthritis. *Ann Rheum Dis*, **68**(6), 914–921.

47. Smolen, J.S., Emery, P., Fleischmann, R., van Vollenhoven, R.F., Pavelka, K., Durez, P., *et al.* (2014). Adjustment of therapy in rheumatoid arthritis on the basis of achievement of stable low disease activity with adalimumab plus methotrexate or methotrexate alone: the randomised controlled OPTIMA trial. *Lancet*, **383**(9914), 321–332.

48. Soubrier, M., Puechal, X., Sibilia, J., Mariette, X., Meyer, O., Combe, B., *et al.* (2009). Evaluation of two strategies (initial methotrexate monotherapy vs its combination with adalimumab) in management of early active rheumatoid arthritis: data from the GUEPARD trial. *Rheumatology (Oxford)*, **48**(11), 1429–1434.

49. Detert, J., Bastian, H., Listing, J., Weiss, A., Wassenberg, S., Liebhaber, A., *et al.* (2013). Induction therapy with adalimumab plus methotrexate for 24 weeks followed by methotrexate monotherapy up to week 48 versus methotrexate therapy alone for DMARD-naive patients with early rheumatoid arthritis: HIT HARD, an investigator-initiated study. *Ann Rheum Dis*, **72**(6), 844–850.

50. Horslev-Petersen, K., Hetland, M.L., Junker, P., Podenphant, J., Ellingsen, T., Ahlquist, P., *et al.* (2014). Adalimumab added to a treat-to-target strategy with methotrexate and intra-articular triamcinolone in early rheumatoid arthritis increased remission rates, function and quality of life. The OPERA Study: an investigator-initiated, randomised, double-blind, parallel-group, placebo-controlled trial. *Ann Rheum Dis*, **73**(4), 654–661.

51. Emery, P., Burmester, G.R., Bykerk, V.P., Combe, B.G., Furst, D.E., Barre, E., *et al.* (2015). Evaluating drug-free remission with abatacept in early rheumatoid

arthritis: results from the phase 3b, multicentre, randomised, active-controlled AVERT study of 24 months, with a 12-month, double-blind treatment period. *Ann Rheum Dis*, **74**(1), 19–26.

52. Smolen, J.S., Nash, P., Durez, P., Hall, S., Ilivanova, E., Irazoque-Palazuelos, F., *et al.* (2013). Maintenance, reduction, or withdrawal of etanercept after treatment with etanercept and methotrexate in patients with moderate rheumatoid arthritis (PRESERVE): a randomised controlled trial. *Lancet*, **381**(9870), 918–929.

53. Emery, P., Hammoudeh, M., FitzGerald, O., Combe, B., Martin-Mola, E., Buch, M.H., *et al.* (2014). Sustained remission with etanercept tapering in early rheumatoid arthritis. *N Engl J Med*, **371**(19), 1781–1792.

54. Grigor, C., Capell, H., Stirling, A., McMahon, A.D., Lock, P., Vallance, R., *et al.* (2004). Effect of a treatment strategy of tight control for rheumatoid arthritis (the TICORA study): a single-blind randomised controlled trial. *Lancet*, **364**(9430), 263–269.

55. Verstappen, S.M., Jacobs, J.W., van der Veen, M.J., Heurkens, A.H., Schenk, Y., ter Borg, E.J., *et al.* (2007). Intensive treatment with methotrexate in early rheumatoid arthritis: aiming for remission. Computer Assisted Management in Early Rheumatoid Arthritis (CAMERA, an open-label strategy trial). *Ann Rheum Dis*, **66**(11), 1443–1449.

56. Smolen, J.S., Aletaha, D., Bijlsma, J.W., Breedveld, F.C., Boumpas, D., Burmester, G., *et al.* (2010). Treating rheumatoid arthritis to target: recommendations of an international task force. *Ann Rheum Dis*, **69**(4), 631–637.

57. Smolen, J.S., Braun, J., Dougados, M., Emery, P., Fitzgerald, O., Helliwell, P., *et al.* (2014). Treating spondyloarthritis, including ankylosing spondylitis and psoriatic arthritis, to target: recommendations of an international task force. *Ann Rheum Dis*, **73**(1), 6–16.

58. van Vollenhoven, R.F., Mosca, M., Bertsias, G., Isenberg, D., Kuhn, A., Lerstrom, K., *et al.* (2014). Treat-to-target in systemic lupus erythematosus: recommendations from an international task force. *Ann Rheum Dis*, **73**(6), 958–967.

INDEX

5-aminosalicylic acid
   (5-ASA, mesalazine), 199
abatacept, 7, 80, 81, 90, 153, 354
Actemra/Roactemra, 296
acute interstitial pneumonia, 258,
   273
adalimumab, 80, , 81, 115, 200, 207
adjuvant, 333, 334
alemtuzumab, 31, 46, 294, 295, 299,
   354
allergen-derived synthetic peptides,
   329
allergen-microarray technology, 335
allergen-specific immunotherapy,
   311, 334
allergen-specific T cells, 312
allergic diseases, 311
allergy vaccines, 337
ambrisentan, 262
anakinra, 7, 80, 81, 85
anaphylaxis, 311
ankylosing spondylitis, 5, 109

anti-CD4, 354
anti-CD20, 44
anti-CD20 therapy, 32
anti-CD22, 353, 354
anti-CD28, 355
anti-CD52, 354
anti-drug antibodies, 206
anti-GMCSF, 353
anti-IL4,
anti-IL17,
anti-TNF, 200
anti-TNF-antibodies, 205
apremilast, 93
Arzerra, 293
asthma, 5
atacicept, 152, 154
atherosclerosis, 5
atopic dermatitis, 5, 225
Aubagio, 289
autoimmune diseases, 4
autoinflammatory diseases, 86, 220
autoinflammatory syndromes, 7

axial SpA, 109
azathioprine, 145, 146, 148

B1 cells, 35
B2 cells, 35
BAFF, 43
bardoxolone, 267
bariticinib, 92
Bath Ankylosing Spondylitis
  Metrology index (BASMI), 110
B cell, 31, 32, 224
BCR complex, 40
bee venom allergy, 328
Behçet's Syndrome, 5
belimumab, 7, 32, 39, 49, 149, 152
biologic agents, 80
Biologic DMARDs, 81, 82
biologic-free remission, 98, 99
biomarker discovery, 24
biomarkers, 19, 201
biosimilars, 210, 211, 358
blinatumomab, 46
blisibimod, 151, 152
blistering skin diseases, 223
BLyS/BAFF, 37
bosentan, 262
brodalumab, 82, 86
bronchoalveolar lavage, 257
bullous pemphigoid, 4

Campath-1H, 354
canakinumab, 7, 86
CD19, 46
CD20-antagonists, 293, 294, 299
CD22, 35, 46
cell-based therapy, 212
certolizumab, 115, 200
certolizumab pegol, 80, 81
chloroquine, 145

chronic autoimmune hepatitis, 5
chronic uveitis, 5
classification criteria, 170
clazakizumab, 82, 85
clinical manifestations, 172
combination of several biomarkers, 19
comparative effectiveness research, 10
concept, 259
Crohn's disease, 3, 5, 199
cryptogenic organising pneumonia,
  258, 273
cutaneous lupus, 4, 5
cutaneous lupus erythematosus, 133,
  134, 237
  ACLE, 241, 242, 244
  acute cutaneous LE (ACLE), 237
  chilblain LE (CHLE), 237
  CHLE, 246
  chronic cutaneous LE (CCLE),
    237
  discoid LE (DLE), 237
  DLE, 241, 242, 244, 246
  intermittent cutaneous LE
    (ICLE), 237
  LE panniculitis (LEP), 237, 246
  LE tumidus (LET), 237, 241
  subacute cutaneous LE (SCLE),
    237, 241, 244, 246, 248
cyclophosphamide, 145, 148
cyclosporine, 200
cytokines, 80

daclizumab, 295, 296
dactylitis, 109
data mining, 23
dendritic cell (DC), 65, 68, 220
desquamative interstitial pneumonia,
  258, 272
development for NMO, 296

dimethylfumarate, 290 , 291, 298
disease modifying antirheumatic
  drugs (DMARDs), 80, 110, 111
dupilumab, 7, 352
dysbiosis, 199

early intervention, 202
early treatment, 359, 360
ectopic germinal centers, 39
eculizumab, 296
enthesitis, 109
epicutaneous immunotherapy, 332
epratuzumab, 47, 48, 150, 151, 153,
  354
Epstein-Barr Virus, 131
etanercept, 80, 81, 115, 262
etrolizumab, 210
EUSCLE, 243
EUSCLE Core Set Questionnaire, 239
everolimus, 269
exercise, 110
EXPLORER, 45

familial Mediterranean fever, 86
fingolimod, 288, 289, 298
Fostamatinib, 93
FOXP3, 69, 70
fragmentation approach, 328
future prospects, 351

Genomics, 21
Gilenya, 288
glatiramer acetate, 287, 288, 289,
  290, 298
golimumab, 80, 81, 115, 200, 210

haematopoietic stem cell
  transplantation (HSCT), 212, 297,
  299

histiocytosis, 258
HLA, 130
hydroxychloroquine, 93, 144
hypoallergenic recombinant allergens,
  326

idiopathic myocarditis, 5
Idiopathic non specific interstitial
  pneumonia, 272
idiopathic pulmonary fibrosis (IPF),
  5, 258, 259
IgE antibodies, 312
IL-1b, 220
IL-1 receptor antagonist, 85
IL17, 86
imatinib, 262
immune-mediated inflammatory
  diseases, 4
immune tolerance, 311
immunotherapy, 326, 328
induction-maintenance, 359, 360
inflammasome, 220
inflammatory bowel disease (IBD), 4,
  5, 199
inflammatory diseases, 4
inflammatory myopathies, 4
inflammatory reflex, 356
infliximab, 80, 81, 114, 200, 206,
  207
interferon (IFN), 287
  IFNb, 287–290, 292, 294–296,
    298
  IFNb-1a, 286, 287
  IFNb-1b, 286
  IFNbs, 287
  interferon-beta 1b, 286
  interferon-α, 353
interleukin 6 (IL-6), 84
interleukin-17, 115

interstitial lung diseases (ILD), 257
ixekizumab, 82, 86

Jaccoud's syndrome, 133
JAK, 91
JC virus, 292, 293
juvenile inflammatory arthritis, 5

Keratinocytes, 220
kinoids, 352, 353

laquinimod, 154, 291, 298
libman–sacks endocarditis, 137
livedo reticularis, 133, 135
löfgren's syndrome, 273
LUNAR, 45
lung transplantation, 266, 273
lupus, 129
lupus nephritis, 135, 136
lupus pernio, 5
lymphangioleyomiomatosis, 258, 266
lymphocytic interstitial pneumonia, 258

Mabthera/Rituxan, 293
macitentan, 263
macrophages, 65, 68, 69
magnetic resonance imaging (MRI), 284, 287, 288, 289, 290, 291, 294, 295, 298, 299
mast cells, 312
mavrilimumab, 352
mesenchymal stem cell transplantation (MSCT), 212, 297
mesenchymal stromal cells, 63–65, 353, 356
metabolomics, 22

methotrexate (MTX), 93, 112, 200, 202
microbiota, 213, 221
microRNA, 213
microscopic colitis, 5
mosaic strategies, 328
mucosal healing, 202
mucosal tolerance, 331
multiple sclerosis (MS), 4, 5, 283–295, 297–299, 354
mycophenolate mofetil, 146, 148

NAC, 262
N-acetylcysteine, 260
natalizumab, 7, 210, 286, 292, 293, 298
nerventra, 291
neurofilament-light (NF-L), 286
neuromyelitis optica (NMO), 284, 293, 296, 297
NF-L, 286
nintedanib, 261–265
NMDA receptor encephalitis, 284, 296, 297
non-radiographic axial SpA, 116
nonspecific Interstitial Pneumonia, 258
non-steroidal anti-inflammatory drugs (NSAIDs), 110

obituzumab, 45
ocrelizumab, 45, 89, 293, 294, 298
ofatumumab, 45, 82, 89, 293, 294
olokizumab, 82, 85
oral immunotherapy, 331

patient stratification, 17
pemphigoid, 223
pemphigus, 4, 223

periodic fever, 86
peripheral SpA, 109
personalized medicine, 17, 204
Pharmacogenomics, 201
photoprotection, 239
photosensitivity, 239
pirfenidone, 261–264
pleurisy, 138
pneumonitis, 138
polymyositis-dermatomyositis, 271
pre-natal therapy, 337
prevention, 239
primary progressive MS (PPMS),
    285, 289, 291, 294
primary sclerosing cholangitis, 5
progressive multifocal leukoencepha-
    lopathy, 7, 292, 293
progressive systemic sclerosis, 4
proliferative lymphoid nodules
    (PLN), 43
proteomics, 21
psoriasis, 3–5, 228
psoriatic arthritis, 4, 5
pulmonary alveolar proteinosis, 258,
    269
pyoderma gangrenosum, 5

quinacrine, 145

Raynaud's phenomenon, 133
recombinant allergens, 316
regulatory myeloid cell, 65, 67
regulatory T cell, 63–65, 69, 212, 355
relapsing-remitting (RRMS) disease,
    283
remission, 201, 202
respiratory bronchiolitis, 272
respiratory bronchiolitis interstitial
    lung disease, 258

revised cutaneous lupus
    erythematosus disease area and
    severity index (RCLASI), 247, 248
rheumatic autoimmune/inflammatory
    diseases (RAID), 31, 32, 44, 50
rheumatoid arthritis (RA), 3–5, 31,
    32, 79
rilonacept, 7
RIM, 45
rituximab, 7, 43, 45, 80, 81, 87, 150,
    152, 293, 294, 296, 297
rontalizumab, 153–155
RRMS, 285–295, 297, 298

sarcoidosis, 5, 273
sarilumab, 82, 85
schnitzler, 221
secondary progressive MS (SPMS),
    285, 291
secukinumab, 7, 82, 86, 115
sex hormones, 131
shrinking lung syndrome (SLS), 138
sifalimumab, 153, 154
sildenafil, 262
sirolimus, 268, 269
sirukumab, 82, 85, 154
Sjögren's syndrome, 5
skin, 219
skin inflammation, 225
smoking, 239
soliris, 296
spondyloarthropathies/
    spondyloarthritis, 4, 5, 109
step-up approach, 202
Stevens-Johnsons syndrome, 225
strategies, 200, 201
subcutaneous injection
    immunotherapy, 313
sublingual immunotherapy, 331

sulphasalazine, 93, 111
sun exposure, 239
sunscreens, 239
switching, 95, 96
    between biologics, 85
Syk, 93
synthetic hypoallergenic peptides, 330
systemic lupus erythematosus (SLE), 4, 5, 129
systemic sclerosis (SSc), 165, 169, 179, 180, 182–184, 271
systemic treatment in CLE, 243
    antimalarials, 243
    belimumab, 247
    dapsone, 246
    fumaric acid esthers (FAEs), 247
    further immunosuppressive agents (azathioprine, cyclosporine, cyclophosphamide), 247
    methotrexate (MTX), 244
    mycophenolate mofetil (MMF) and mycophenolate sodium (EC-MPS), 246
    retinoids, 245
    rituximab, 248
    sirukumab (anti-il6) and tocilizumab (anti-il6r), 249
    systemic corticosteroids (CS), 244
systemic vasculitis, 5

tabalumab, 151, 152
T cell dependent (TD) B cell activation, 33
T cell-independent manner (TI responses), 35
T cells, 220

tecfidera, 290
teriflunomide, 289, 290, 298
tetrathiomolyb, 267
TGFβ, 213
TGN1412, 353, 355
thalidomide, 267
therapeutic drug monitoring, 200, 204
therapeutic strategies, 207
therapy, 165, 178, 179
therapy strategy, 203
thiopurines, 200, 201, 204
tissue resident immune system, 226
TNF, 80, 81
TNF-blockers, 114, 119
TNF-receptor associated periodic syndrome, 86
tocilizumab, 7, 81, 84, 85, 153, 154, 296
tofacitinib, 91, 210, 211
topical treatment in CLE, 240
    calcineurin inhibitors (CI), 241
    other topical treatment options, 242
    R-salbutamol (ASF-1096), 242
    topical corticosteroids (CS), 240
toxic epidermal necrolysis, 225
Tr1, 69, 71
transforming growth factor, 260
translational science, 26
treatment algorithm in CLE, 240
treatment strategies, 93, 95, 358, 359
treat to target, 359, 363
tregalizumab, 353, 355
triggered, 239
trigger factors
    drug-induced LE (DI-LE), 240
    smoking, 244
triple therapy, 93, 94, 260, 272

type 1 (autoimmune) diabetes, 5
Tysabri, 292

ulcerative colitis, 5, 199
ultraviolet (UV) light, 239
ustekinumab, 115, 210, 211
usual interstitial pneumonia, 260
uveitis, 109, 117, 118

veltuzumab, 45, 210
VX-509, 93

wild-type recombinant allergen,
  325
window of opportunity, 201

zileuton, 267

www.ingramcontent.com/pod-product-compliance
Lightning Source LLC
Chambersburg PA
CBHW050536190326
41458CB00007B/1799